Fundamentals of
Body CT

Fundamentals of Body CT

SECOND EDITION

W. Richard Webb, M.D.

Professor of Radiology
University of California, San Francisco
San Francisco, California

William E. Brant, M.D.

Associate Professor of Radiology
University of California, Davis
Sacramento, California

Clyde A. Helms, M.D.

Professor of Radiology
Duke University Medical Center
Durham, North Carolina

W.B. SAUNDERS COMPANY

An Imprint of Elsevier Science
Philadelphia   London   New York   St. Louis   Sydney   Toronto

W. B. SAUNDERS COMPANY
An Imprint of Elsevier Science
The Curtis Center
Independence Square West
Philadelphia, PA 19106

Library of Congress Cataloging-in-Publication Data

Webb, W. Richard (Wayne Richard) Fundamentals of body CT / W. Richard Webb,
William E. Brant, Clyde A. Helms.—2nd ed.

p.   cm.

Includes bibliographical references and index.

ISBN 0–7216–6862–3

1. Tomography.   I. Brant, William E.   II. Helms, Clyde A.   III. Title.
    [DNLM: 1. Tomography, X-Ray Computed.   WN 160 W368f 1998]

RC78.7.T6W433 1998   616.07′572—dc21

DNLM/DLC   97-5450

FUNDAMENTALS OF BODY CT   ISBN 0–7216–6862–3

Printed in the United States of America.

Last digit is the print number: 9   8   7   6

This book is dedicated to our families,
for their continued support.

Norma, Teresa, Emma, Sonny, and Andy
W.R.W.

Daniel, Ryan, Jonathan, and Rachel
W.E.B.

Mrs. F.L. Helms, Nancy, Caroline, Jeremy,
Allyson, Jason, and Benjamin
C.A.H.

Preface

Writing the preface to a second edition is a pleasure for three reasons. First, it means the first edition was successful, and the publishers are willing to go through the whole process again; second, it means that you're finally done with the rewriting; and last, and most important, a second edition gives you the chance to add new material, correct mistakes, and bring things up to date.

The five years or so since this book was first published have seen a number of innovations and advances in CT technique, most notably the development of spiral/helical CT. In this edition, we have updated our descriptions of CT techniques to include various spiral/helical CT protocols now accepted in clinical practice for the diagnosis of chest, abdominal, and musculoskeletal abnormalities, and have included some discussion of the role of spiral CT, 3D CT, and CT angiography. Other recent CT developments are also reviewed in this edition. For example, the section on high-resolution lung CT has been significantly expanded in a fashion paralleling the expanded clinical use of this technique, and new topics and new illustrations have been added to all chapters. At the same time, we have tried to keep things simple and have condensed some of the text in favor of lists and tables. We hope you enjoy and profit from our efforts.

W. RICHARD WEBB
WILLIAM E. BRANT
CLYDE A. HELMS

Preface to the First Edition

Our goal is to have this book cut from the same cloth as *Fundamentals of Skeletal Radiology,* the "Cliff's Notes" of skeletal radiology, recently published by Clyde Helms to great acclaim (to hear him tell it, W.R.W.).

Instead of writing a text intended to record everything that is known about body CT or even everything that we know about body CT, we have attempted to write one that *teaches* how to perform and read body CT scans. In doing this, we have tried to limit ourselves to discussing what is key to understanding body CT from a practical clinical standpoint—the key anatomy, the key concepts, the key diseases, and the key controversies. We have done this at the risk of leaving a few things out, but it isn't necessary to read about everything when you are first learning a subject. In other words, *Fundamentals of Body CT* is not intended to provide more than the best CT texts on the market do, but rather less, with a different emphasis, and in a more manageable package.

Each of us has written a different part of this book, obviously depending on our areas of expertise. Since each of us teaches in a slightly different way, each of the three sections of the book—the thorax, the abdomen, and the musculoskeletal system—is somewhat different in approach. We hope that by preserving our individual styles we have made the book more interesting to read, and for us, it certainly made this book easier to write.

W. RICHARD WEBB
WILLIAM E. BRANT
CLYDE A. HELMS

Contents

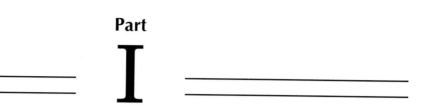

Part

I

The Thorax

1

Techniques of Thoracic CT

W. Richard Webb, M.D.

ROUTINE CHEST CT

In most patients, chest CT is performed using a standard protocol. This technique is designed to provide useful (although not necessarily optimal) information about the lungs, mediastinum, hila, pleura, and chest wall and therefore is valuable in the diagnosis of a variety of conditions or diseases, and in the assessment of diseases such as lung cancer, that involve each of these regions. Somewhat different CT techniques are often employed in specific clinical settings or to look for specific abnormalities (e.g., aortic dissection, pulmonary embolism, lung disease). These are reviewed in subsequent sections of this book.

Chest CT is usually obtained from the level of the lung apices (or suprasternal notch) to the level of the posterior costophrenic angles; these scans also encompass the diaphragm and a part of the upper abdomen. Routinely, patients are scanned (1) supine, (2) during suspended respiration, and (3) at full lung volume (total lung capacity).

Scans can be performed with or without the administration of contrast media, depending on the indication for the study and, to some extent, on one's level of knowledge or confidence. For example, if you are not confident about mediastinal vascular and node anatomy, by all means administer contrast medium, so that vessels can be distinguished from other structures. If you are experienced, contrast is not always necessary. (If you are experienced, why are you reading this book?)

Once the scans have been performed, the scan data are reconstructed using an algorithm that determines some characteristics of the resulting image. For routine chest imaging, a high-resolution algorithm has been shown to be advantageous. However, a standard or soft tissue algorithm, which produces a smoother image, can also be used.

In chest CT, the scans must be viewed using two different window settings. These settings are appropriately named "lung" and "soft tissue" (or "mediastinal") windows, names that also describe their primary use. Lung windows typically have a window mean of -600 to -700 H and a window width of 1000 to 1500 H. Lung windows best demonstrate lung anatomy and pathology, contrasting soft tissue structures to surrounding air-filled lung. Mediastinal or soft tissue windows (window mean 20 to 40 H, width 450 to 500 H) demonstrate soft tissue anatomy in the mediastinum and other areas of the thorax, allowing the differentiation of fat, fluid, tissue, calcium, and, if contrast medium has been administered, opacified vessels. This window is also of value in providing information about consolidated lung, the hila, pleural disease, and structures of the chest wall. More specific uses of these two windows are discussed in subsequent chapters.

The protocols used for routine chest CT

vary depending on the type of scanner employed.

Conventional CT Technique

On a conventional CT scanner, standard chest CT is often performed using contiguous 8- to 10-mm collimation from the lung apices to bases. A useful alternative is to obtain contiguous 5-mm collimated scans through the pulmonary hila, to provide better definition of hilar anatomy and bronchi, with contiguous 8- to 10-mm collimation at other levels.

When one is using a conventional scanner, a slow drip infusion of 100 mL of contrast medium during scanning often provides sufficient opacification for diagnosis, but divided boluses of contrast medium administered at 1 mL/sec can also be used (i.e., three separate small boluses given in the upper mediastinum, hilar regions, and at the level of the heart).

Spiral CT Technique

If you have the option of using spiral CT, you should always use it. As with many important rules there is one exception. In the diagnosis of chest diseases, the exception is high-resolution CT (HRCT).

Spiral CT is advantageous in scanning the chest because a number of levels can be studied during a single breath hold. Although spiral (helical) CT greatly simplifies the CT examination, it offers a great number of options, with numerous possible variations in collimation, pitch, and reconstruction interval. However, similar results can be obtained using a variety of different techniques, and no one technique should be considered "correct" to the exclusion of others.

When spiral CT is used, a helpful routine technique is to obtain scans with 5- to 7-mm collimation and a pitch* of 1. With a gantry rotation time of 1 second, which is used on most scanners, this protocol allows about half of the chest to be imaged during a single breath hold of 20 to 30 seconds. Most patients can hold their breath for 20

$$\text{*Pitch} = \frac{\text{table excursion (mm) in 1 sec} \times \text{gantry rotation time (sec)}}{\text{collimation (mm)}}$$

seconds; thus, one can routinely use 7-mm collimation, a pitch of 1, and two 20-second breath holds to scan the chest (with a 12-second delay between breaths) (Table 1–1); the two scan sequences are overlapped by 5 mm so that nothing is missed.

One alternative is to time the patient's breath hold before scanning, varying the collimation or pitch to cover the chest in a single breath hold; the distance the scans need to encompass can be determined from the scout view. Increasing the collimation or pitch increases the distance covered during a specific time interval. For example, increasing the pitch from 1 to 1.7 increases the area scanned in a given time interval by 70%. A similar increase in the area scanned can be achieved by increasing the scan collimation. However, a general rule with spiral CT is that it is better to increase the pitch to cover a given area, up to a pitch of 2, than it is to increase the collimation; increasing the pitch rather than the collimation generally results in better resolution. For example, doubling the pitch results in an increase in effective slice thickness by only about 30% when a 180° interpolation algorithm is used; doubling the collimation results in a doubling of the effective slice thickness. The downside of increasing pitch or collimation is that resolution is reduced. Examples of possible scan protocols are given in the Table 1–1.

Spiral technique has several advantages. First, spiral CT ensures the volumetric acquisition of data. This means that nothing is missed: you can accurately relate anatomy on one scan to the next, and you can do three-dimensional reconstructions if you want. Second, because the scan data are acquired in a relatively short period of time, you can get excellent contrast opacification of vessels with a relatively small dose of contrast medium.

With a spiral scanner, giving contrast medium at 1.5 to 2.5 mL/sec and beginning the injection 20 to 30 seconds before the scanning begins, and for the duration of the scan series, provides excellent opacification of vascular structures. The amount, rate, and scan delay can vary with the indication for the study and with the protocol used (see Table 1–1).

TABLE 1–1. **Examples of Possible Variations in Spiral CT Protocols**

Indication	Collimation and Pitch	Effective Slice Thickness	Breath Hold	Area Scanned	Scan Delay	Amount of Contrast Medium Needed
Routine chest	7-mm collimation pitch of 1	7 mm	2 breath holds, 20 seconds each	28 cm	30 sec	120 mL at 1.5 mL/sec
	7-mm collimation pitch of 1	7 mm	1 breath hold, 40 seconds	28 cm	30 sec	105 mL at 1.5 mL/sec
	7-mm collimation pitch of 1.7	8.5 mm	1 breath hold, 24 seconds	28 cm	30 sec	80 mL at 1.5 mL/sec
	5-mm collimation pitch of 2	6.5 mm	1 breath hold, 28 seconds	28 cm	30 sec	80 mL at 1.5 mL/sec
Pulmonary embolism	3-mm collimation pitch of 2	4 mm	1 breath hold, 20 seconds	12 cm (hila only)	20 sec	100 mL at 2.5 mL/sec
	5-mm collimation pitch of 1	5 mm	1 breath hold, 20 seconds	10 cm (hila only)	20 sec	100 mL at 2.5 mL/sec

VASCULAR LESIONS AND DYNAMIC CT

In some patients, CT is performed for the diagnosis of a vascular lesion, suggested either on the basis of clinical symptoms or radiographic findings. Also, sometimes, a standard CT is inconclusive as to what an abnormality is, and additional scans are performed to evaluate the possibility of a vascular lesion. If this is the case, dynamic CT is performed with the bolus injection of contrast medium.

The term *dynamic CT* means that a number of scans are performed in rapid sequence, usually during suspended respiration. Because spiral scanning is continuous, it is a dynamic technique, but dynamic scanning can also be performed using a conventional scanner.

Dynamic CT can be performed at the same level or at adjacent levels *(dynamic incremental CT)*. Because contrast medium is simultaneously injected, the rapid sequence of scans shows progressive opacification of vessels or vascular lesions at the levels scanned, clearly demonstrate the vascular nature of masses, and can provide some information regarding the rapidity of blood flow through the abnormal area. Scans of this sort are used, for example, for the diagnosis of aortic aneurysm and dissection and pulmonary embolism and are also valuable in the diagnosis of hilar or mediastinal masses, in which distinction of mass and vessels is essential. Dynamic CT during forced expiration can also be used in the detection of air trapping.

HIGH-RESOLUTION LUNG CT

In diagnosing certain abnormalities, such as diffuse lung disease or a solitary nodule, HRCT is used to optimize the spatial resolution of scans and is advantageous or essential in diagnosis. Individual scans are obtained at selected levels, to sample lung anatomy, without table motion if a spiral scanner is used. Because the goal of HRCT is to optimize resolution, using spiral technique would be counterproductive. This technique is described further in Chapter 6, Lung Disease.

Necessary techniques for obtaining high-resolution CT include the following:

1. *Thin collimation (1–2 mm)*. With 10-mm, 7-mm, or even 5-mm collimation, the volume averaging that occurs in the plane of scan significantly reduces the ability of CT to resolve small structures. Volume averaging means that various different densities present in the same slice volume (voxel) are averaged together, thus obscuring details or edges that may be important in di-

agnosis. Thin collimation allows anatomic detail to be clearly seen.

2. *A sharp (high-resolution) reconstruction algorithm.* With conventional body CT, scan data are often reconstructed with a relatively low spatial frequency algorithm (i.e., "standard" or "soft tissue" algorithm), which smoothes the image, reduces visible image noise, and improves contrast resolution. Reconstruction using a sharp or high-resolution algorithm (i.e., "bone" algorithm) reduces image smoothing and increases spatial resolution, making structures appear sharper. Although using a sharp algorithm also increases image noise, only rarely does this create a problem in interpretation.

Optional techniques for improving spatial resolution include

1. *Targeted reconstruction.* Using a smaller field of view for image reconstruction than was used to scan the patient reduces image pixel size and, thus, increases its spatial resolution. However, this is time consuming and not often necessary for diagnosis.

2. *Increased kilovolts peak (kVp) and milliampere (mA) settings.* On HRCT, image noise decreases when scan technique (kVp and mA) is increased to levels higher than those used for routine chest CT. However, the improvement in image quality that results from increased scan technique is minimal, and with state-of-the-art scanners this is not necessary. In fact, excellent HRCT can be obtained with lower than normal milliampere settings.

Suggested Reading

Costello P, Dupuy DE, Ecker CP, Tello R. Spiral CT of the thorax with reduced volume of contrast material: a comparative study. Radiology 1992; 185:663–666.

Dillon EH, van Leeuwen MS, Fernandez MA, Mali WPTM. Spiral CT angiography. AJR 1993; 160:1273–1278.

Glazer GM, Francis IR, Gebarski K, et al. Dynamic incremental computed tomography in evaluation of the pulmonary hila. J Comput Assist Tomogr 1983; 7:59–64.

Heiken JP, Brink JA, Vannier MW. Spiral (helical) CT. Radiology 1993; 189:647–656.

Kalender WA, Seissler W, Klotz E, Vock P. Spiral volumetric CT with single-breath-hold technique, continuous transport, and continuous scanner rotation. Radiology 1990; 176:181–183.

Mayo JR. The high-resolution computed tomography technique. Semin Roentgenol 1991; 26:104–109.

Mayo JR, Webb WR, Gould R, et al. High-resolution CT of the lungs: an optimal approach. Radiology 1987; 163:507–510.

Paranjpe DV, Bergin CJ. Spiral CT of the lungs: optimal technique and resolution compared with conventional CT. AJR 1994; 162:561–567.

Remy-Jardin M, Remy J, Giraud F, Marquette CH. Pulmonary nodules: detection with thick-section spiral CT versus conventional CT. Radiology 1993; 187:513–520.

Zwirewich CV, Mayo JR, Müller NL. Low-dose high-resolution CT of lung parenchyma. Radiology 1991; 180:413–417.

2

Mediastinum—Introduction and Normal Anatomy

W. Richard Webb, M.D.

CT is commonly used in patients suspected of having a mediastinal mass or vascular abnormality (such as an aortic aneurysm), because its ability to image mediastinal anatomy is far superior to that of conventional radiographic techniques. In general, CT of the mediastinum is obtained in two situations.

First, CT is almost always performed in patients who have an abnormality visible on plain radiographs that is suggestive or indicative of mediastinal pathology. It is quite unusual in current medical practice for a patient with a mediastinal abnormality visible on plain films to have surgery or even mediastinoscopy without having CT first. In patients with a visible mass, CT can be helpful in confirming the presence of a significant lesion (mediastinal contour abnormalities seen, or imagined, on plain films do not always reflect a real abnormality); defining its location; determining the relationship of the lesion to vascular or non-vascular structures from which it may be arising or is involving; showing other, unrecognized mediastinal lesions; and characterizing the mass as solid, cystic, vascular, enhancing, calcified, inhomogeneous, fatty, and so on. Although CT may not be able to diagnose a lesion with certainty, it may be possible to limit the differential diagnosis to a few entities, and this may determine the most appropriate next step, be it percutane-

ous biopsy, mediastinoscopy, surgery, arteriography, or nothing.

Second, CT is often used to evaluate the mediastinum in patients who have normal chest radiographs but who also have a clinical reason that makes one suspect mediastinal disease. Chest films are relatively insensitive to mediastinal abnormalities. One example would be a patient with lung cancer in whom mediastinal nodes might be detected using CT despite a normal chest radiograph. Another example would be a patient with myasthenia gravis who, therefore, has a significant chance of having a thymoma (approximately 15%) that may be detected on CT.

NORMAL MEDIASTINAL ANATOMY

The mediastinum can be thought of as the tissue compartment situated between the lungs, marginated on each side by the mediastinal pleura, anteriorly by the sternum and chest wall, and posteriorly by the spine and chest wall. It contains the heart, great vessels, trachea, esophagus, thymus, considerable fat, and a number of lymph nodes, grouped together in specific regions. Many of these structures can be reliably identified on CT by their location, appearance, and attenuation.

In general, the mediastinum can be thought of as consisting of three almost equal divisions, the first beginning at the thoracic inlet and the third ending at the diaphragm. In adults, each of these divisions is made up of about 7 contiguous 10-mm slices, or 10 contiguous 7-mm slices. For lack of official anatomic names, these can be remembered as follows:

1. The *supraaortic mediastinum*—from the thoracic inlet to the top of the aortic arch
2. The *subaortic mediastinum*—from the aortic arch to the level of the heart
3. The *paracardiac mediastinum*—from the heart to the diaphragm

In each of these compartments, specific structures are consistently seen, and these need to be evaluated in every patient. Although very detailed mediastinal anatomy can be seen using CT, this description of normal anatomy is limited to structures that have some diagnostic value. If a more detailed knowledge of mediastinal anatomy is desired, there are a number of excellent atlases of cross-sectional anatomy. I do not think that a more detailed knowledge is usually necessary in interpreting CT. My main goal here is to provide an approach to viewing the mediastinum.

Supraaortic Mediastinum

In evaluating a CT scan of this part of the mediastinum, it is a good idea to localize the trachea before you do anything else (Fig. 2–1A). The trachea is easy to recognize because it contains air, is seen in cross section, and has a reasonably consistent round or oval shape. It is relatively central in the mediastinum, from front to back and from right to left, and it serves as an excellent reference point. Many other mediastinal structures maintain a consistent relationship to it. If you cannot find the trachea in looking at a scan of this part of the mediastinum, I would suggest giving up right now.

At or near the thoracic inlet, the mediastinum is relatively narrow from front to back. The esophagus lies posterior to the trachea at this level (see Fig. 2–1), but depending on the position of the trachea relative to the

spine, the esophagus can be displaced to one side or the other, usually the left. It is usually collapsed and appears as a flattened structure of soft tissue attenuation, but small amounts of air or air and fluid are often seen in its lumen.

In the supraaortic mediastinum, the great arterial branches of the aortic arch and the great veins are the most important structures to recognize. At or near the thoracic inlet, the brachiocephalic veins are the most anterior and lateral vascular branches visible, lying immediately behind the clavicular heads (see Fig. 2–1A and B). Although they vary in size, their positions are relatively constant. The great arterial branches (innominate, left carotid, and left subclavian arteries) are posterior to the veins and lie adjacent to the anterior and lateral walls of the trachea. They can be reliably identified by their relative positions.

Below the thoracic inlet, anterior to the arterial branches of the aorta, the left brachiocephalic vein crosses the mediastinum from left to right (see Fig. 2–1C), to join the right brachiocephalic vein, thus forming the superior vena cava (see Fig. 2–1C and 2–1D). The left subclavian artery is most posterior and is situated adjacent to the left side of the trachea, at 3 or 4 o'clock relative to the tracheal lumen. The left carotid artery is anterior to the left subclavian artery, at 1 or 2 o'clock, and is somewhat variable in position. The innominate artery is usually anterior and somewhat to the right of the tracheal midline (11 o'clock), but it is the most variable of all the great vessels and can have a number of different appearances in different patients or in the same patient at different levels (see Fig. 2–1D).

Near its origin from the aortic arch, the innominate artery is usually oval, being somewhat larger than the other aortic branches. As it ascends toward the thoracic outlet, it may appear oval or elliptical, because of its orientation or because of its bifurcation into the right subclavian and carotid arteries. Also, this vessel can be quite tortuous and can appear double if both limbs of a U-shaped part of the vessel are imaged in the same slice. Usually, these vessels can be traced from their origin at the aortic arch to the point they leave the chest, if there is any doubt as to what they represent.

Other than the great vessels, trachea, and esophagus, little is usually seen in the supraaortic mediastinum. Some lymph nodes are sometimes visible. Small vascular branches, particularly the internal mammary veins, can be seen in this part of the mediastinum but are rarely important in diagnosing disease. In some patients, the thyroid gland may extend into this portion of the mediastinum and the right and left thyroid lobes may be visible on each side of the trachea. This appearance is not abnormal and does not imply thyroid enlargement or "substernal thyroid." On CT, the thyroid can be distinguished from other tissues or masses because its attenuation is greater than that of soft tissue (because of its iodine content).

Subaortic Mediastinum

Like the supraaortic region, in adults, the subaortic mediastinum consists of approximately seven 10-mm (or ten 7-mm) scans, extending from the aortic arch to the upper heart (Fig. 2–2). Whereas the supraaortic region largely contains arterial and venous branches of the aorta and vena cava, this compartment contains many of the undivided mediastinal great vessels, such as the aorta, superior vena cava, and pulmonary arteries. This compartment also contains most of the important lymph nodes groups, which may be abnormal in patients with lung cancer, infectious diseases, or lymphoma. In other words, on most CT studies of the mediastinum, this is where the action is. There are a few key levels in this part of the mediastinum that need to be discussed in detail.

Aortic Arch Level

In the upper portion of this compartment, the aortic arch is easily seen and has a characteristic but somewhat variable appearance (see Fig. 2–2A and B). The anterior aspect of the arch is seen anterior to the trachea, with the arch itself passing to the left of the trachea, and the posterior arch is usually lying anterior and lateral to

the spine. Usually the aortic arch is about the same diameter in its anterior and midportion, although the posterior arch is typically a little smaller. The position of the anterior and posterior aspects of the arch can vary in the presence of atherosclerosis and aortic tortuosity; in patients with a tortuous aorta, the anterior arch moves anteriorly and to the right, whereas the posterior aorta moves more laterally and posteriorly, to a position to the left of the spine.

At this level, the superior vena cava is visible anterior and to the right of the trachea, usually being oval (see Fig. 2–2A through *D*). The esophagus appears the same as at higher levels and is variable in position. Often it lies somewhat to the left of the midline of the trachea (and of course is behind the trachea).

The aortic arch on the left, the superior vena cava and mediastinal pleura on the right, and the trachea posteriorly serve to define a roughly triangular space (with the apex of the triangle directed anteriorly), which has been named the *pretracheal* or *anterior paratracheal* space (see Fig. 2–2A, *B*, and *D*). This fat-filled space is important because it contains middle mediastinal lymph nodes in the pretracheal chain, commonly involved in various lymph node diseases. Whenever you view the mediastinum for the diagnosis of lymphadenopathy, you should look here first. Other mediastinal node groups are closely related to this group both spatially and in regard to lymphatic drainage. It is not uncommon to see a few normal-sized lymph nodes (diameter < 1 cm) in the pretracheal space, but this is discussed in detail when mediastinal lymphadenopathy is reviewed.

Anterior to the great vessels (aorta and superior vena cava) is another roughly (very roughly) triangular space called the *prevascular* space (see Fig. 2–2A, *B*, and *D*). This compartment represents the anterior mediastinum and primarily contains the thymus, lymph nodes, and fat. The apex of this triangular space represents the anterior junction line, sometimes visible on chest radiographs.

In young patients, usually in their teens or early twenties, CT shows the thymus to be of soft tissue attenuation and bilobed or

Text continued on page 14

Normal Mediastinal Anatomy. The following illustrations are largely from a single normal patient who had contrast medium–enhanced CT of the thorax. Some structures indicated in the accompanying diagrams are not visible in the scans. Scans were obtained using spiral technique with 7-mm collimation and 7-mm reconstruction.

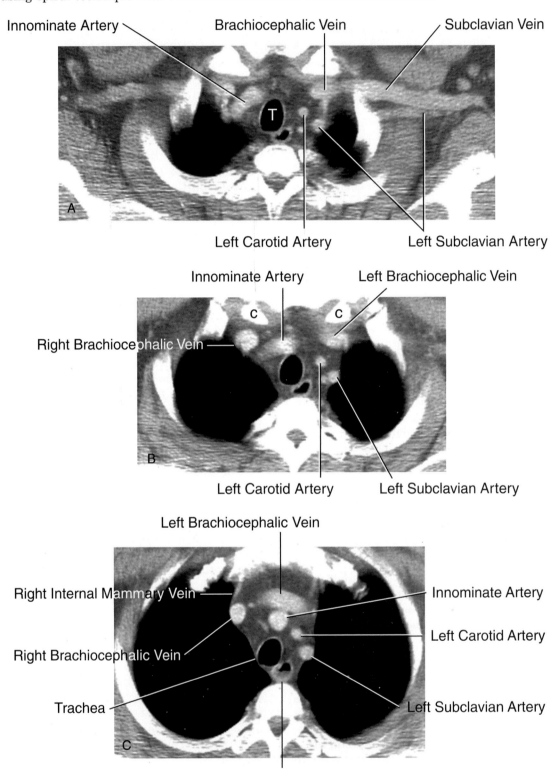

Figure 2–1 *See legend on opposite page*

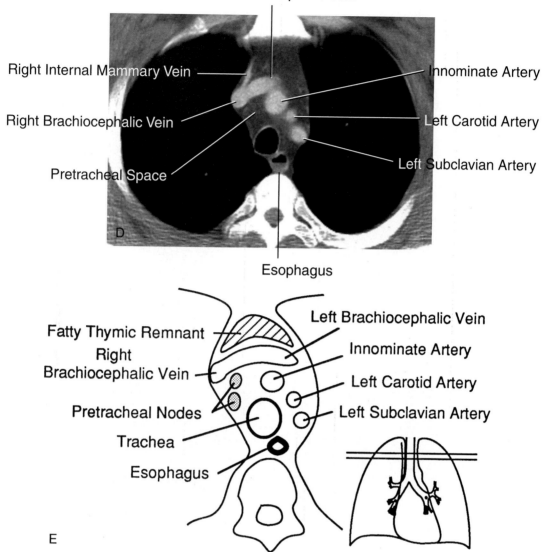

Figure 2–1. Supraaortic mediastinum. *(A)* At the thoracic inlet, the trachea (T) is clearly seen, with the air-filled esophagus posterior and to the left of it. The right and left brachiocephalic veins are anterior and lateral, being seen behind the clavicular heads. At this level the axillary veins are also visible (within the axilla). The great arterial branches (innominate, left carotid, and left subclavian arteries) are posterior to the veins, lying adjacent to the anterior and lateral walls of the trachea. The innominate artery appears elliptical because of its orientation in the plane of scan. *(B)* At 7 mm below *A*, the brachiocephalic veins are visible posterior to the clavicular heads (C). The left subclavian artery is most posterior and is situated lateral to the left tracheal wall, at 3 or 4 o'clock relative to the tracheal lumen, and contacting the mediastinal pleura. The left carotid artery is anterior to the left subclavian artery, at about 2 o'clock, and is somewhat variable in position. The innominate artery is usually anterior and to the right of the tracheal midline. *(C)* At 7 mm below *B*, the left brachiocephalic vein is visible crossing the mediastinum from left to right. The subclavian, carotid, and innominate arteries maintain the same relative positions as in *B*. The right internal mammary vein is visible arising from the right brachiocephalic vein. The esophagus contains a small amount of fluid in its lumen, with an air–fluid level visible. *(D)* At 7 mm below *C*, the left brachiocephalic vein joins the right brachiocephalic vein, forming the superior vena cava. The major aortic branches are again clearly seen. The pretracheal space is anterior to the trachea and posterior to the arteries and veins. *(E)* Diagram of supraaortic anatomy at the level of *D*. The location of pretracheal lymph nodes is shown, although these are not visible in the scan. Also, although not well seen in *D*, the location of the thymic remnant is marked. The approximate level of the scan in *D* is indicated by horizontal lines.

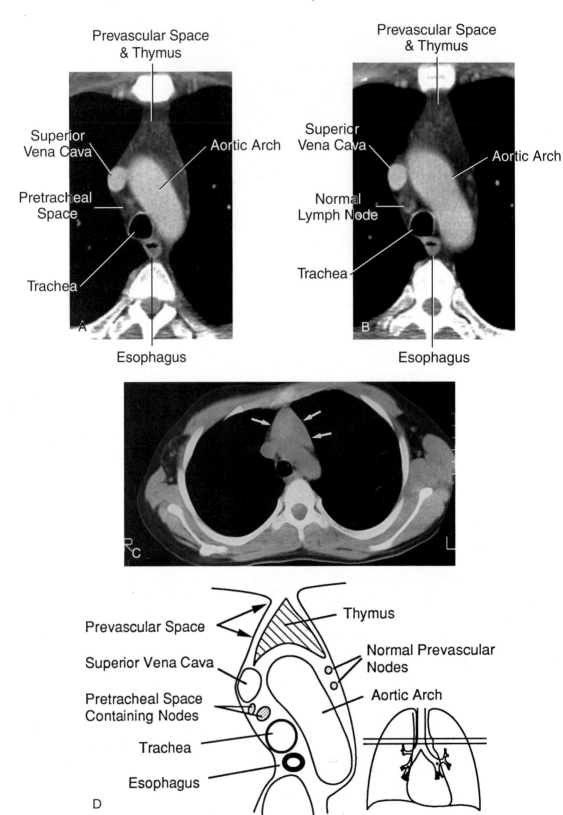

Figure 2–2 *See legend on opposite page*

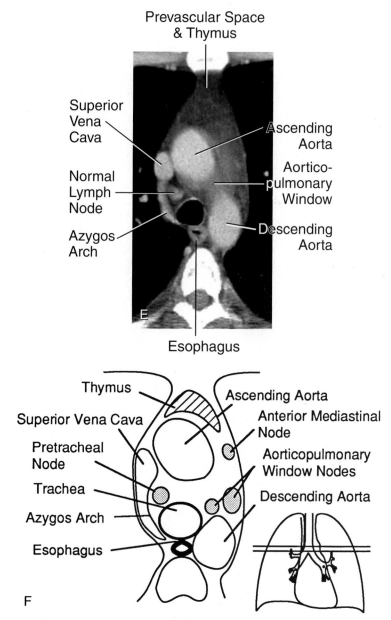

Figure 2–2. Subaortic mediastinum. *(A)* **Aortic arch level.** The aortic arch extends from a position anterior to the trachea, to the left, with the posterior part of the arch usually lying anterior and lateral to the spine. The superior vena cava contacts the right mediastinal pleura and along with the aortic arch delineates the anterior aspect of the pretracheal space. The prevascular space is anterior to the great vessels and contains the thymus, which is largely replaced by fat in this patient. *(B)* The locations of the pretracheal node-bearing space and prevascular space, containing the thymic remnant, are indicated. A normal pretracheal node is visible. *(C)* A large normal thymus *(arrows)* in a young patient occupies most of the prevascular space. *(D)* Diagram of the anatomy at the aortic arch level. *(E)* **Azygos arch and aorticopulmonary window level.** The azygos arch is visible arising from the posterior aspect of the superior vena cava, contacting the right mediastinal pleura, and forming the lateral margin of the pretracheal space. Fat visible under the aortic arch *(arrow)* is in the aorticopulmonary window. *(F)* The locations of lymph nodes in the pretracheal space, aorticopulmonary window, and anterior mediastinum at this level are shown, although they are not visible in *E*.

Illustration continued on following page

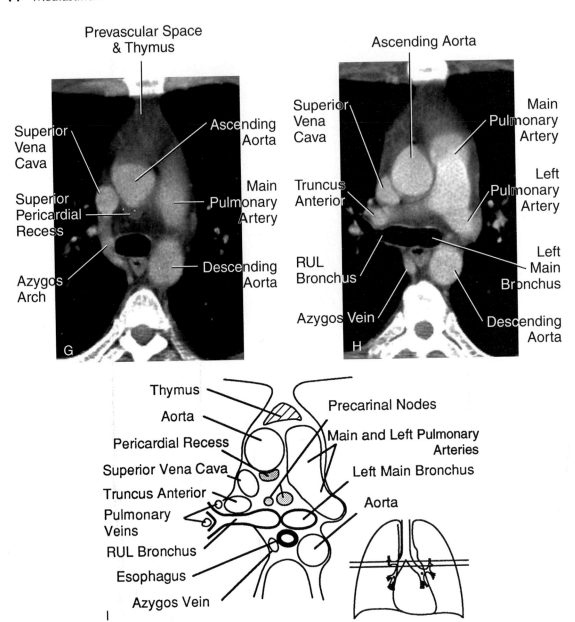

Figure 2–2 *Continued. (G)* At the tracheal carina, the trachea assumes an oval shape. The azygos arch remains visible. The upper aspect of the main pulmonary artery, which marginates the caudal aspect of the aorticopulmonary window, should not be confused with a mass lesion. *(H and I)* Scan and diagram at the level of the left pulmonary artery and right upper lobe bronchus. The superior pericardial recess posterior to the aorta appears larger in *I* than in *H*.

arrowhead shaped, with each of the two lobes (the right and left) contacting the mediastinal pleura. Each lobe usually measures 1 to 2 cm in thickness (measured perpendicular to the pleura), but this is variable (see Fig. 2–2C). In adulthood, the thymus involutes, with soft tissue being replaced by fat. In patients older than 30,

the prevascular space appears primarily fat filled, with thin wisps of tissue passing through the fat. Most of this, including the fat, actually represents the thymus. At higher levels, the thymus is sometimes visible anterior to the brachiocephalic arteries and veins, also within the prevascular space.

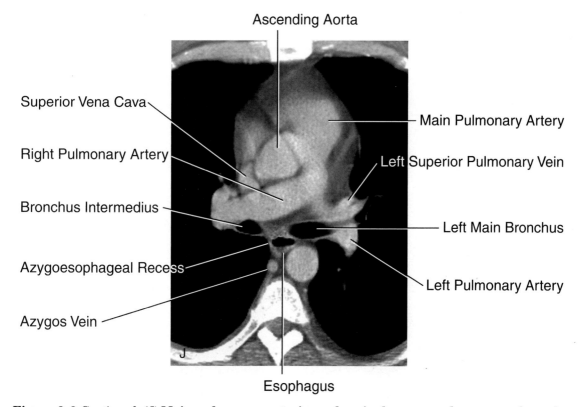

Ascending Aorta

Superior Vena Cava

Right Pulmonary Artery

Bronchus Intermedius

Azygoesophageal Recess

Azygos Vein

Main Pulmonary Artery

Left Superior Pulmonary Vein

Left Main Bronchus

Left Pulmonary Artery

Esophagus

Figure 2–2 *Continued.* *(J)* **Main pulmonary arteries, subcarinal space, and azygoesophageal recess level.** Slightly below the tracheal carina, the right pulmonary artery is visible crossing the mediastinum, filling the pretracheal and precarinal space. A small amount of fat is visible in the subcarinal space, slightly anterior to the esophagus, azygos vein, and azygoesophageal recess.

Illustration continued on following page

Azygos Arch and Aorticopulmonary Window Level

At a level slightly below the aortic arch, the ascending aorta and descending aorta are visible as separate structures. Characteristically, the ascending aorta (25–35 mm in diameter) is slightly larger than the descending aorta (20–30 mm).

At or near this level, the trachea bifurcates into the right and left main bronchi. Near the carina, the trachea commonly assumes a somewhat oval or triangular shape (see Fig. 2–2*G*). The carina itself is usually visible on CT. On the right side, the arch of the azygos vein (*azygos,* incidentally, means "unpaired") arises from the posterior wall of the superior vena cava, passes over the right main bronchus (thus it is seen at a higher level than the bronchus itself), and continues posteriorly along the mediastinum, to lie to the right and anterior of the

spine (see Fig. 2–2*E* through *G*). (Below the level of the azygos arch, the azygos vein remains visible in this position). The azygos arch is often visible on one or two adjacent slices and sometimes appears nodular. However, its characteristic location is usually sufficient to correctly identify this structure. When the azygos arch is visible, it marginates the right border of the pretracheal space.

On the left side of the mediastinum, under the aortic arch, but above the main pulmonary artery, is the region termed the *aorticopulmonary window.* The aorticopulmonary window contains fat, lymph nodes (middle mediastinal), the recurrent laryngeal nerve, and the ligamentum arteriosum (the latter two are usually invisible) (see Fig. 2–2*E* and *F*). Aorticopulmonary window lymph nodes freely communicate with those in the pretracheal space, and, in fact, it may be difficult to distinguish nodes in the

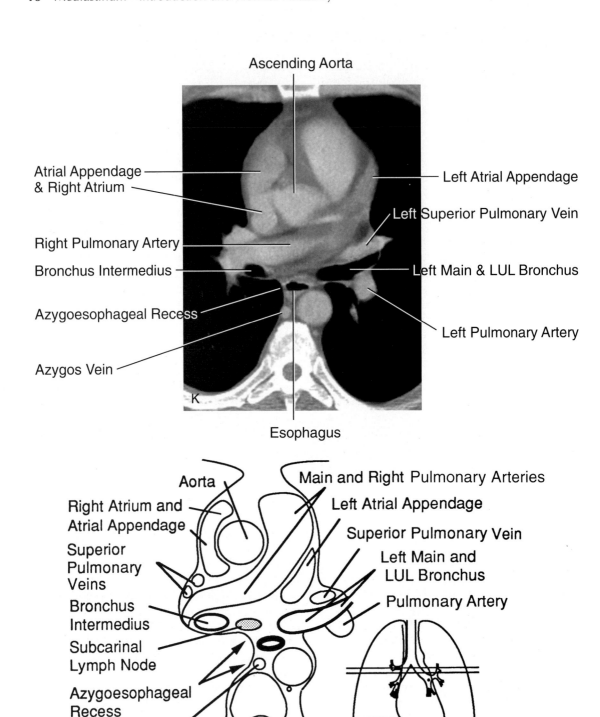

Ascending Aorta

Atrial Appendage & Right Atrium

Left Atrial Appendage

Left Superior Pulmonary Vein

Right Pulmonary Artery

Bronchus Intermedius

Left Main & LUL Bronchus

Azygoesophageal Recess

Left Pulmonary Artery

Azygos Vein

K

Esophagus

Aorta

Main and Right Pulmonary Arteries

Right Atrium and Atrial Appendage

Left Atrial Appendage

Superior Pulmonary Veins

Superior Pulmonary Vein

Left Main and LUL Bronchus

Bronchus Intermedius

Pulmonary Artery

Subcarinal Lymph Node

Azygoesophageal Recess

Azygos Vein

L

Figure 2–2 *Continued. (K and L)* Scan and diagram at the level of the azygoesophageal recess. The recess appears concave laterally, with the mediastinal pleura closely related to the azygos vein and esophagus.

medial aorticopulmonary window from those in the left part of the pretracheal space. In some patients, the aorticopulmonary window is not well seen, with the main pulmonary artery lying immediately below the aortic arch. In such patients, it is usually difficult to distinguish lymph nodes from volume averaging of the adjacent aorta and pulmonary artery (see Fig. 2–2G), and caution should be exercised. However, sometimes scans with thin collimation are helpful in distinguishing nodes from volume averaging.

At or slightly below the aorticopulmonary window, at the level of the ascending aorta is first clearly seen in cross section (i.e., it is round or nearly round), a portion of the pericardium, usually containing a small amount of pericardial fluid, extends up from below into the pretracheal space and immediately behind the ascending aorta. This part of the pericardium is called the *superior pericardial recess* (see Fig. 2–2G through *I*). Although it can sometimes be confused with a lymph node, its typical location, immediately behind and hugging the aortic wall, its oval or crescentic shape, and its relatively low (water) attenuation allow it to be distinguished from a significant abnormality. Another part of the pericardial recess can sometimes be seen anterior to the ascending aorta and pulmonary artery.

Main Pulmonary Arteries, Subcarinal Space, and Azygoesophageal Recess

Below the level of the carina and azygos arch (see Fig. 2–2H through *L*), the medial aspect of the right lung tucks into the posterior portion of the middle mediastinum, in close association with the azygos vein and esophagus. This part of the mediastinum, reasonably called the *azygoesophageal recess*, is important because of the adjacent subcarinal lymph nodes and its close relationship to the esophagus and main bronchi. The contour of the azygoesophageal recess is concave laterally in the large majority of normal subjects, and a convexity in this region indicates the possibility of an underlying pathologic process. However, a convexity in this region may be produced by a normal esophagus or azygos vein. Of course, the great value of CT is that we do not need to rely on contours, as we do on plain radiographs, to make a diagnosis of mediastinal disease. If a contour abnormality is detected (usually on lung window scans, which best show mediastinal contours), a close look at the mediastinal windows should be sufficient to delineate the cause of the abnormal contour. If the contour abnormality does not reflect the esophagus or azygos vein, then it is abnormal and subcarinal node enlargement is the usual culprit.

In many subjects, the azygoesophageal recess is somewhat posterior to the node-bearing subcarinal space, which lies between the main bronchi. Normal nodes are commonly visible in this space, being larger than normal nodes in other parts of the mediastinum and up to 1.5 cm in diameter. The esophagus is usually seen immediately behind the subcarinal space, and distinguishing nodes and esophagus may be difficult, unless the esophagus contains air or contrast material. At levels below the subcarinal space, the appearance of the azygoesophageal recess is relatively constant, although it narrows somewhat in a retrocardiac region.

Also at or near this level, the main pulmonary artery divides into its right and left branches. The left pulmonary artery (see Fig. 2–2G through *I*) is somewhat higher than the right, usually being seen 1 cm above it, and appears to be the continuation of the main pulmonary artery, directed posterolaterally and to the left. The right pulmonary artery arises at an angle of nearly 90° to the main and left pulmonary artery and crosses the mediastinum, anterior to the carina or main bronchi. In this location, the right pulmonary artery effectively fills in the pretracheal space.

At the point the main bronchi and pulmonary arteries exit the mediastinum, the pulmonary hila are entered (see Chapter 5).

Paracardiac Mediastinum

As we progress caudad through the mediastinum, the origins of the great vessels from the cardiac chambers can be seen to a variable degree. Although CT is not commonly used to diagnose cardiac abnormalities

Text continued on page 22

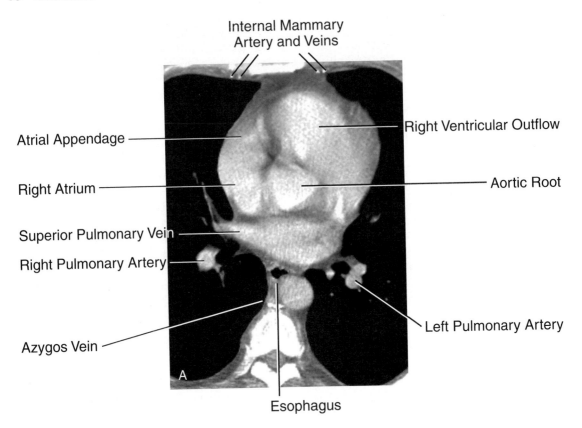

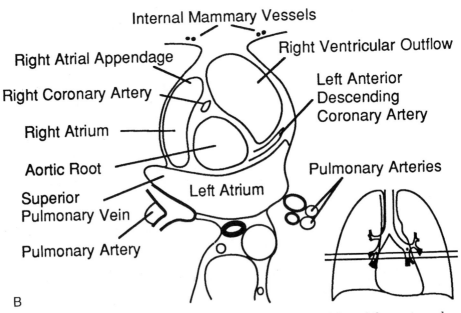

Figure 2–3. Paracardiac mediastinum. *(A)* Most cephalad, the origins of the aorta and pulmonary artery are visible, with the aortic root being central. The right ventricular (pulmonary) outflow tract or main pulmonary artery are anterior and to the left of the aortic root at this level. The right atrium, with its appendage extending anteriorly, border the right mediastinal pleura. The superior pulmonary veins enter the upper aspect of the left atrium at this level or slightly above. Anteriorly, the right internal mammary vessels are visible *(arrow)*. *(B)* Diagram at the level of *A*. The positions of left and right coronary arteries are shown.

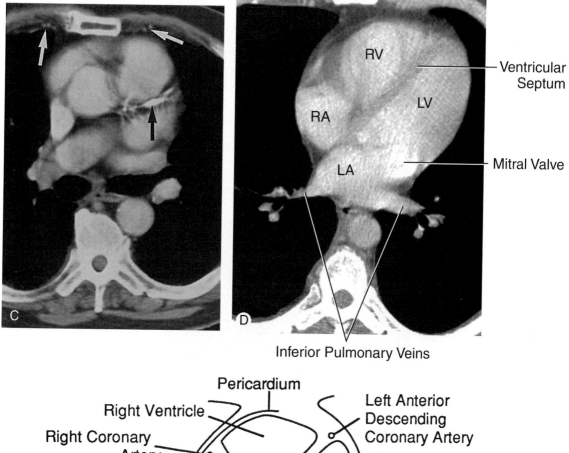

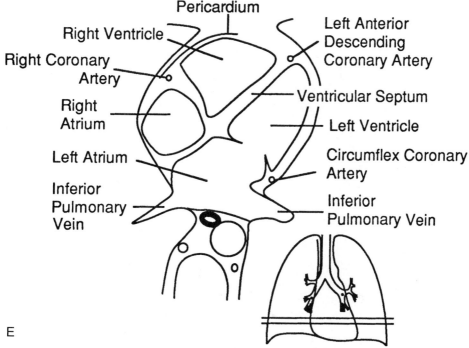

Figure 2–3 *Continued. (C)* In another subject, calcification of the left anterior descending coronary artery *(black arrow)* is easily seen. The left coronary artery arises from the posterolateral aortic root. The internal mammary vessels *(white arrows)* are also visible. *(D and E)* At a lower level, the right and left atria and ventricles are visible. The right ventricle is located anterior and to the right of the left ventricle. At this level, the inferior pulmonary veins enter the left atrium.

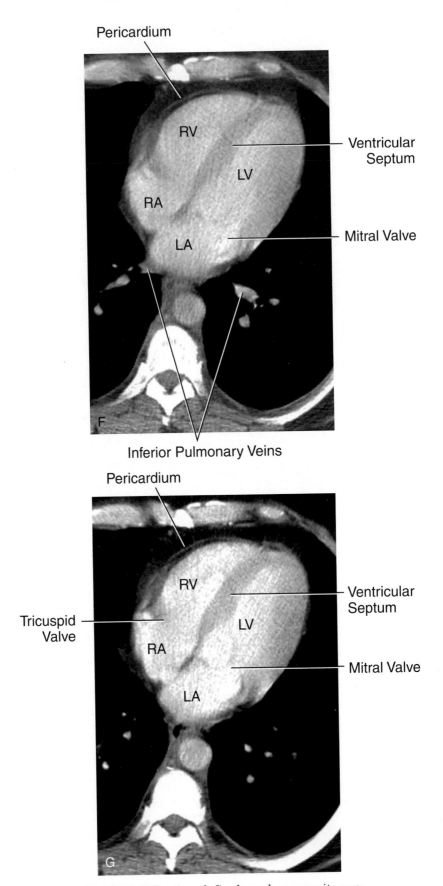

Figure 2–3 *Continued. See legend on opposite page*

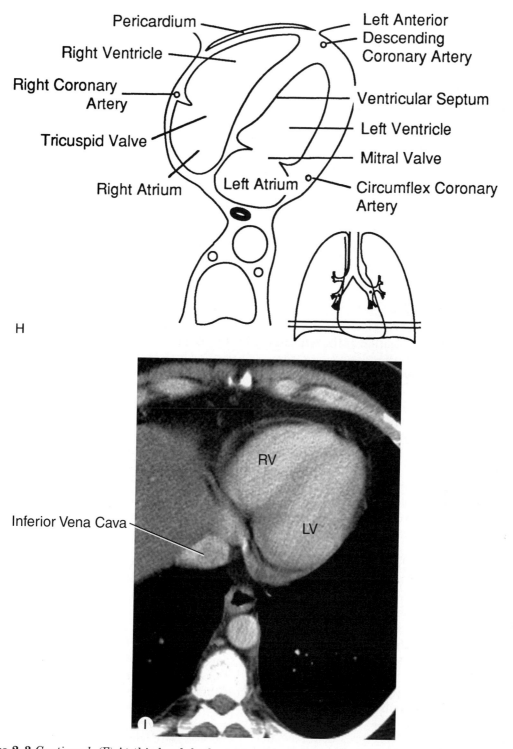

Figure 2–3 *Continued.* *(F)* At this level, both atria and ventricles are visible. The ventricular septal and left ventricular walls are thicker than the right ventricular wall, and the septum is convex toward the right ventricle. *(G and H)* All four chambers are visible, and the location of both tricuspid and mitral valves can be identified. The interventricular septum and free wall of the left ventricle are considerably thicker than the wall of the right ventricle. The pericardium is visible as a thin white line surrounded by mediastinal fat. It should appear as 1 to 2 mm in thickness. *(I)* Near the diaphragm, the inferior vena cava is visible as a separate structure, below the level of the right atrium.

(echocardiography or magnetic resonance imaging is usually preferred), some simple understanding of cardiac anatomy on CT can be helpful in diagnosis.

The main pulmonary artery is most anterior, arising from the right ventricle, which can be seen at lower levels to be anterior and to the right of the left ventricle (Fig. 2–3A and B). The superior vena cava enters the right atrium, which is elliptical or crescentic. The right atrial appendage extends anteriorly from the upper atrium, bordering the right mediastinal pleura.

Between the right atrium and the main pulmonary artery or pulmonary outflow tract, the aortic root enters the left ventricle. At this level it is common in adults to see some coronary artery calcification (see Fig. 2–3C), and, occasionally, uncalcified coronary arteries are visible surrounded by mediastinal fat. Calcification of the left coronary artery, left anterior descending coronary artery, circumflex coronary artery, and right coronary artery can be identified. The left atrium is posteriorly located, appearing larger than the right. The left atrial appendage extends anteriorly and to the left and is visible below the left pulmonary artery, bordering the pleura. On each side, superior and inferior pulmonary veins can be seen entering the left atrium (see Fig. 2–3A, B, D, and E). These are discussed further in Chapter 5.

Near the level of the diaphragm, the inferior vena cava is visible as on oval structure extending caudad from the posterior right atrium. It is easy to identify.

The only other structures of consequence at this level that need to be mentioned are the esophagus, which lies in a retrocardiac location, the azygos vein, which is often still visible in the same relative position as at higher levels, and the hemiazygos vein, which is usually smaller than the azygos, and on the opposite side, behind the descending aorta. Paravertebral nodes lie in association with the azygos and hemiazygos veins but are not normally visible.

NORMAL CARDIAC ANATOMY

Without the injection of contrast medium, little cardiac anatomy is discernible on CT,

but some differentiation of cardiac chambers is possible because of the presence of epicardial fat collections. When contrast medium is used, additional features of cardiac anatomy are visible, depending on the amount and rapidity of contrast medium injection; the myocardium opacifies less than the intracardiac blood and is often visible as a relatively low-attenuation band after rapid infusion of a large contrast medium bolus. The interventricular septum is usually visible if contrast medium has been infused; it is typically oriented at an angle of about 2 o'clock to the vertical and is convex anteriorly because of the higher left ventricular pressure (see Fig. 2–3). However, other segments of the myocardium may be difficult to appreciate as distinct from the opacified cardiac chambers on clinical scans, unless contrast medium is rapidly infused. The lateral or "free" left ventricular wall is about three times thicker (it is about 1 cm in thickness) than the right ventricular wall.

Cardiac anatomy is easiest to understand if we start with a scan near the cardiac apex (and diaphragm). At this level, the left ventricle is elliptical, with its long axis directed laterally and anteriorly (see Fig. 2–3F through H). Being the highest pressure chamber, it dominates cardiac anatomy, and the other cardiac chambers mold themselves to its shape. The right ventricle, which is anterior and to the right, is triangular. On scans at this level or slightly above, the line of the interventricular septum, if continued posteriorly and to the right, separates the lower right atrium anteriorly (and in contiguity with the right ventricle), from the lower left atrium posteriorly. The mitral and tricuspid valves are located at or near this level and can be seen if there is good contrast opacification of the cardiac chambers.

At higher levels (see Fig. 2–3A and B), the left ventricular outflow tract and aortic valve are centrally located within the heart. The right ventricular outflow tract is directed toward the left and is visible anterior or to the left of the left ventricular outflow tract. In other words, because of twisting of the heart during development, the left ventricular outflow tract is directed rightward and the right ventricular outflow tract is directed leftward. This accounts for the location of the aorta on the right and the pulmonary artery on the left. The aortic and pulmonary valves are located near this level and are invisible in normal subjects.

The Normal Pericardium

The normal pericardium (the visceral and parietal pericardium and pericardial contents) is visible as a 1- to 2-mm stripe of soft tissue attenuation paralleling the heart and outlined by mediastinal fat (outside the pericardial sac) and epicardiac fat. It is best seen near the diaphragm, along the anterior and lateral aspects of the heart, where the fat layers are thickest (Fig. 2–3*F* through *H*). As stated earlier, extensions of the pericardium into the upper mediastinum can also be seen in normal subjects.

THE RETROSTERNAL SPACE

In a retrosternal location, the internal mammary arteries and veins are normally visible 1 or 2 cm lateral to the edge of the sternum on good CT scans (see Fig. 2–3*A* through *C*); up to three vessels can be seen on each side (one artery, two veins). These vessels are not of much diagnostic significance, although the veins commonly enlarge in patients with superior vena caval obstruction, but they are important because they serve to localize the internal mammary

chain of lymph nodes. Although normal nodes can be seen in several areas of the mediastinum (most notably the pretracheal space, aorticopulmonary window, and subcarinal space), normal internal mammary nodes are not large enough to be recognized. A lymph node in this region that is large enough to be visible should be regarded as abnormal. Internal mammary node enlargement is most common in patients with breast cancer or lymphoma.

Suggested Reading

Aronberg DJ, Peterson RR, Glazer HS, Sagel SS. The superior sinus of the pericardium: CT appearance. Radiology 1984; 153:489–492.

Francis I, Glazer GM, Bookstein FL, Gross BH. The thymus: reexamination of age-related changes in size and shape. AJR 1985; 145:249–254.

Glazer HS, Aronberg DJ, Sagel SS. Pitfalls in CT recognition of mediastinal lymphadenopathy. AJR 1985; 144:267–274.

Kiyono K, Sone S, Sakai F, et al. The number and size of normal mediastinal lymph nodes: a postmortem study. AJR 1988; 150:771–776.

Müller NL, Webb WR, Gamsu G. Paratracheal lymphadenopathy: radiographic findings and correlation with CT. Radiology 1985; 156:761–765.

Müller NL, Webb WR, Gamsu G. Subcarinal lymph node enlargement: radiographic findings and CT correlation. AJR 1985; 145:15–19.

Zylak CJ, Pallie W, Pirani M, et al. Anatomy and computed tomography: a correlative module on the cervicothoracic junction. Radiographics 1983; 3:478–530.

Mediastinum—Vascular Abnormalities

W. Richard Webb, M.D.

On any thoracic CT in a patient with a mediastinal mass, the first objective is often to prove that the mass is or is not vascular in origin.

AORTIC ABNORMALITIES

A variety of aortic arch and great arterial abnormalities are visible on CT, and CT is commonly used to diagnose aortic disease when it is suspected clinically or when chest radiographs are abnormal.

Congenital Anomalies

Congenital abnormalities of the aorta and its mediastinal branches are easily diagnosed using CT, and no other study is usually needed unless the anomaly is complex or associated with congenital heart disease. Magnetic resonance imaging is often used to study coarctation.

Anomalous Right Subclavian Artery

This relatively common anomaly (1 in 100 individuals) does not usually produce a recognizable mediastinal abnormality on chest radiographs and, thus, is usually detected incidentally on CT scans obtained for another reason. Its main significance is that it should not be misinterpreted as something

else. In patients with this anomaly, the aortic arch is often somewhat higher than normal. The anomalous artery arises from the medial wall of the aorta, as its last branch (Fig. 3–1). It passes to the right, behind the esophagus, and then ascends on the right toward the thoracic outlet. It lies much more posterior than is normal for the subclavian artery, often anterolateral to the spine. At its point of origin, the artery may be dilated, or if you wish to think of it in a more complicated way, the artery may arise from an aortic diverticulum (diverticulum of Kommerell). This may cause compression of the esophagus and symptoms of dysphagia. In some patients, the diverticulum or the anomalous artery becomes aneurysmal (Fig. 3–2).

Right Aortic Arch

There are two main types of right aortic arch—*mirror image right arch* and *right arch associated with anomalous left subclavian artery.* Mirror image right arch is relatively uncommon and is almost always (98%) associated with congenital heart disease (usually complex anomalies such as tetralogy of Fallot). The CT appearance of a mirror image arch is well described by its name—it is the mirror image of a normal left arch, with a left innominate artery being present. Right arch with an anomalous left subclavian artery is present in about 1

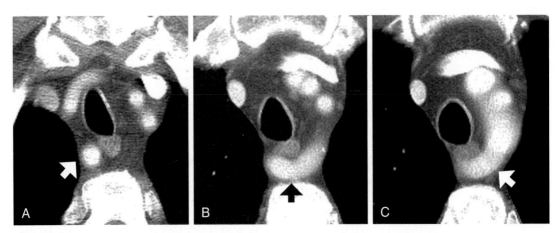

Figure 3–1. Anomalous right subclavian artery. *(A)* An anomalous right subclavian artery *(arrow)* is located posteriorly in the right superior mediastinum. *(B)* At a level 7 mm below *A,* the anomalous artery *(arrow)* passes posterior to the esophagus. *(C)* At 7 mm below *B,* the origin *(arrow)* of the anomalous artery from the posterior superior aortic arch is visible.

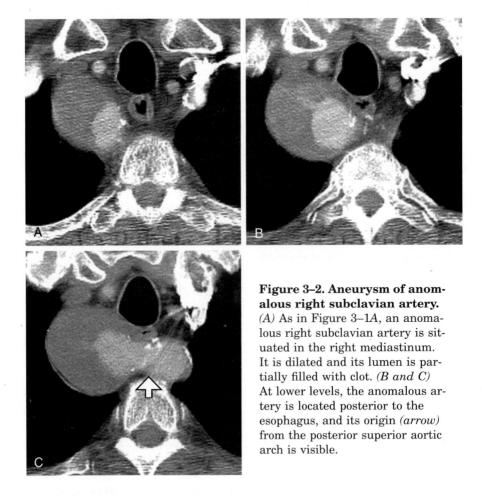

Figure 3–2. Aneurysm of anomalous right subclavian artery. *(A)* As in Figure 3–1A, an anomalous right subclavian artery is situated in the right mediastinum. It is dilated and its lumen is partially filled with clot. *(B and C)* At lower levels, the anomalous artery is located posterior to the esophagus, and its origin *(arrow)* from the posterior superior aortic arch is visible.

in 1000 subjects. It is the reverse of a left arch with an anomalous right subclavian artery, although the presence of an aortic diverticulum is more common in the presence of a right arch (Fig. 3–3). With this anomaly, there is a low frequency (5%–10%) of associated congenital heart lesions, and they are usually simple, such as atrial septal defect. With both types of right arch the descending aorta is usually left sided, crossing from right to left in the lower mediastinum.

Double Aortic Arch

Double aortic arches are relatively uncommon, but because the plain radiograph shows a mediastinal abnormality they are often evaluated using CT. This anomaly is uncommonly associated with congenital heart disease, but because a complete vascular ring is present, symptoms of dysphagia are common. In this anomaly, the ascending aorta splits into right and left halves. The right arch, which is usually higher and larger than the left, passes to the right of the trachea and esophagus, crosses behind these structures, and rejoins the left arch, which occupies a relatively normal position (Fig. 3–4). Each arch is smaller than normal and smaller than the descending aorta. Also, each arch gives rise

to a subclavian and carotid artery and no innominate artery is present. This results in a symmetric appearance to the great vessels in the supraaortic mediastinum that is highly suggestive of the diagnosis.

Coarctation and Pseudocoarctation

Coarctation, and its variant pseudocoarctation, can be diagnosed using CT, but even if this is possible, catheterization is usually necessary to measure intraarterial pressures and, thus, the significance of the vascular obstruction. Some believe that the use of the term *pseudocoarctation* is inappropriate, considering this lesion to be a coarctation and not "pseudo," but the CT and clinical findings in these two entities are different. They will be considered separately if for no other reason than the term *pseudocoarctation* is in common usage.

The site of narrowing in coarctation is generally at the aortic isthmus, distal to the origin of the left subclavian artery and near the ligamentum arteriosum (juxtaductal coarctation). On CT, the narrowed segment is often visible, being decidedly smaller than the aorta above and below this level (Fig. 3–5). This size difference not only reflects the narrowed segment at the coarctation but also reflects some dilation of the prestenotic and poststenotic aorta. Reconstructed

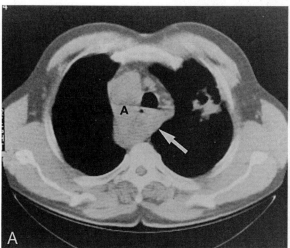
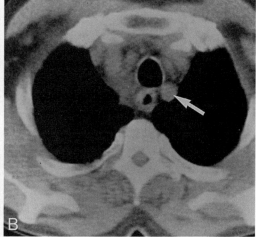

Figure 3–3. Right aortic arch with anomalous left subclavian artery. *(A)* In a patient with no evidence of congenital heart disease, and a right aortic arch (A), an anomalous left subclavian artery arises from a retroesophageal aortic diverticulum *(arrow)*. The position of the esophagus is marked by air in its lumen. *(B)* At a higher level, the anomalous left subclavian artery *(arrow)* is visible.

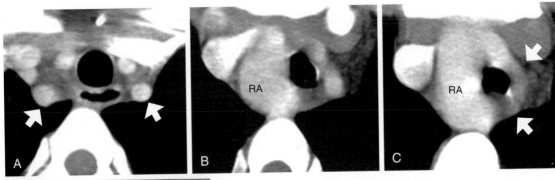

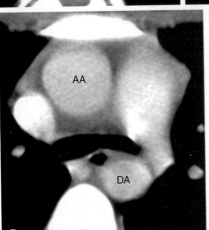

Figure 3–4. Double aortic arch. *(A)* In the upper mediastinum, the subclavian *(arrows)* and carotid arteries appear bilaterally symmetric. *(B)* At a level below *A,* the right arch (RA) is visible to the right of the trachea. On the left side of the mediastinum, the left carotid and subclavian arteries, which arise from the left arch, are visible. The right arch is characteristically higher and larger than the left. *(C)* At a level below *B,* the left arch *(arrows)* is now visible. It appears smaller than the right arch (RA). *(D)* At a level below *C,* the ascending aorta (AA) and descending aorta (DA) appear normal.

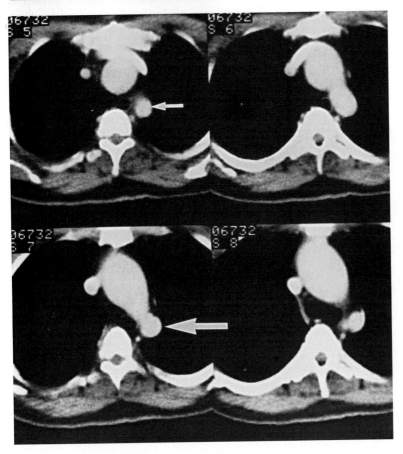

Figure 3–5. Aortic coarctation. CT scan with bolus contrast medium enhancement at four levels in a patient with coarctation. The proximal descending aorta, at the level of the coarctation *(large arrow),* is significantly smaller than the ascending aorta. The coarctation is distal to the origin of the left subclavian artery *(small arrow),* which is large because of collateral blood flow.

CT in the plane of the aortic arch can show the coarctation to better advantage; with spiral CT, excellent re-formations or three-dimensional reconstructions can be obtained. One word of caution: the degree of narrowing at the site of coarctation may be overestimated if the reformatted plane is slightly off the sagittal plane of the aorta. A long narrowing of the aortic arch (hypoplasia) is less common. Dilatation of internal mammary arteries or intercostal arteries (usually the third through eighth) acting as collateral pathways can be seen.

In pseudocoarctation, the aortic arch is kinked anteriorly and its lumen is somewhat narrowed, but a significant pressure gradient across the kink and collateral vessels are not present. The CT appearance of this anomaly is characteristic but sometimes confusing. The aortic arch is higher than normal and initially descends in an abnormally anterior position, well in front of the spine. At a level near the carina, however, it again angles posteriorly, forming a second arch, and assumes its normal position anterolateral to the spine. This anomaly is usually unassociated with symptoms and is usually detected incidentally on chest radiographs. Its plain film appearance may also be characteristic.

Both coarctation and pseudocoarctation are associated with congenital bicuspid aortic valve (30%–85% of patients with coarctation); this may result in aortic stenosis. In some patients, CT shows aortic valve calcification, allowing this diagnosis to be suggested.

Aortic Aneurysm

CT is of great value in diagnosing aortic aneurysm and distinguishing it from soft tissue mediastinal mass. If the ascending aorta measures more than 4 cm in diameter, it is usually referred to as dilated or ectatic. Although a diagnosis of "aortic dilatation" as opposed to "aortic aneurysm" is somewhat arbitrary, I use "aortic dilatation" or "ectasia" to refer to a generalized dilatation of relatively mild degree (4 cm), with the implication that it is not necessarily a serious problem. "Aneurysm," on the other hand, is used to refer to a more focal abnor-

mality or more severe dilatation of the entire aorta (5 cm). If the aorta is more than 6 cm, treatment is usually necessary. In other words, for the aorta, 4 cm = dilated; 5 cm = aneurysm; and 6 cm = surgery.

In some patients with an (atherosclerotic) aortic aneurysm, the diagnosis can be made and the aneurysm distinguished from a solid mass because of peripheral intimal calcification visible on unenhanced scans. In most patients, however, this diagnosis requires contrast medium infusion, and the best opacification is achieved if a rapid bolus of contrast agent is given with dynamic scanning at one or more levels in the area of abnormality. With a bolus technique, the lumen of the aorta and the aneurysm and the thickness of the aortic wall can be clearly defined (Fig. 3–6).

With atherosclerotic aneurysms, the aortic wall is thickened and calcification is commonly visible. There may be visible areas of plaque or thrombus in the lumen of the aorta that occasionally show some calcification as well. The plaque often appears low in attenuation relative to soft tissue or aortic wall because of its fat content or because of some opacification of the aortic wall itself. Plaque can also be seen in patients with atherosclerosis who do not have aortic dilatation. Mycotic aneurysms are usually focal and may be associated with periaortic inflammation or abscess, and air bubbles within soft tissues may be seen.

Trauma

Conventional CT has a limited role in the diagnosis of acute aortic injuries, such as aortic rupture or laceration. Although conventional CT is good for demonstrating the mediastinal hematoma that occurs in association with aortic laceration, the tear itself is often not visible. However, it is suggested that a normal CT in a patient with trauma, with no evidence of mediastinal blood, effectively excludes aortic laceration. In patients with mediastinal hematoma, aortography is usually required.

Spiral CT, on the other hand, because of volumetric acquisition and dense aortic enhancement, is reported to be of considerable

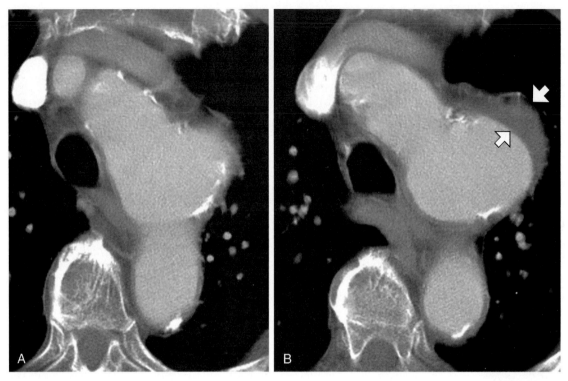

Figure 3–6. Aortic aneurysm. *(A and B)* A focal, saccular aneurysm of the aortic arch shows some clot lining its lumen *(arrows, B).*

value in diagnosing aortic laceration, with a sensitivity of 100% in detecting the tear itself. It has been suggested that aortography is not needed if (1) no mediastinal hematoma is visible or (2) no aortic abnormality is seen in patients with hematoma. Aortography would still be necessary in patients with inadequate CT studies or questionable CT findings or in some patients before surgery.

Posttraumatic false aneurysms are usually located in the region of the aorticopulmonary window, below the takeoff of the left subclavian artery (Fig. 3–7). Because these represent a contained aortic rupture, and they are not marginated by aortic wall, peripheral calcification is unusual. Aneurysmal dilatation of the ductus or ductus diverticulum (ductus aneurysm) can occur in the same region.

Dissection

CT has revolutionized the diagnosis of dissection and to a large extent has replaced arteriography. The goal in diagnosing dissection, using any technique, is the demonstration of an intimal flap, displaced inward from the edge of the aorta, separating the true and false channels. CT is ideally suited to this because of its cross-sectional format.

Two schemes for the classification of dissections have been proposed by Daily and DeBakey. Daily's classification (also known as the Stanford classification) is most frequently used because of its simplicity and relevance to treatment.

Using this classification, aortic dissections are divided into types A and B. Type A dissections involve the ascending aorta (Fig. 3–8); approximately two thirds of acute dissections are type A. Because of the possibility of retrograde dissection and rupture into the pericardium (resulting in tamponade) or occlusion of the coronary or cephalic arteries, these dissections are usually treated surgically with grafting of the region of the tear. Type B dissections do not involve the aortic arch but typically arise distal to the left subclavian artery (Fig. 3–9). These are generally treated medically instead of surgically.

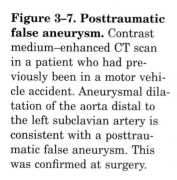

Figure 3–7. Posttraumatic false aneurysm. Contrast medium–enhanced CT scan in a patient who had previously been in a motor vehicle accident. Aneurysmal dilatation of the aorta distal to the left subclavian artery is consistent with a posttraumatic false aneurysm. This was confirmed at surgery.

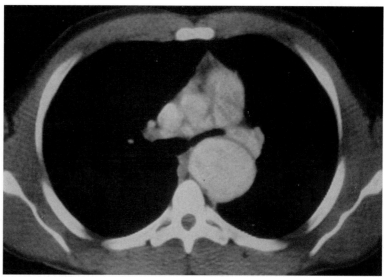

DeBakey's classification has three types. Type I (involvement of the entire aorta, both ascending and descending) is most common. Type II dissections, which are often associated with Marfan's syndrome, involve the ascending aorta only and along with type I correspond to Daily's type A. Type III dissections involve the descending aorta only and are often related to trauma; these are equivalent to Daily's type B.

Because CT is quite accurate in diagnosing dissection and in determining its location and type (it is better than arteriography), CT is an excellent screening procedure in patients with a suggestive clinical presentation. CT is the only imaging procedure performed in most patients with suspected dissection, although an aortogram or magnetic resonance image may be obtained before surgery in patients shown to have a type A dissection. Also, CT or magnetic resonance imaging can be used to follow pa-

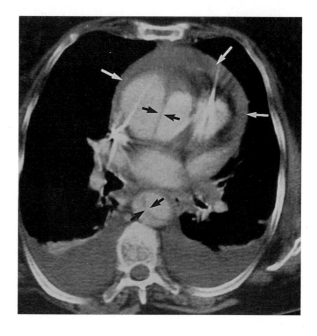

Figure 3–8. Type A aortic dissection. A patient with acute chest pain shows a type A dissection involving the ascending and descending aorta. The intimal flaps *(black arrows)* are lower in attenuation than the contrast medium–opacified blood. The ascending aorta is also dilated. Pleural and pericardial hemorrhage *(white arrows)* are present as a complication of the dissection. Streak artifacts reflect the presence of a catheter in the superior vena cava and pulmonary artery.

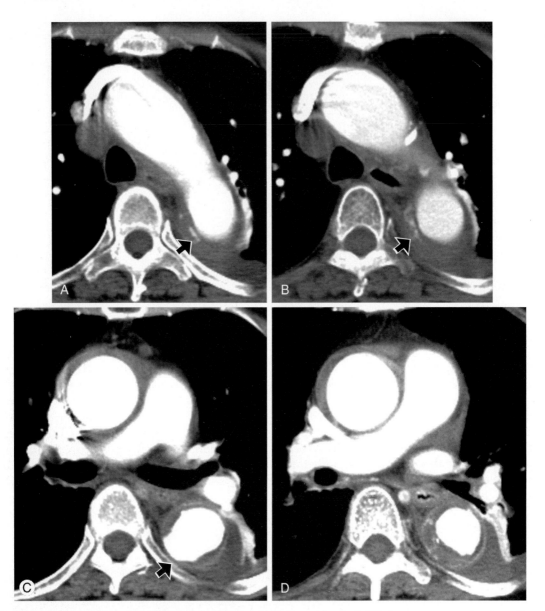

Figure 3–9. Type B aortic dissection. *(A and B)* Enhanced spiral CT shows some contrast medium dissecting into the aortic wall *(arrows)*. Artifacts mimic an intimal flap in the ascending aorta. *(C)* At a lower level, the site of communication between the false and true channels can be seen *(arrow)*. *(D)* At a level below *C,* the aortic wall appears thickened. This appearance can be referred to as "penetrating ulcer."

tients with dissection after treatment to watch for redissection or extension of the dissection.

In patients with suspected dissection, CT should be performed with bolus contrast medium enhancement, dynamic scanning, and spiral technique if available. Using spiral technique, it is easy to scan through the great vessels, aortic arch, and descending aorta (7 mm collimation, pitch 1) during contrast infusion (at 2 mL/sec, 30-second delay) and continue the scans into the abdomen, with one or two breath holds; this is my preferred technique.

With a conventional scanner, several techniques can be used. Sequential scans can be obtained at three levels during rapid infusion of contrast medium. These levels are

(1) the aortic arch, (2) the proximal aortic root and descending aorta near the level of the right pulmonary artery, and (3) the more distal descending thoracic aorta. If a dissection is present, it will involve one of these levels. Generally, the injection of 25 mL of contrast medium at each level will be sufficient, if rapid infusion is used along with sequential dynamic scanning. After scanning these levels, and if a dissection is present, the remainder of the aorta, including its major abdominal branches, can be studied using a drip infusion of contrast medium and obtaining scans every 1 or 2 cm. Alternatively, scanning at contiguous levels in the region of the aortic arch during the infusion of contrast medium can also be diagnostic.

In a patient with dissection, the intimal flap is usually delineated by contrast medium filling both the true and false channels. Slow flow in one of the channels, usually the false channel, may require that late images be used to make this diagnosis, if bolus contrast medium enhancement has been used. Other findings that can be associated with dissection are an abrupt change in aortic caliber, with a long dilated segment, and thickening of the aortic wall, but these are nonspecific and insufficient to make a definite diagnosis.

Streak artifacts, arising because of motion or vascular pulsations, may mimic an intimal flap. They are usually seen in the descending aorta, adjacent to the left heart border. Typically they are less sharply defined than a true intimal flap, extend beyond the edges of the aorta, and are inconsistently seen from one level to the next. On spiral CT, the appearance of the ascending aorta may mimic a dissection because of motion, but an intimal flap will not be seen. If any question exists as to the reality of an intimal flap, repeating the scan with a reinfusion of contrast medium may be helpful.

Intramural (dissecting) hematoma results from hemorrhage into the aortic wall. As with dissection, it may be associated with acute chest pain. It is thought to occur because of bleeding from vasa vasora, although in some cases it may represent a sealed-off dissection. Intramural hematoma

may progress to frank dissection (by rupture into the aortic lumen) or aneurysmal dilatation or may resolve. On contrast medium–enhanced scans, intramural hematoma appears as an eccentric, or less commonly, concentric thickening of the aortic wall (Fig. 3–10). On unenhanced scans, the intramural hematoma appears denser than blood in the aortic lumen. Inward displacement of intimal calcification can also be seen. Intramural hematoma is indistinguishable from thrombosed dissection, but the presence of chest pain suggests an acute hemorrhage. Thrombus lining an aneurysm can also mimic intramural hematoma but is usually more irregular in contour. Treatment is similar to that of dissection.

In some institutions, non–contrast CT is obtained before enhanced scans in patients with acute chest pain to assess the possibility of intramural hematoma; delayed scans can also be obtained after contrast medium enhancement.

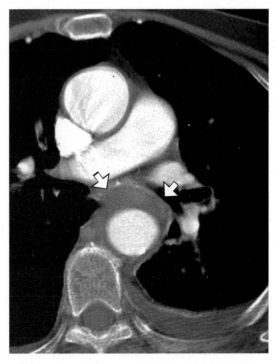

Figure 3–10. Intramural (dissecting) hematoma. In a woman with acute chest pain, contrast medium–enhanced spiral CT shows thickening of the aortic wall *(arrows)* due to intramural hemorrhage. Unenhanced scan showed the thick aortic wall to be high in attenuation, consistent with this diagnosis.

SUPERIOR VENA CAVA AND GREAT VEINS

Congenital Abnormalities

Azygos Lobe

An azygos lobe is a common anomaly and is present in about 1 in 200 patients. Azygos lobe results in a typical appearance on plain radiographs and CT that is easily recognized and produces a characteristic alteration in normal mediastinal anatomy. In patients with this anomaly, the azygos arch is located more cephalad than normal, at or near the junction of the brachiocephalic veins. Above this level, the azygos fissure is visible within the lung, marginating the azygos lobe (Fig. 3–11).

Persistent Left Superior Vena Cava

The only other frequent venous anomaly is persistent left superior vena cava, representing failure of the embryonic left anterior cardinal vein to regress. This anomaly is difficult to recognize on plain films, but in some patients there is a slight prominence of the left superior mediastinum. It is present in 0.3% of normal subjects, approximately the same frequency as an azygos lobe; is usually without symptoms or associated abnormalities; and occurs in 4.4% of patients with congenital heart disease.

On CT in patients with this anomaly, the left superior vena cava is positioned lateral to the left common carotid artery in the supraaortic mediastinum (Fig. 3–12). It descends along the left mediastinum, passing downward, anterior to the left hilum, to enter the coronary sinus posterior to the left atrium. In most subjects, a right vena cava is also present and the two vessels will be about the same size and in the same relative position, on opposite sides of the mediastinum. In 65% of patients, the left brachiocephalic vein is absent. If it is also present, joining the right and left superior venae cavae, the right superior vena cava will be larger than the left.

A left superior vena cava will densely opacify after contrast medium injection into the left arm. If contrast medium is injected on the right and the vein does not opacify, its tubular shape and characteristic position are usually enough for a definite diagnosis.

Azygos or Hemiazygos Continuation of the Inferior Vena Cava

The embryogenesis of the inferior vena cava is one of the most complicated sequences I know of, and several vessels must develop and regress in turn for it to form normally. During fetal development, the vessels that form the azygos and hemiazygos veins normally communicate with the suprarenal inferior vena cava, but this communication usually breaks down. If it does not, then azygos or hemiazygos continuation of the inferior vena cava is said to be present.

These lesions may be associated with other congenital anomalies, including polysplenia (in patients with hemiazygos communication) or asplenia (with azygos communication), or they may be isolated abnormalities. Typical findings include marked dilatation of the azygos arch and

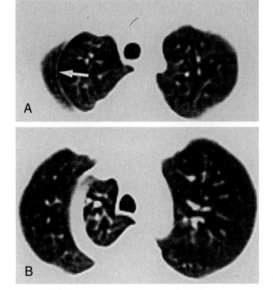

Figure 3–11. Azygos lobe. *(A)* Within the upper lung, the azygos fissure *(arrow)* distinguishes the azygos lobe medially from the remainder of the upper lobe. *(B)* At a lower level, the azygos arch passes from anterior to posterior. The posterior azygos vein is characteristically more laterally placed than normal.

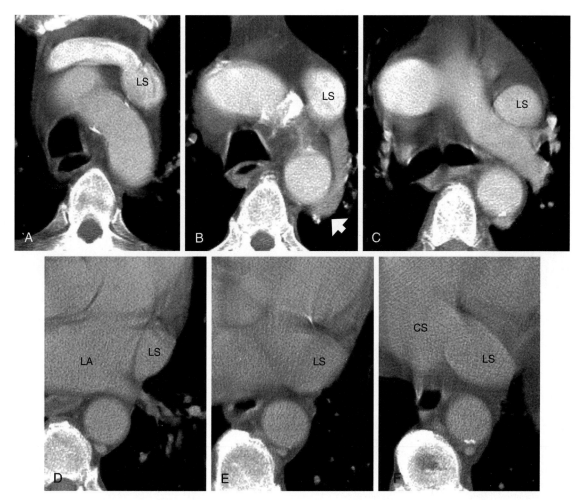

Figure 3–12. Persistent left superior vena cava with a hemiazygos arch. The course of the left superior vena cava is visible at six different levels. *(A)* The right vena cava is absent, and injection into the right arm results in dense opacification of the left brachiocephalic vein, because its only drainage is by means of the left SVC (LS). *(B)* At a lower level, the left SVC (LS) gives rise to a hemiazygos arch *(arrow)*, derived from the left superior intercostal vein. The azygos arch is absent, along with the right SVC. *(C)* Inferior to *B*, the left SVC (LS) passes anterior to the left pulmonary artery. *(D through F)* Adjacent to the heart, the left SVC (LS) passes anterior to the inferior pulmonary vein, lateral to the left atrium (LA), and enters the coronary sinus (CS).

posterior azygos vein (Fig. 3–13). If hemiazygos continuation is present, the dilated azygos vein will be seen to cross the mediastinum, from right to left, behind the descending aorta, to communicate with a dilated hemiazygos vein. A normal-appearing inferior vena cava is very often visible at the level of the heart and diaphragm, draining the hepatic veins. Either anomaly may be associated with duplication of the abdominal inferior vena cava. Rarely, a dilated hemiazygos vein drains into the left brachiocephalic vein instead of joining the azygos.

Superior Vena Cava Syndrome

Obstruction of the superior vena cava, or either of the brachiocephalic veins, is a common clinical occurrence, and symptoms of venous obstruction may lead to CT. Also, in some patients having CT for the diagnosis of mediastinal mass, CT will show findings of vena cava obstruction. CT has replaced other methods of making this diagnosis, because it not only shows the vascular abnormality but also shows the responsible mass, if one happens to be present.

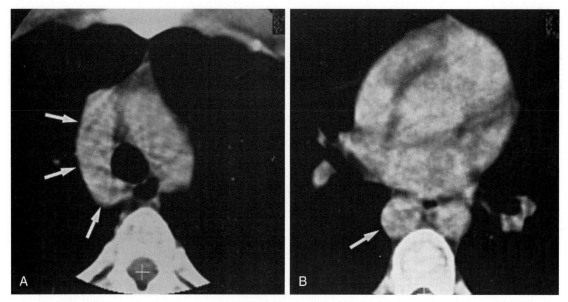

Figure 3–13. Azygos continuation of the inferior vena cava. *(A and B)* The azygos arch *(arrows, A)* and the posterior azygos vein *(arrow, B)* are markedly dilated. (From Webb WR, Gamsu G, Speckman JM, et al. CT demonstration of mediastinal venous anomalies. AJR 1982; 159:157–161. With permission.)

Superior vena cava obstruction can be seen in a variety of diseases, most commonly bronchogenic carcinoma, although in some parts of the country, granulomatous mediastinitis as a result of histoplasmosis is a very common cause. Because of the frequent use of subclavian catheters, venous thrombosis resulting in obstruction is not uncommon.

On CT in patients who have superior vena cava obstruction (Figs. 3–14 and 3–15), a number of characteristic findings are pres-

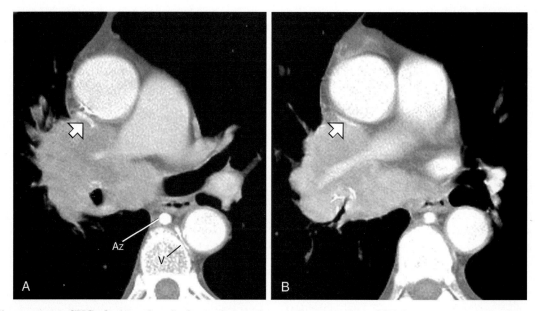

Figure 3–14. SVC obstruction in bronchogenic carcinoma. *(A and B)* In a patient with a large right hilar mass and mediastinal invasion, the superior vena cava *(arrows)* is nearly obstructed. The azygos vein (Az) and a left intercostal vein (V) are opacified, as they are serving as collateral pathways to bypass the obstruction.

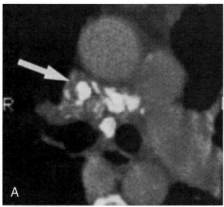

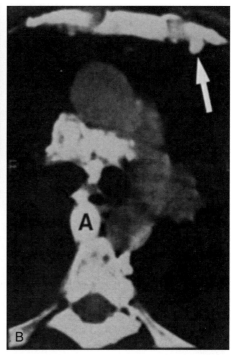

Figure 3–15. Superior vena cava syndrome. *(A)* CT without contrast medium enhancement in a patient with granulomatous mediastinitis from histoplasmosis shows calcified mediastinal lymph nodes. The superior vena cava contains calcified clot *(arrow).* (Modified from Putman CE, Ravin CE [eds]. Textbook of Diagnostic Imaging, 2nd ed. Philadelphia, WB Saunders, 1994.) *(B)* After contrast medium infusion, there is opacification of a dilated azygos vein (A) and internal mammary vein *(arrow).*

ent. Beginning peripherally as the contrast medium bolus is injected, it is common to see opacification of a number of small venous collateral vessels in the shoulder, upper chest wall, and upper mediastinum. However, this finding is not always abnormal; some filling of small veins in the chest wall and axilla can be seen in the absence of a venous abnormality (perhaps because of poor positioning of the patient's arm for injection). Unless other evidence of venous obstruction is present, this finding should not be of great concern.

In patients with obstruction of the superior vena cava, flow of contrast medium from the arm is delayed and the scan sequence must be delayed accordingly, or mediastinal vascular opacification will be poor. Some characteristic collateral vessels are often seen in patients with obstruction of the superior vena cava. These include a number of veins that drain into the azygos system and thus bypass the area of obstruction. These veins commonly include the internal mammary veins, left superior intercostal vein (which results in the "aortic nipple" sometimes visible on chest radiographs), in-

tercostal veins, and the hemiazygos vein. In addition to dilatation of these veins because of increased flow, they opacify after contrast medium infusion.

In patients with thrombosis of the superior vena cava or brachiocephalic veins, thrombus is sometimes visible in the vessel lumen, outlined by contrast medium. One word of caution, however: if contrast medium is injected into only one arm, as is typical, streaming of unopacified blood from one brachiocephalic vein into the superior vena cava can mimic the appearance of vena cava clot. This problem can be avoided by injecting contrast medium into both arms at the same time.

PULMONARY ARTERIES

Pulmonary artery anomalies are very rare, but some may be diagnosed using CT. Dilatation of the pulmonary artery as a result of pulmonic stenosis or pulmonary hypertension is much more common than congenital lesions. A main pulmonary artery diame-

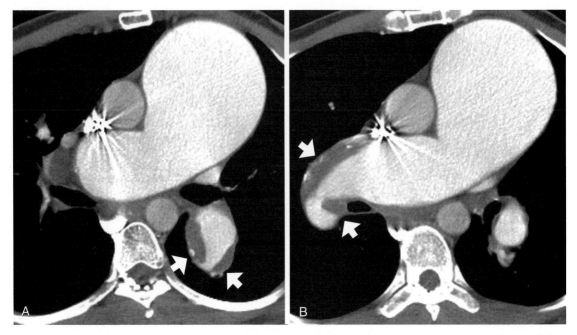

Figure 3–16. Chronic pulmonary embolism and pulmonary hypertension in a patient with Marfan's syndrome. *(A and B)* The main pulmonary artery is dilated because of pulmonary hypertension. Thrombus *(arrows)* is adherent to the vessel wall. Some calcification of the vessel wall is also seen.

ter exceeding 2.9 cm suggests pulmonary hypertension (Fig. 3–16). With pulmonic stenosis, the main and left pulmonary arteries will be dilated, whereas the right pulmonary artery is relatively normal in size. With pulmonary hypertension, both pulmonary arteries are large.

Pulmonary Embolism

Contrast medium–enhanced CT can be used to diagnose pulmonary embolism or thrombosis (Figs. 3–16 and 3–17). Until the advent of spiral CT, this was most often done in patients with suspected chronic emboli

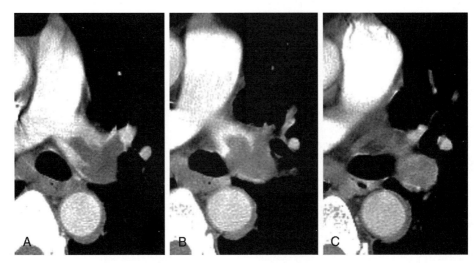

Figure 3–17. Acute pulmonary embolism, main pulmonary artery. *(A through C)* Clot fills the left main pulmonary artery and is outlined by contrast medium in *A.*

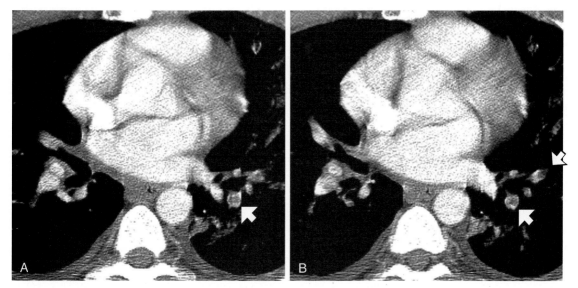

Figure 3–18. Acute pulmonary embolism, segmental. *(A and B)* Small clots *(arrows)* are visible within segmental pulmonary artery branches. They are outlined by contrast medium.

and pulmonary hypertension, and a definite diagnosis was usually limited to large central artery branches. However, spiral CT is now commonly done to diagnose acute pulmonary embolism, and it is beginning to replace angiography in some patients. An appropriate spiral CT technique would be to scan using (1) 3-mm collimation; (2) a pitch of 2; (3) a single breath hold of 20 seconds; (4) contrast medium injection at a rate of 2 to 3 mL/sec, with the injection started 20 seconds before scanning; and (5) reconstruction at 3-mm intervals. This technique allows scanning of 12 cm during the breath hold, sufficient to cover all the segmental pulmonary artery branches.

A filling defect visible within the pulmonary artery is usually diagnostic of pulmonary embolism (see Figs. 3–16 and 3–17). An acute pulmonary embolism is often outlined by the contrast agent (see Fig. 3–17); a chronic pulmonary embolism is usually adherent to the vessel wall (see Fig. 3–16). Pulmonary artery webs can indicate prior emboli. The sensitivity and specificity of spiral CT in diagnosing acute pulmonary embolism in the main pulmonary artery branches is 100% (see Figs. 3–16 and 3–17), with an overall sensitivity of about 90% when branches to the segmental level are included (Fig. 3–18); however, its sensitivity for subsegmental emboli is considerably

less. Large intraluminal masses can be seen with pulmonary artery sarcoma. The role of CT in diagnosing pulmonary embolism remains to be elucidated.

Suggested Reading

Bechtold RE, Wolfman NT, Karstaedt N, Choplin RH. Superior vena caval obstruction: detection using CT. Radiology 1985; 157:485–487.

Costello P, Dupuy DE, Ecker CP, Tello R. Spiral CT of the thorax with reduced volume of contrast material: a comparative study. Radiology 1992; 185:663–666.

Costello P, Ecker CP, Tello R, Hartnell GG. Assessment of the thoracic aorta by spiral CT. AJR 1992; 158:1127–1130.

Dillon EH, van Leeuwen MS, Fernandez MA, Mali WPTM. Spiral CT angiography. AJR 1993; 160:1273–1278.

Gavant ML, Flick P, Menke P, Gold RE. CT aortography of thoracic aortic rupture. AJR 1996; 166:955–961.

Gavant ML, Menke PG, Fabian T, et al. Blunt traumatic aortic rupture: detection with helical CT of the chest. Radiology 1995; 197:125–133.

Gefter WB, Hatabu H, Holland GA, et al. Pulmonary thromboembolism: recent developments in diagnosis with CT and MR imaging. Radiology 1995; 197:561–574.

Goodman LR, Curtin JJ, Mewissen MW, et al. Detection of pulmonary embolism in patients with unresolved clinical and scintigraphic diagnosis: helical CT versus angiography. AJR 1995; 164:1369–1374.

Goodman LR, Lipchik RJ. Diagnosis of pulmonary embolism: time for a new approach (editorial). Radiology 1996; 199:25–27.

Parish JM, Marschke RF, Dines DE, et al. Etiologic considerations in superior vena cava syndrome. Mayo Clin Proc 1981; 56:407–413.

Remy-Jardin M, Remy J, Wattinne L, Giraud F. Central pulmonary thromboembolism: diagnosis with spiral volumetric CT with the single-breath-hold technique: comparison with pulmonary angiography. Radiology 1992; 185:381–387.

Schnyder P, Chapuis L, Mayor B, et al. Helical CT angiography for traumatic aortic rupture: correlation with aortography and surgery in five cases. J Thorac Imaging 1996; 11:39–45.

Tello R, Costello P, Ecker C, et al. Spiral CT evalua-

tion of coronary artery bypass graft patency. J Comput Assist Tomogr 1993; 17:253–259.

Trerotola SO. Can helical CT replace aortography in thoracic trauma (editorial)? Radiology 1995; 197:13–15.

Webb WR, Gamsu G, Speckman JM, et al. CT demonstration of mediastinal aortic arch anomalies. J Comput Assist Tomogr 1982; 6:445–451.

Webb WR, Gamsu G, Speckman JM, et al. CT demonstration of mediastinal venous anomalies. AJR 1982; 159:157–161.

White RD, Dooms GC, Higgins CB. Advances in imaging thoracic aortic disease. Invest Radiol 1986; 21:761–778.

Zeman RK, Berman PM, Silverman PM, et al. Diagnosis of aortic dissection: value of helical CT with multiplanar re-formations and three-dimensional rendering. AJR 1995; 164:1375–1380.

Chapter

4

Mediastinum—Lymph Node Abnormalities and Masses

W. Richard Webb, M.D.

LYMPH NODE GROUPS

The detection and diagnosis of mediastinal lymph node enlargement is important in the evaluation of a number of thoracic diseases, particularly bronchogenic carcinoma. Mediastinal lymph nodes are generally classified by location, and most descriptive systems are based on a modification of Rouvière's classification of lymph node groups.

Anterior Mediastinal Nodes

Internal mammary nodes are located in a retrosternal location near the internal mammary artery and veins (Fig. 4–1). They drain the anterior chest wall, anterior diaphragm, and medial breasts.

Paracardiac nodes (diaphragmatic, pericardial) surround the heart on the surface of the diaphragm and communicate with the lower internal mammary chain (Fig. 4–2). Like internal mammary nodes, they are most commonly enlarged in patients with lymphoma and metastatic carcinoma, particularly breast cancer.

Prevascular nodes lie anterior to the great vessels (Fig. 4–3). They may be involved in a variety of diseases, notably lymphoma, but their involvement in lung cancer is unusual.

Middle Mediastinal Nodes

Lung diseases (e.g., lung cancer, sarcoidosis, tuberculosis, fungal infections) that second-arily involve lymph nodes typically involve middle mediastinal lymph nodes.

Pretracheal or paratracheal nodes occupy the pretracheal (or anterior paratracheal) space (Figs. 4–3 and 4–4A and B). The most inferior node in this region is the so-called azygos node. These nodes form the final pathway for lymphatic drainage from most of both lungs (excepting the left upper lobe). Because of this, they are commonly abnormal regardless of the location of the lung disease.

Aorticopulmonary nodes are considered by Rouvière to be in the anterior mediastinal group, but because they serve the same function as right paratracheal nodes, I prefer to consider them here (see Figs. 4–3C and 4–4C). The left upper lobe drains by means of this node group.

Subcarinal nodes are located in the subcarinal space, between the main bronchi (see Fig. 4–4D), and drain the inferior hila and both lower lobes. They communicate in turn with the right paratracheal chain.

Tracheobronchial nodes surround the main bronchi on each side. They communicate with bronchopulmonary (hilar), subcarinal, and paratracheal nodes.

Posterior Mediastinal Nodes

Paraesophageal nodes lie posterior to the trachea and/or are associated with the

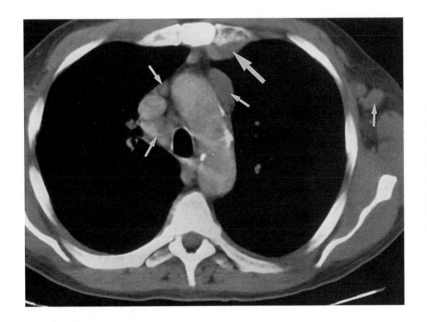

Figure 4–1. Internal mammary node enlargement from Hodgkin's lymphoma. A left internal mammary node *(large arrow)* is enlarged, as are pretracheal, prevascular, and axillary nodes *(small arrows)*.

Figure 4–2. Paracardiac node enlargement. In a patient with lymphoma, enlargement of paracardiac nodes *(large arrows)* is visible. The pericardium *(small arrows)* and inferior vena cava (v) are also seen. (From Putman CE, Ravin CE [eds]. Textbook of Diagnostic Imaging, 2nd ed. Philadelphia, WB Saunders, 1994.)

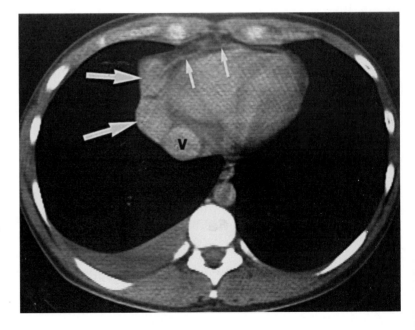

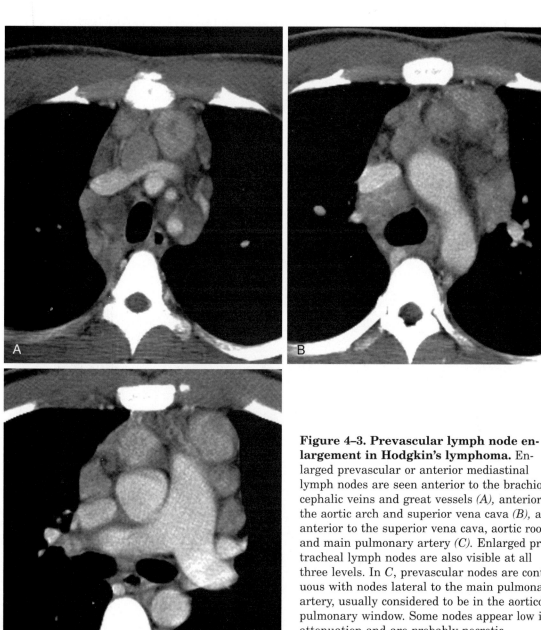

Figure 4–3. Prevascular lymph node enlargement in Hodgkin's lymphoma. Enlarged prevascular or anterior mediastinal lymph nodes are seen anterior to the brachiocephalic veins and great vessels *(A)*, anterior to the aortic arch and superior vena cava *(B)*, and anterior to the superior vena cava, aortic root, and main pulmonary artery *(C)*. Enlarged pretracheal lymph nodes are also visible at all three levels. In *C*, prevascular nodes are contiguous with nodes lateral to the main pulmonary artery, usually considered to be in the aorticopulmonary window. Some nodes appear low in attenuation and are probably necrotic.

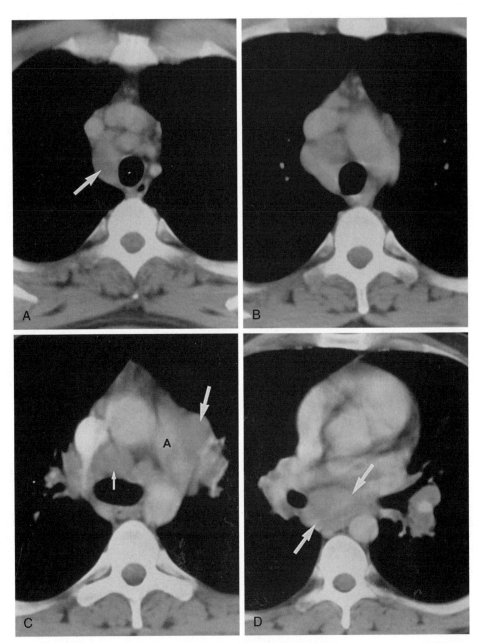

Figure 4–4. Lymph node enlargement in a patient with sarcoidosis. *(A and B)* Pretracheal or paratracheal nodes. *(A)* Enlarged nodes *(arrow)* are anterolateral relative to the trachea and posterior to the brachiocephalic veins. *(B)* At a lower level, they displace the vena cava anteriorly. *(C)* Aortico-pulmonary, precarinal, and tracheobronchial nodes. Extensive mediastinal adenopathy is present. The superior aspect of the left pulmonary artery (A) mimics adenopathy *(large arrow)* in the aorticopulmo-nary window. A large precarinal node *(small arrow)* is also visible. Tracheobronchial and peribron-chial nodes lie adjacent to the main bronchi. *(D)* Subcarinal nodes. A large convex mass *(arrows)* is present in the azygoesophageal recess and subcarinal space. The right pulmonary artery anterior to the mass is slightly compressed.

esophagus (Fig. 4–5). Subcarinal nodes are not included in this group.

Inferior pulmonary ligament nodes are located below the pulmonary hila, medial to the inferior pulmonary ligament. On CT, they are usually seen adjacent to the esophagus on the right and descending aorta on the left. Below the hila, they are difficult to distinguish from paraesophageal nodes. Along with the paraesophageal nodes, they drain the medial lower lobes, esophagus, pericardium, and posterior diaphragm.

Paravertebral nodes lie lateral to the vertebral bodies, posterior to the aorta on the left (see Fig. 4–5). They drain the posterior chest wall and pleura. They are most commonly involved, along with retrocrural or retroperitoneal abdominal nodes, in patients with lymphoma or metastatic carcinoma.

American Thoracic Society Node Stations

The American Thoracic Society (ATS) has developed a numerical system of lymph node localization for use in lung cancer staging. In the ATS system, nodes are classified as belonging to one of a number of "node stations," for which mediastinoscopic, surgical, and CT criteria have been established (Table 4–1). Clinically, this system is not often used for the description of lymph node abnormalities in diseases other than lung cancer, and not all intrathoracic lymph node groups are included in the ATS system.

It is not usually necessary to precisely localize enlarged nodes on the basis of detailed ATS criteria when interpreting scans for clinical purposes. From a practical standpoint, if you are asked about the ATS station of a node, some simple landmarks can be easily remembered and used to localize nodes with sufficient accuracy (Table 4–2).

CT APPEARANCE OF LYMPH NODES

Lymph nodes are generally visible as discrete, round or elliptical, soft tissue attenu-

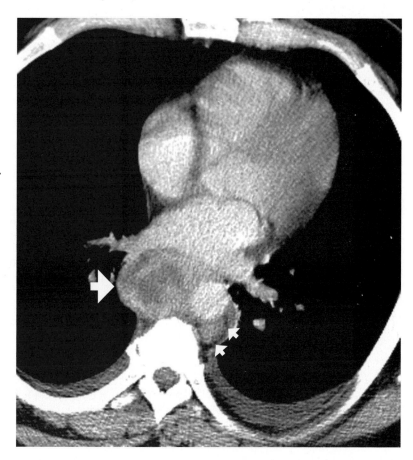

Figure 4–5. Paravertebral lymph node enlargement in metastatic testicular carcinoma. Very large lymph nodes on the right *(large arrow)* can be considered paraesophageal or inferior pulmonary ligament. They appear inhomogeneous and are necrotic. An enlarged left paravertebral lymph node *(small arrows)* is also visible posterior to the aorta.

TABLE 4–1. **American Thoracic Society (ATS) Lymph Node Stations**

Node Group	ATS Node Station(s)	ATS Node Station: Anatomic Criteria
Pretracheal (paratracheal)	2R	Right upper paratracheal nodes, between the caudal margin of the innominate artery and the apex of lung
	2L	Left upper paratracheal nodes, between the top of the aortic arch and the apex of lung
	4R	Right lower paratracheal nodes, between the cephalic margin of the azygos arch and below the innominate artery
	4L	Left upper paratracheal nodes, between the carina and the top of the aortic arch and medial to ligamentum arteriosum
Aorticopulmonary	5	Subaortic and paraaortic nodes, lateral to the ligamentum arteriosum or aorta or left pulmonary artery, proximal to the first branch of left pulmonary artery
Prevascular	6	Anterior mediastinal nodes anterior to aortic arch or innominate artery
Subcarinal	7	Nodes caudal to the carina but not associated with the lower lobe bronchi or pulmonary arteries
Paraesophageal	8	Nodes dorsal to the posterior wall of trachea, and on either side of the esophagus, not including subcarinal nodes
Inferior pulmonary ligament	9	Nodes in relation to right or left inferior pulmonary ligaments
Tracheobronchial	10R	Nodes to the right of the tracheal midline, between the cephalic border of the azygos arch and the right upper lobe bronchus
Peribronchial	10L	Nodes to the left of the tracheal midline, between the carina and the left upper lobe bronchus, medial to the ligamentum arteriosum
Intrapulmonary (hilar)	11	Nodes removed at pneumonectomy or distal to the mainstem bronchi or secondary carina
Internal mammary	—	—
Paracardiac	14	—
Paravertebral	—	—

TABLE 4–2. **Simple Criteria for ATS Node Stations**

ATS Node Station(s)	ATS Node Station: Easily Remembered and Sufficiently Accurate CT Criteria
2R or 2L	Paratracheal nodes above the aorta, to the right (R) or left (L) of the tracheal midline
4R or 4L	Paratracheal nodes between the aorta and carina, to the right (R) or left (L) of the tracheal midline
5	Aorticopulmonary window nodes, lateral to the aorta or left pulmonary artery
6	Prevascular nodes, anterior to the great vessels (aorta and its branches, brachiocephalic veins, vena cava, or pulmonary artery)
7	Subcarinal nodes between the main bronchi
8	Nodes posterior to the trachea (rare)
8 or 9	Nodes below the carina, on either side, adjacent to the esophagus or aorta
10R or 10L	Nodes adjacent to the right or left main bronchi, but not subcarinal
11	Hilar nodes distal to the main-stem bronchi

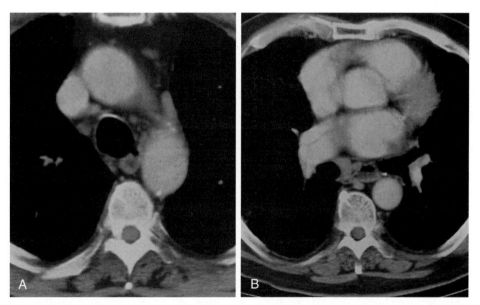

Figure 4–6. Normal mediastinal nodes. *(A)* Small lymph nodes are visible in the pretracheal and prevascular spaces and in the aorticopulmonary window. A lymph node in the lateral aorticopulmonary window measures 20 × 7 mm. The least node diameter is the best measurement to use. *(B)* A normal subcarinal lymph node is visible. Subcarinal nodes larger than 1 cm are common.

ation structures, surrounded by mediastinal fat and distinguishable from vessels by their location. They often occur in clusters (Fig. 4–6*A* and *B*). In some locations, nodes that contact vessels may be difficult to identify without contrast medium infusion.

Internal mammary nodes, paracardiac nodes, and paravertebral nodes are not usually seen on CT in normal subjects, but in other areas of the mediastinum, normal nodes are often visible. The expected size of normal nodes varies with their location, and a few general rules apply. Subcarinal nodes (ATS station 7) can be quite large in normal patients. Pretracheal nodes are also commonly visible, but these nodes are typically smaller than normal subcarinal nodes. Nodes in the supraaortic mediastinum (ATS station 2) are usually smaller than lower pretracheal nodes (ATS station 4), and left paratracheal nodes are usually smaller than right paratracheal nodes.

Measurement of Lymph Node Size

The *short axis* or *least diameter* (i.e., the smallest node diameter seen in cross section) is generally used when measuring the size of a lymph node. Measuring the short axis is better than measuring the *long axis* or *greatest diameter* because it more closely reflects actual node diameter when nodes are obliquely oriented relative to the scan plane and shows less variation among normal subjects.

Different values for the upper limits of normal short-axis node diameter have been found for different mediastinal node groups (Table 4–3). However, except for the subcarinal regions, a short-axis node diameter of 1 cm or less is generally considered normal

TABLE 4–3. Upper Limits of Normal for Short-Axis Node Diameter

Node Group	ATS Node Station	Short-Axis Node Diameter (mm)*
Supraaortic pretracheal	2	7
Subaortic pretracheal	4	9
Aorticopulmonary window	5	9
Prevascular	6	8
Subcarinal	7	12
Paraesophageal	8	8

*Mean normal node diameter plus two standard deviations.

for clinical purposes. In the subcarinal region, 1.5 cm is usually considered to be the upper limits of normal.

Lymph Node Enlargement

Except in the subcarinal space, lymph nodes are considered to be enlarged if they have a short-axis diameter greater than 1 cm. In most cases, they are outlined by fat and visible as discrete structures. However, in the presence of inflammation or neoplastic infiltration, abnormal nodes can be matted together, giving the appearance of a single large mass or resulting in infiltration and replacement of mediastinal fat by soft tissue opacity. The diagnosis of mediastinal infiltration may be difficult to make unless the attenuation of mediastinal soft tissues (which should be the same as fat) is compared with the attenuation of subcutaneous fat on the same scan.

The significance given to the presence of an enlarged lymph node must be tempered by knowledge of the patient's clinical situation. For example, if the patient is known to have lung cancer, then an enlarged lymph node has a 70% likelihood of being involved by tumor. However, the same node in a patient without lung cancer is much less likely to be of clinical significance. In the absence of a known disease, an enlarged node must be regarded as likely to be hyperplastic or postinflammatory.

DIFFERENTIAL DIAGNOSIS OF MEDIASTINAL LYMPH NODE ENLARGEMENT

Lung Cancer

The most common cause of mediastinal node enlargement is metastatic lung cancer, and the use of CT in making this diagnosis is discussed here in detail.

Approximately 35% of patients diagnosed with lung cancer have mediastinal node metastases. Lung cancer most often involves the middle mediastinal node groups. Left upper lobe cancers typically metastasize to aorticopulmonary window nodes, whereas tumors involving the lower lobes on either side tend to metastasize to the subcarinal and right paratracheal groups. Right upper lobe tumors typically involve paratracheal nodes.

Lung Cancer Staging

In patients with non–small cell bronchogenic carcinoma, although the cell-type and histologic characteristics of the tumor affect prognosis, the anatomic extent of the tumor (tumor stage) is usually most important in determining the therapeutic approach. The most widely used anatomic staging classification is the TNM classification of the American Joint Committee on Cancer Staging (AJCC).

This classification is based on a consideration of (1) the location and extent of the primary tumor (T); (2) the presence or absence of lymph node metastases (N); and (3) the presence or absence of distant metastases (M) (Table 4–4). On the basis of this classification, excellent correlations are found between tumor stage and survival after treatment.

For radiologic purposes, precise classification of tumor stage is not usually necessary. However, differentiation of resectable disease (stages I–IIIa) and unresectable disease (stages IIIb–IV) is important (see Table 4–4). The criteria for resectability listed in Table 4–4 are not written in stone; different surgeons can have different criteria as to what is resectable. In particular, the resectability of some stage IIIa tumors is controversial.

The impact of mediastinal lymph node metastases and mediastinal invasion on lung cancer staging is discussed next. Other aspects of lung cancer staging are discussed in subsequent chapters.

Mediastinal Node Metastases in Lung Cancer

In the TNM lung cancer staging system, ipsilateral mediastinal node metastases and subcarinal node metastases are termed *N2* and are considered potentially resectable (although this is not always the case); contralateral nodes are termed *N3* and are considered unresectable (Fig. 4–7).

In patients with lung cancer, the likeli-

TABLE 4–4. **TNM Staging of Lung Cancer***

T (primary tumor)
T0	No evidence of primary tumor
T1	Tumor 3 cm or less in greatest diameter, limited to lung, with no invasion proximal to lobar bronchus
T2	Tumor > 3 cm; tumor that invades visceral pleura or produces collapse or consolidation of less than entire lung; tumor must be > 2 cm distal to the carina
T3	Tumor focally invading parietal pleura, chest wall, diaphragm, or mediastinal pleura or pericardium; tumor < 2 cm from the carina or producing collapse or consolidation of entire lung
T4	*Tumor of any size involving heart, great vessels, trachea, esophagus, vertebral body, or carina, or producing malignant pleural effusion*

No (nodal involvement)
N0	No node metastases
N1	Metastases to ipsilateral hilar nodes
N2	Metastases to ipsilateral mediastinal nodes or subcarinal nodes
N3	*Metastases to contralateral hilar or mediastinal lymph nodes or scalene or supraclavicular lymph nodes*

M (distant metastases)
M0	Metastases absent
M1	*Metastases present*

Resectable stages
Stage I	T1–2; N0; M0
Stage II	T1–2, N1; M0
Stage IIIa	T2, 3 and/or N2; M0

Unresectable stages
Stage IIIb	*T4 and/or N3; M0*
Stage IV	*M1; any T or N*

*Italics indicate unresectability.

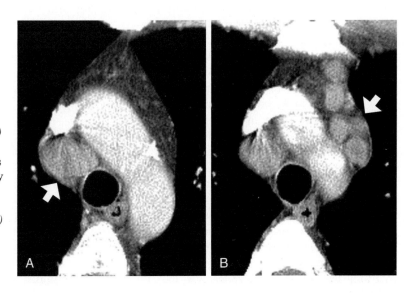

Figure 4–7. Lymph node enlargement in a patient with a right-sided bronchogenic carcinoma. *(A)* Lymph node enlargement in the pretracheal space *(arrow)* is ipsilateral, N2, and potentially resectable. These nodes are very large and, thus, very likely involved by tumor. *(B)* Lymph node enlargement in the prevascular space *(arrow)* is contralateral, N3, and is considered unresectable.

hood that a mediastinal node is involved by tumor is directly proportional to its size. Thus, although large nodes are most likely to be involved by tumor (see Fig. 4–7), they can be benign; similarly, although small nodes are usually normal, they can harbor metastases. Although a short-axis measurement of greater than 1 cm is used in clinical practice to identify abnormally enlarged nodes, it is important to realize that no node diameter clearly separates benign nodes from those involved by tumor.

Using a short-axis node diameter of 1 cm as the upper limit of node size, CT will detect mediastinal lymph node enlargement in about 60% of patients who have node metastases (its sensitivity), whereas about 70% of patients with normal nodes will be called normal on CT (its specificity). Although CT is not highly accurate in diagnosing node metastases, it is commonly used to guide subsequent procedures or treatment.

In patients who do not have node enlargement on CT, thoracotomy is often performed without prior mediastinoscopy, although this will vary with the surgeon. Although some of these patients will be found to have microscopic or small intranodal metastases, their presence does not necessarily indicate that surgery was inappropriate. Some patients with ipsilateral intranodal mediastinal metastases (N2) can be cured after surgical excision of nodes and radiation.

On the other hand, if mediastinal lymph node enlargement is seen on CT, about 70% of patients will have node metastases; benign hyperplasia of mediastinal lymph nodes accounts for the other 30%. Patients with large mediastinal nodes usually have node sampling at mediastinoscopy or by CT-guided needle biopsy before surgery. If node metastases are found at mediastinoscopy, surgery is not generally performed, even though the nodes would be classified as N2; it has been shown that patients with node metastases diagnosed at mediastinoscopy have a poor prognosis after surgery. It should be kept in mind that in patients with enlarged nodes on CT and mediastinal lymph node metastases, the metastases are not always in the nodes that appear large. In other words, in some cases, CT can be right for the wrong reason.

Mediastinoscopy is slightly more sensitive than CT, has a much higher specificity (100%—no normals are called abnormal based on mediastinoscopy), and a higher accuracy for diagnosing mediastinal node metastases. However, the mediastinoscopist cannot evaluate all mediastinal compartments or lymph node groups, and a significant percentage (up to 25%) of patients with bronchogenic carcinoma, who have a negative mediastinoscopy, are found to have mediastinal nodal metastases at surgery. Through a standard transcervical approach, the mediastinoscopist can only evaluate pretracheal lymph nodes, nodes in the anterior subcarinal space, and lymph nodes extending anterior to the right main bronchus. Lymph nodes in the anterior mediastinum (prevascular space), aorticopulmonary window, and posterior portions of the mediastinum (e.g., posterior subcarinal space, azygoesophageal recess) are inaccessible using this technique, although some can be evaluated using a left parasternal mediastinoscopy (Chamberlain procedure). CT, on the other hand, allows evaluation of all these areas, shows where any enlarged nodes are, and can serve to guide needle aspiration biopsy or parasternal mediastinotomy if enlarged lymph nodes are visible in areas that cannot be evaluated using a standard approach.

In patients with small, peripheral lung nodules, mediastinal metastases are uncommon, and thoracotomy may be warranted without prior CT or mediastinoscopy, but this is controversial. Most surgeons obtain CT in this situation.

Mediastinal Invasion by Lung Cancer

In addition to mediastinal node metastasis, bronchogenic carcinoma can involve the mediastinum by direct extension, so-called mediastinal invasion. In current surgical practice, invasion of the mediastinal pleura, termed *T3* in the lung cancer staging system, does not prevent surgery. However, significant invasion of mediastinal fat or other mediastinal structures, such as the trachea or esophagus, does prevent resection; such lesions are termed *T4* (Fig. 4–8).

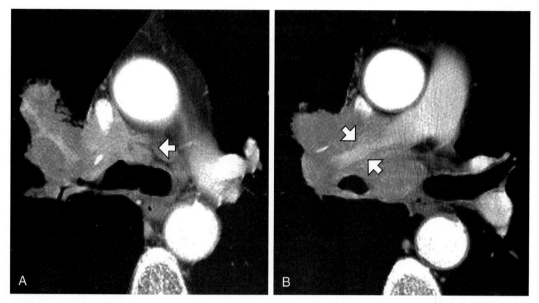

Figure 4–8. Mediastinal invasion by bronchogenic carcinoma. A right hilar tumor has resulted in extensive mediastinal invasion, anterior to the carina *(arrow, A)* and surrounding and narrowing the right pulmonary artery *(arrows, B)*. There is extensive replacement of fat by tumor; the tumor surrounds and compresses the pulmonary artery and compresses the vena cava; and fat planes are invisible adjacent to the great vessels.

How accurate is CT in predicting mediastinal invasion? Obviously, you can be sure that a lung mass not contacting the mediastinum is not invasive, and this is an important use of CT.

CT findings of mediastinal invasion (see Fig. 4–8) include

1. Replacement of mediastinal fat by soft tissue attenuation tumor

2. Compression or displacement of mediastinal vessels by tumor

3. Tumor contacting more than 90° of the circumference of a structure such as the aorta, pulmonary artery, and so on (the greater the extent of circumferential contact, i.e., 180°, the greater the likelihood of invasion)

4. Obliteration of the mediastinal fat plane normally seen adjacent to most mediastinal structures

5. Tumor contacting more than 3 cm of the mediastinum

6. Obtuse angles where tumor contacts the mediastinum

7. Mediastinal pleural or pericardial thickening

A definite diagnosis of invasion can be made if tumor is visible infiltrating mediastinal fat. Other findings of mediastinal invasion are less accurate. If none of these findings are present, the tumor is likely resectable.

Lymphoma and Leukemia

Mediastinal lymph nodes are commonly involved in patients with lymphoma. A small percentage of patients are first recognized because of mediastinal masses noted on chest films, but these patients will often have systemic signs and symptoms, including fever, night sweats, weight loss, weakness, and fatigue.

Hodgkin's Disease

Hodgkin's disease has a predilection for thoracic involvement, both at the time of diagnosis and if the disease recurs. Hodgkin's disease occurs in all ages but peaks in incidence in the third and fifth decades.

More than 85% of patients with Hodgkin's disease eventually develop intrathoracic disease, typically involving the superior mediastinal (prevascular, pretracheal, and aorticopulmonary) lymph nodes (Table 4–5;

TABLE 4–5. **Mediastinal Lymph Node Enlargement in Hodgkin's Disease**

Site	% Abnormal	% Visible on CT	% Visible on Radiographs
Pretracheal	64	64	57
Aorticopulmonary window	62	62	48
Subcarinal	46	44	9
Internal mammary	38	38	4
Posterior medial	18	12	11
Paracardiac	13	10	7

Fig. 4–9; see also Fig. 4–3). An important rule is that intrathoracic lymphadenopathy unassociated with superior mediastinal node enlargement is unlikely to be Hodgkin's lymphoma.

In one study, it was uncommon for CT to show evidence of mediastinal adenopathy if the chest radiograph was normal, but if the chest film was abnormal, CT detected additional sites of adenopathy in many cases (see Table 4–5). CT was most helpful in diagnosing subcarinal, internal mammary,

and aorticopulmonary window node enlargement. Cardiophrenic angle (paracardiac) lymph nodes are present in about 10% of patients and are well seen on CT. Adenopathy in this location is less common in other diseases. In a significant percentage of patients, the additional node involvement shown by CT changes therapy.

Enlargement of a single node group can be seen with Hodgkin's disease, most commonly in the prevascular mediastinum. This often indicates the presence of nodular

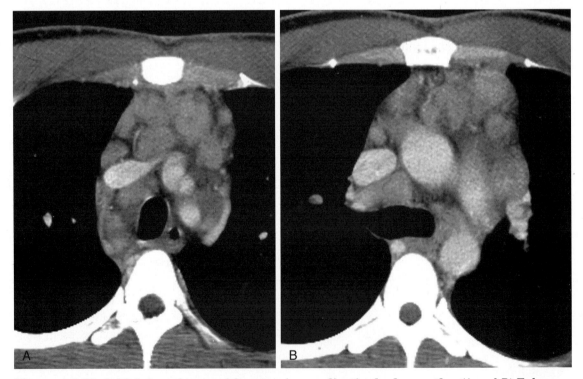

Figure 4–9. Hodgkin's lymphoma with extensive mediastinal adenopathy. *(A and B)* Enlargement of anterior mediastinal nodes in the prevascular space is visible at two levels. Large pretracheal lymph nodes are also visible. Involvement of these node groups in the superior mediastinum is common in Hodgkin's lymphoma.

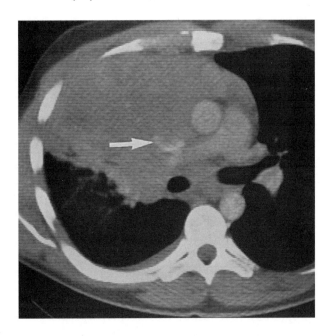

Figure 4–10. Hodgkin's lymphoma with mediastinal mass. Enlargement of anterior mediastinal nodes is compressing the superior vena cava *(arrow)* posteriorly. Extensive right hilar and subcarinal node enlargement is also present. Discrete nodes are not visible as they are in Figure 4–9, suggesting infiltration of the mediastinum. Lung involvement is also present. This is the same patient as shown in Figure 4–2.

sclerosing histology, which accounts for 50% to 80% of adult Hodgkin's disease. In patients with lymphoma, mediastinal lymph nodes may become matted, being visible as a single large mass (Fig. 4–10) rather than individual discrete nodes. Mediastinal nodes or masses in patients with Hodgkin's lymphoma can appear cystic or fluid filled on CT (Fig. 4–11). Calcification is unusual

and of limited extent, except after treatment.

Non-Hodgkin's Lymphoma

Non-Hodgkin's lymphoma is a diverse group of diseases that vary in radiologic manifestation, clinical presentation, course, and prognosis. In comparison to Hodgkin's dis-

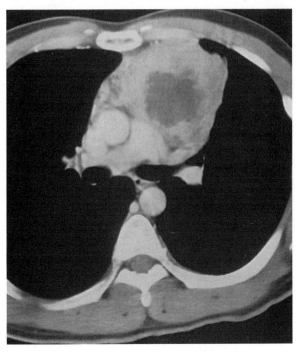

Figure 4–11. Cystic or necrotic Hodgkin's lymphoma. The anterior mediastinal mass contains an irregular area of cystic necrosis.

ease, these tumors are less common and occur in an older group (40–70 years). At the time of presentation the disease is often generalized (85% are stages III or IV) and chemotherapy is most appropriate. Because of this, precise anatomic staging is less crucial than with Hodgkin's disease.

In one series, 43% had intrathoracic disease and 40% had involvement of only one node group—much more common than in patients with Hodgkin's disease. Also, posterior mediastinal nodes were more frequently involved. Lung involvement was present in only 4%; in some patients, lung infiltration may be rapid.

CT, as in patients with Hodgkin's disease, can show evidence of intrathoracic disease when it is unrecognizable on plain radiographs and can affect management in patients with localized (stage I or II) disease.

Leukemia

Leukemia, particularly the lymphocytic varieties, can cause hilar or mediastinal lymph node enlargement, pleural effusion, and occasionally infiltrative lung disease. Lymphadenopathy is generally confined to the middle mediastinum, and the larger masses seen with some lymphomas generally do not occur.

Metastases

Extrathoracic primary tumors can result in mediastinal node enlargement, either with or without hilar or lung metastases. Node metastases can be present because of inferior extension from neck masses (thyroid carcinoma, head and neck tumors) extension along lymphatic channels from below the diaphragm (testicular carcinoma [see Fig. 4–5], renal cell carcinoma, gastrointestinal malignancies), or dissemination by other routes (breast carcinoma, melanoma). Middle mediastinal (paratracheal) or paravertebral mediastinal nodes are most commonly involved when the tumor is subdiaphragmatic. With breast carcinoma, internal mammary node metastases occur. Occasionally, lymph node metastases can appear cystic (Fig. 4–12).

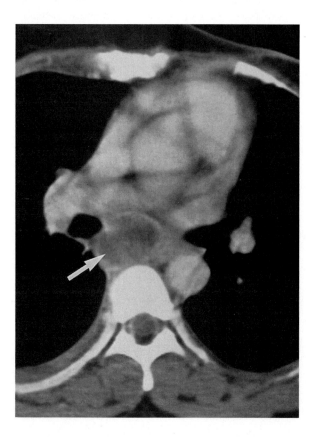

Figure 4–12. Cystic lymph node metastasis. In a patient with metastatic carcinoma, a subcarinal node mass *(arrow)* is cystic, with an enhancing rim and low attenuation center.

Sarcoidosis

Mediastinal lymph node enlargement is very common in patients with sarcoidosis, occurring in 60% to 90% of cases. Typically, node enlargement is extensive, involving the hila as well as the mediastinum, and masses appear bilateral and symmetric in the large majority of patients (see Fig. 4–4); this sometimes allows the differentiation of sarcoid from lymphoma, which is more typically asymmetric. Also, lymph nodes can be quite large in patients with sarcoidosis, but large isolated masses, as seen in some patients with lymphoma, do not occur. Paratracheal lymph nodes are typically involved. Even though it is commonly stated that sarcoidosis does not involve anterior mediastinal lymph nodes, this is often visible on CT; paravertebral node enlargement is occasionally seen.

An important rule is that in patients with sarcoid it is uncommon for mediastinal lymph nodes to be enlarged without hilar node enlargement.

Infections

A variety of infectious agents can cause mediastinal lymph node enlargement during the acute stage of the infection. These include a number of fungal infections (commonly histoplasmosis and coccidioidomycosis), tuberculosis, bacterial infections, and viral infections. Typically, there will be symptoms and signs of acute infection, and chest radiographs will show evidence of pneumonia.

The lymph node enlargement will often be asymmetric, involving hilar and middle mediastinal nodes. In patients with tuberculosis, enlarged nodes typically show rim enhancement and central necrosis after contrast medium injection; this appearance is nearly diagnostic in patients with an appropriate history. Lymph node calcification occurs in patients with chronic fungal or tuberculous infection.

Castleman's Disease (Angiofollicular Lymph Node Hyperplasia)

This unusual disease, of unknown cause, occurs in two forms. The more common localized form is characterized by enlargement of hilar or mediastinal lymph nodes, with mediastinal nodes, usually middle or posterior. A single smooth or lobulated mass, which can be large, is typically visible on CT, and dense opacification after contrast medium infusion is commonly visible. Localized Castleman's disease is usually asymptomatic and has a benign course.

The rare diffuse form of Castleman's disease results in generalized lymph node enlargement, involving mediastinal and hilar nodes, and often axillary, abdominal, and inguinal node groups (Fig. 4–13). It is often associated with systemic symptoms and has a progressive course despite treatment. As with the localized form, marked node enhancement can be seen.

DIAGNOSIS OF MEDIASTINAL MASSES

The differential diagnosis of a mediastinal mass on CT is usually based on several characteristics of the mass, and on the presence or absence of several findings. These include the mass' location, whether it is single or multifocal (involves several areas of the mediastinum), its shape (round or lobulated), whether it appears cystic, its attenuation (fat, fluid, tissue, or a combination of these, the presence of calcification and its character and amount), and additional findings such as pleural effusion.

Attenuation

The attenuation of a mass can be very helpful in differential diagnosis. The variety of densities that can be seen in a mediastinal mass and their frequency are shown in Table 4–6.

Localization of Mediastinal Masses

Mediastinal masses result in alterations of normal mediastinal contours and displacement or compression of mediastinal structures. Recognizing these findings can be valuable in diagnosis and in suggesting the site of origin of the mass. Although most mediastinal masses can occur in different

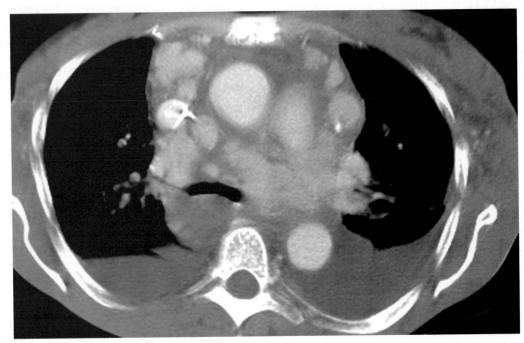

Figure 4–13. Diffuse Castleman's disease. Extensive, enhancing mediastinal lymphadenopathy in a patient with the diffuse form of Castleman's disease. The enhancement is typical. Enlarged axillary, abdominal, and inguinal lymph nodes were also visible. Bilateral pleural effusions are also present.

TABLE 4–6. **Attenuation Characteristics of Mediastinal Masses**

Mass	Air	Fat	Water	Tissue	> Tissue	Calcium
Thymoma	N	N	O	A	N	O
Thymolipoma	N	A	N	C	N	N
Lymphoma (thymic)	N	N	O	A	N	R
Dermoid/teratoma	N	O	O	A	N	O
Germ-cell tumor	N	N	R	A	N	R
Thyroid tumor	N	N	O	A	C	C
Lipoma	N	A	N	N	N	N
Hygroma	N	C	C	C	N	N
Cysts (congenital)	R	N	C	O	N	R
Hernia	O	O	N	O	N	N
Lung cancer (nodes)	N	N	O	A	N	N
Tuberculosis (nodes)	N	N	C	A	N	C
Sarcoid (nodes)	N	N	R	A	N	O
Castleman's (nodes)	N	N	N	A	N	O
Neurogenic tumor	N	O	C	C	N	O
Neurenteric cyst	R	N	A	N	N	N
Meningocele	N	N	A	N	N	N
Hematopoiesis	N	N	N	A	N	N

"ACORN": A = always; C = common; O = occasionally; R = rare; N = never ("never" does not mean it never happens but that it is so unlikely that practically, you should "never" consider the diagnosis, and if you turn out to be wrong, you will "never" be blamed).

parts of the mediastinum, most have characteristic locations.

PREVASCULAR SPACE MASSES

Masses in this compartment, when large, tend to displace the aorta and great arterial branches posteriorly (see Fig. 4–10), but distinct compression or narrowing of these relatively thick-walled structures is unusual. Within the supraaortic mediastinum, displacement, compression, or obstruction of the brachiocephalic veins is not uncommon. In the subaortic mediastinum, posterior displacement or compression of the superior vena cava is typical only with right-sided masses. On the left, compression of the main pulmonary artery can be seen. Mediastinal contours in this region are not particularly helpful in diagnosing masses. The anterior junction line is rather variable in thickness and cannot be relied on as abnormal unless grossly thickened. The lateral mediastinal pleural contours are often convex laterally, although a marked convexity may suggest mass. The differential diagnosis of masses arising in this area include thymoma and other thymic tumors, lymphoma, germ cell tumors, thyroid masses, parathyroid masses, cysts, fatty masses, and lymphangioma (hygroma).

THYMIC TUMORS

Tumors of various histology arise from cells of thymic origin and therefore can be called thymomas. However, it is most appropriate to reserve the term *thymoma* for tumors derived from thymic epithelial or lymphocytic tissues. Other thymic tumors include thymic carcinoma, thymic carcinoid, thymolipoma, thymic cyst, lymphoma, and leukemia.

Thymoma

Thymoma is a common anterior mediastinal mass occurring primarily in adults. Occasionally, these lesions arise in the middle or posterior mediastinum. It is extremely difficult to determine if thymomas are benign or malignant by histologic criteria. Local invasion is a much more reliable sign, and the term *invasive thymoma* is preferable to *malignant thymoma*. Approximately 30% of thymomas are pathologically and surgically invasive. Invasion of mediastinal structures or the pleural space is most typical. Distant metastases are not common.

From 10% to 30% of patients with myasthenia gravis will be found to have a thymoma, whereas a larger percentage of patients with thymoma (30% to 50%) have myasthenia. Other syndromes associated with thymoma include red cell hypoplasia and hypogammaglobulinemia.

On CT, thymomas are usually visible in the prevascular space (Fig. 4–14), but they can also be seen in a paracardiac location. They are detected as a localized bulge or mass distorting or replacing the normally arrowhead-shaped thymus. Typically they are unilateral. Calcification and cystic degeneration can be present. On CT, bilaterality, large size, lobulated contour, poor definition of the tumor's margin, and associated pleural effusion or nodules suggest the presence of an invasive thymoma, but a definite diagnosis is difficult to make.

In patients suspected of having a thymoma because of myasthenia gravis, CT can demonstrate tumors that are invisible using plain radiographs. However, very small thymic tumors may not be distinguished from a normal or hyperplastic gland with CT.

Thymic Carcinoma

Like invasive thymoma, thymic carcinoma arises from thymic epithelial cells. However, unlike invasive thymoma, thymic carcinoma can be diagnosed as malignant on the basis of histology. This tumor is aggressive and more likely to result in distant metastases than invasive thymoma. Thymic carcinoma cannot be distinguished from thymoma on CT.

Thymic Carcinoid Tumor

Thymic carcinoid tumors are usually malignant and aggressive. This lesion does not differ significantly from thymoma in its CT

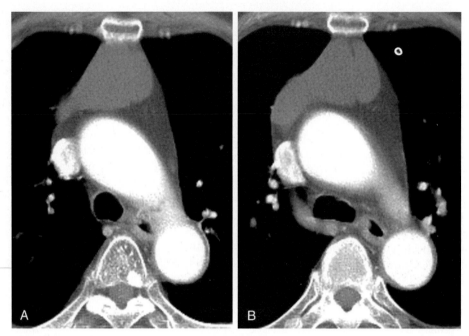

Figure 4–14. Thymoma. *(A and B)* At two levels, a large but well-marginated mass involves the right thymic lobe. A noninvasive thymoma was found at surgery. The left thymic lobe is replaced by fat.

appearance but has a worse prognosis. Approximately 40% of patients have Cushing's syndrome as a result of tumor secretion of adrenocorticotropic hormone, and nearly 20% have been associated with multiple endocrine neoplasia syndromes I and II.

Thymolipoma

Thymolipoma is a rare, benign thymic tumor, consisting primarily of fat but also containing strands or islands of thymic tissue. The tumor is generally unaccompanied by symptoms and can be large when first detected, usually on routine chest radiographs. Because of its fatty content and pliability, it tends to drape around the heart and can simulate cardiac enlargement. On CT, its fatty composition, with wisps of soft tissue within it, can permit a preoperative diagnosis (Fig. 4–15).

Thymic Cyst

Thymic cysts, either congenital or acquired, can be diagnosed using CT if their contents have an attenuation close to that of water, but in some cases, they will show soft tissue attenuation. Calcification of the cyst margin

can occur. It is important to note that thymoma can have cystic components but will also demonstrate solid areas or a thick or irregular wall.

An important general rule in diagnosing mediastinal masses is that cysts can appear solid, and solid (malignant) masses can have cystic or necrotic components. A true cyst has a very thin wall; a mass with cystic degeneration usually has a thick irregular wall.

Thymic Hyperplasia and Thymic Rebound

The thymus may appear enlarged and relatively dense (containing little fat) in patients with thymic hyperplasia, but, in some, it may appear quite normal. In young patients, the thymus may show a significant rebound hyperplasia 3 months to a year after cessation of chemotherapy for malignancy. This can result in a distinctly enlarged thymus.

Lymphoma

Anterior mediastinal lymph node enlargement (see Figs. 4–3 and 4–9) or lymphoma

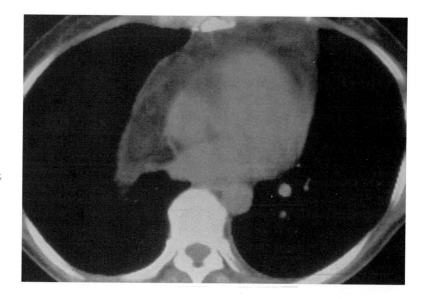

Figure 4–15. Thymolipoma. The large anterior mediastinal mass is composed primarily of fat but also contains strands of soft tissue.

involving the thymus (Fig. 4–16; see also Figs. 4–10 and 4–11) is present in more than half of patients with Hodgkin's disease. In patients with thymic involvement, lymphoma can present as a single spherical or lobulated mass or as thymic enlargement. In such cases, it can be indistinguishable from thymoma or other causes of prevascular mass. However, if it is multifocal (indicating its origin from nodes) or is associated with other sites of lymph node enlargement, the diagnosis is more easily

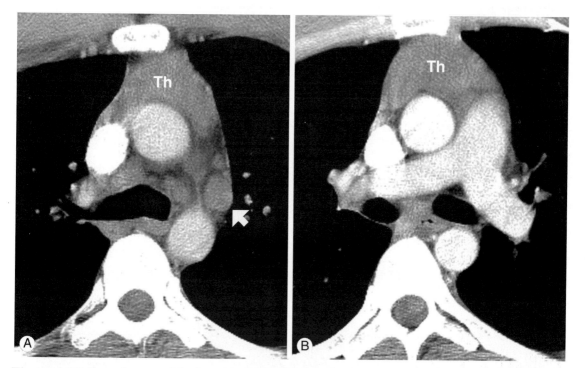

Figure 4–16. Lymphoma with thymic and mediastinal lymph node enlargement. *(A and B)* The thymus (Th) is symmetrically enlarged. This appearance could represent thymoma or other primary thymic tumor. However, enlarged lymph nodes in the aorticopulmonary window *(arrow, A)* and pretracheal space are a clue to the diagnosis.

made (see Fig. 4–16). Cystic areas of necrosis may be visible at CT (see Fig. 4–11). Except in rare cases, calcification does not occur in the absence of radiation. Hodgkin's disease limited to the prevascular mediastinum is typically the nodular sclerosing cell type.

Germ Cell Tumors

Several different tumors, originating from rests of primitive germ cells, can occur in the anterior mediastinum. These include dermoid cysts, teratoma, seminoma, choriocarcinoma, and endodermal sinus tumor. These tumors are somewhat less common than thymoma. Approximately 80% of germ cell tumors are benign.

Dermoid Cyst and Teratoma

These tumors can be cystic or solid and are most commonly benign. Dermoid cyst is a tumor derived from epidermal tissues, whereas a teratoma contains tissues of ectodermal, mesodermal, and endodermal origins.

They occur in a distribution similar to that of thymomas; rarely they originate in the posterior mediastinum. Benign lesions are often round, oval, and smooth in contour (Figs. 4–17 and 4–18) whereas, as with thy-

moma, an irregular, lobulated, or ill-defined margin suggests malignancy. On the average, these tumors are larger than thymomas but can be any size. Calcification can be seen (see Fig. 4–17) but is nonspecific except in the unusual instance when a bone or tooth is present within the mass. They may appear cystic or contain visible fat, a finding of great value in differential diagnosis (see Fig. 4–18). A fat–fluid level can also be seen.

Other Germ Cell Tumors

Seminoma, choriocarcinoma, and endodermal sinus (yolk sac) tumors are other cell types of anterior mediastinal germ cell tumors. They are malignant lesions occurring primarily in young men. They have no distinguishing characteristics on CT but are often large.

Thyroid Masses

A small percentage of patients with a thyroid mass have some extension of the mass into the superior mediastinum, and, rarely, a completely intrathoracic mass can arise from ectopic mediastinal thyroid tissue. In most patients, such masses represent a goiter (Fig. 4–19), but other diseases (Graves' disease, thyroiditis) and neoplasms can re-

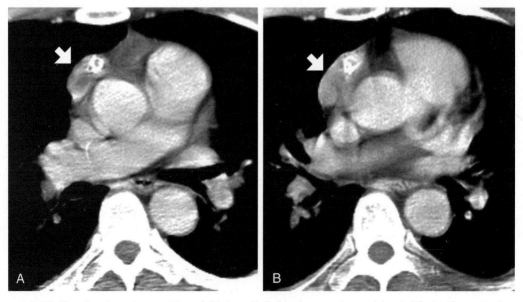

Figure 4–17. Benign teratoma. *(A and B)* A well-defined mass *(arrow)* is visible in the anterior mediastinum containing calcium and some low attenuation, which may represent fat.

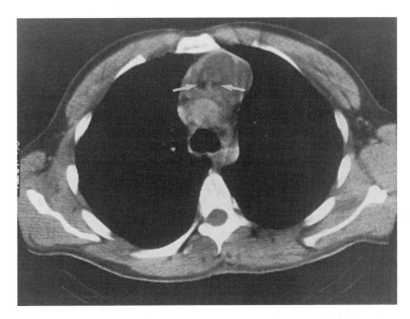

Figure 4–18. Benign teratoma. A lobulated anterior mediastinal mass contains areas of fat *(arrows)*. This appearance strongly suggests teratoma as the diagnosis. (From Webb WR. Computed tomography of the thorax. Radiol Clin North Am 1983; 21:723–739.)

sult in an intrathoracic mass. Masses are often asymmetric. Most patients with intrathoracic goiter are asymptomatic, but symptoms of tracheal or esophageal compression can be present. CT usually shows anatomic continuity with the cervical thyroid gland. The location of the mass at CT is somewhat variable, and they can be anterior or poste-

rior to the trachea. Masses anterior to the trachea splay the brachiocephalic vessels, whereas masses that are primarily posterior and lateral to the trachea displace the brachiocephalic vessels anteriorly. A location anterior to the great vessels is somewhat unusual (see Fig. 4–19). Calcifications and low-attenuation cystic areas are com-

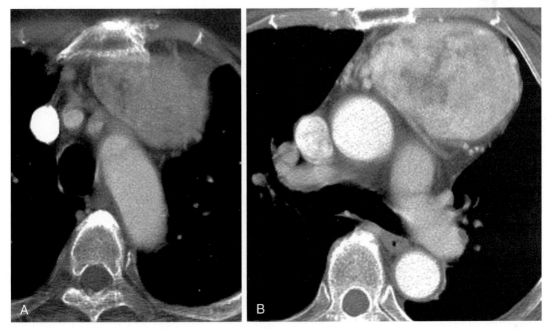

Figure 4–19. Mediastinal goiter. *(A)* A large inhomogeneous mass is visible in the anterior mediastinum. It shows enhancement after contrast medium infusion. *(B)* At higher levels, the mass was contiguous with the inferior thyroid.

mon in patients with goiter. Also, because of their iodine content, the CT attenuation of goiters, Graves' disease, and thyroiditis can be greater than that of soft tissue and thyroid tumors but less dense than normal thyroid tissue.

Mesenchymal Masses

Lipomatosis and Lipoma

A diffuse accumulation of unencapsulated fat in the mediastinum, so-called mediastinal lipomatosis, can occur in patients with Cushing's syndrome, after long-term corticosteroid therapy, or as a result of exogenous obesity. It produces no symptoms. CT shows a generalized increase in anterior mediastinal fat surrounding the great vessels, with some lateral bulging of the mediastinal pleural reflections. On CT, fat has a characteristic low attenuation, measuring from −50 to −100 H.

As with other mesenchymal tumors, lipomas can occur in any part of the mediastinum but are most common anteriorly. Because of their pliability, they rarely cause symptoms. A lipoma, although of the same attenuation as lipomatosis, is localized. Most fatty masses are benign. Liposarcoma, teratoma, and thymolipoma, other masses that can contain fat, also contain soft tissue elements and thus can be distinguished from lipoma or lipomatosis.

Lymphangioma (Hygroma)

Lymphangiomas are classified histologically as simple, cavernous, and cystic. Simple lymphangiomas are composed of small, thin-walled lymphatic channels with considerable connective tissue stroma. Cavernous lymphangiomas consist of dilated lymphatic channels, whereas cystic lymphangiomas (hygromas) contain single or multiple cystic masses filled with serous or milky fluid and having little if any communication with normal lymphatics. Most commonly, these lesions are detected in children and may extend into the neck. However, they can be seen in adults as well. On CT, the mass can appear as a single cyst, can be multicystic, or can envelop, rather than displace, mediastinal structures. Discrete cysts may not be visible; calcification does not occur.

PRETRACHEAL SPACE MASSES

Masses that occupy this compartment characteristically replace or displace the normal pretracheal fat. Because the pretracheal space is limited by the relatively immobile aortic arch anteriorly and to the left, large masses extend preferentially to the right, displacing and compressing the superior vena cava anteriorly and laterally. In the presence of a pretracheal mass, the superior vena cava will appear crescentic, convex laterally, with its concave aspect molding itself to the convex contour of the adjacent mass. This lateral displacement of the superior vena cava results in most of the mediastinal widening visible on plain films. Very large masses also displace the trachea posteriorly, but this is somewhat more difficult to recognize because the tracheal cartilages prevent much tracheal narrowing. Masses in this compartment are almost always of lymph node origin.

The Trachea

The trachea extends inferiorly from the thoracic inlet for a distance of 8 to 10 cm before bifurcating into the right and left main bronchi. The trachea is usually round, or more often oval, and is approximately 2 cm in diameter. In some patients, the trachea appears somewhat triangular, with the apex of the triangle directed anteriorly. This appearance is particularly common at the level of the carina and proximal main bronchi. In some patients, the tracheal cartilage is visible as a relatively dense horseshoe-shaped structure within the tracheal wall, with the open part of the horseshoe being posterior; calcification is common in older patients, particularly women. The tracheal wall should measure no more that 2 or 3 mm in thickness.

Tracheal abnormalities are uncommon and may be asymptomatic unless the tracheal lumen is reduced to a few millimeters. A high degree of suspicion must be maintained if tracheal abnormalities are to be correctly interpreted. Spiral CT, usually with narrow (3–5 mm) collimation is advantageous in imaging tracheal abnormalities. *Saber-sheath trachea* is a relatively com-

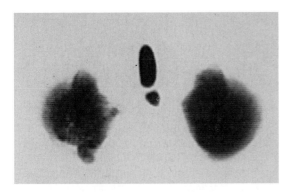

Figure 4–20. Saber-sheath trachea. The trachea is narrowed from side to side, whereas the sagittal diameter is normal or increased. In this patient, the air-filled esophagus is visible posterior to the trachea.

mon tracheal abnormality, occurring in patients with chronic obstructive pulmonary disease, probably because of the repeated trauma of coughing. In this condition there is side-to-side narrowing of the intrathoracic trachea, with the anterior-to-posterior tracheal diameter being preserved or increased (Fig. 4–20); the extrathoracic trachea is normal. A focal segment of the trachea at the thoracic inlet may be involved first. In severe cases, the opposite tracheal walls may touch each other and appear slightly thickened. Saber-sheath trachea should be distinguished from several diseases that produce concentric tracheal narrowing and involve the extrathoracic tra-

chea as well. These include amyloidosis and tracheobronchopathia osteochondroplastica (both of which show thickening and irregular calcification of the tracheal wall), Wegener's granulomatosis, and polychondritis. These are very rare and are not described further.

Tracheal stenosis occurring because of previous intubation is a relatively common abnormality. Narrowing of the tracheal lumen may be associated with intratracheal soft tissue masses of reactive (granulation) tissue or collapse of the tracheal wall because of destruction of the tracheal rings and associated fibrosis. Identifying the shapes of the tracheal cartilages (and therefore the tracheal wall) may be helpful in distinguishing these two types of tracheal stenosis, and this may affect treatment.

Primary tracheal tumors are rare. The most common primary malignancies, occurring in approximately equal numbers, are squamous cell carcinoma (Figs. 4–21 and 4–22) and cylindroma (adenoid cystic carcinoma). In patients with either of these, CT can be helpful in choosing treatment. If there is no mediastinal invasion (as evidenced by a mediastinal mass), then the lesion may be curable with a partial tracheal resection.

The trachea may be compressed, displaced, or invaded by a variety of malignant mediastinal tumors. Unless tumor can be seen within the tracheal lumen, tracheal

Figure 4–21. Tracheal carcinoma (squamous cell). There is narrowing of the tracheal lumen and an intraluminal mass *(large arrow)*, associated with a significant mediastinal mass *(small arrows)*, in a patient with invasive carcinoma. (From Gamsu G, Webb WR. Computed tomography of the trachea: normal and abnormal. AJR 1982; 139:321–326.)

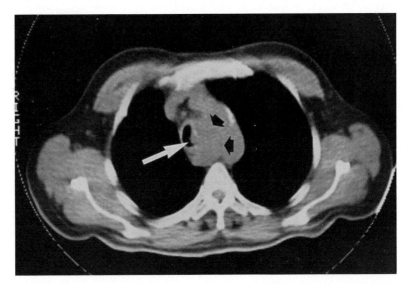

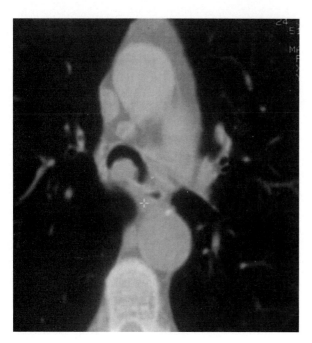

Figure 4–22. Tracheal carcinoma (squamous cell). An intraluminal mass is visible in a patient with squamous cell carcinoma involving the trachea. (From Webb WR. Plain radiography and computed tomography in the staging of bronchogenic carcinoma: a practical approach. J Thorac Imaging 1987; 2:57–65, with permission of Aspen Publishers Inc., © January 1987.)

invasion is difficult to diagnose. The trachea can be involved by lung cancer as a result of direct extension from a tumor arising in a main bronchus; bronchogenic carcinomas involving the trachea or carina are usually considered unresectable (T4). Thickening of the carina or tracheal wall contiguous with a bronchial lesion suggests this diagnosis, but bronchoscopy is usually required for a definite diagnosis.

SUBCARINAL SPACE

Large masses in this location can (1) produce a convexity of the azygoesophageal recess, (2) splay the carina, (3) displace the carina anteriorly, (4) displace the esophagus to the left, and/or (5) displace the right pulmonary artery anteriorly and compress its lumen. The most common masses involving this compartment are lymph node masses, cysts, and esophageal lesions.

Bronchogenic and Esophageal Cysts

Congenital bronchogenic cysts result from anomalous budding of the foregut during development. Most commonly, they are visible in the subcarinal space, but they can occur in any part of the mediastinum. They appear as single, smooth, round, or elliptical masses (Fig. 4–23) and occasionally show calcification of their walls or contents. Air–fluid levels occurring because of communication with the trachea or bronchi are rare. When large, bronchogenic cysts can produce symptoms by compression of mediastinal structures. A rapid increase in size can occur because of infection or hemorrhage.

Esophageal duplication cysts are indistinguishable from bronchogenic cysts. They usually appear as well-defined solitary masses and can also contain an air–fluid level when they communicate with the esophagus.

CT can be of great value in diagnosing a mediastinal cyst. If a mass is thin walled and is of fluid attenuation (approximately 0 H), it can be assumed to represent a benign cyst. However, high CT numbers (40 to 80 H), suggesting a solid mass, can also be found in patients with foregut duplication cysts. These cysts contain a thick gelatinous material or blood. In such patients, surgery is usually required for diagnosis, but magnetic resonance imaging may sometimes help.

Esophageal Lesions

Esophageal lesions are discussed in Chapter 16.

AORTICOPULMONARY WINDOW MASSES

Masses in this region typically replace mediastinal fat; and when large, they displace the mediastinal pleural reflection laterally. Displacement or compression of the aorta, pulmonary artery, and trachea are usually difficult to recognize. Aorticopulmonary window masses are almost always the result of lymph node enlargement.

RETROSTERNAL MEDIASTINUM

Enlargement of internal mammary nodes results in a convexity in the expected position of this node chain (see Fig. 4–1). Other than lymph node enlargement, masses in this region are unusual.

PARAVERTEBRAL MASS

Paravertebral masses may be seen to replace paravertebral fat. On the left, the normal concave mediastinal pleural reflection, posterior to the aorta, becomes convex in the presence of a significant mass. On the right, a paravertebral convexity is visible in a region where little tissue normally exists (see Figs. 4–5 and 4–20).

Neurogenic Tumors

Neurogenic tumors are divided into three groups, arising from peripheral nerves (neurofibroma, neurilemmoma), sympathetic ganglia (ganglioneuroma, neuroblastoma), and paraganglionic cells (pheochromocytoma, chemodectoma). Tumors in each of these three groups may be benign or malignant. Although neurogenic tumors can occur at any age, they are most common in young patients. Neuroblastoma and ganglioneuroma are most common in children, whereas neurofibroma and neurilemmoma more frequently affect young adults.

Radiographically, neurogenic tumors appear as well-defined, round or oval soft tissue masses, typically in a paravertebral location (Fig. 4–24). Although the different tumors are by no means always distinguishable, ganglioneuromas tend to be elongated,

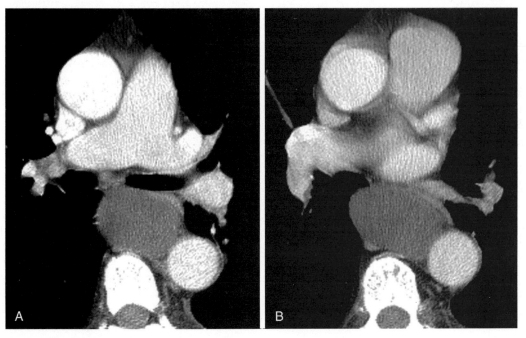

Figure 4–23. Bronchogenic cyst. *(A and B)* A large, oval, low-attenuation cyst is visible in the subcarinal region and azygoesophageal recess. This location is typical.

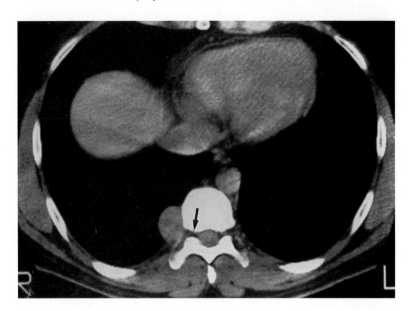

Figure 4–24. Neurofibroma. A smooth paravertebral, posterior mediastinal mass is visible *(arrow)*. The neural foramen is normal. (Modified from Putman CE, Ravin CE [eds]. Textbook of Diagnostic Imaging, 2nd ed. Philadelphia, WB Saunders, 1994.)

lying adjacent to the spine, whereas neurofibromas and neurilemmomas are smaller and more spherical. Although neural tumors are frequently of soft tissue attenuation, they can be low in attenuation because of the presence of (1) lipid-rich Schwann cells, (2) fat, or (3) cystic regions. Although benign tumors tend to be sharply marginated and fairly homogeneous, and malignant tumors tend to be infiltrating and irregular, these findings are not sufficiently reliable for diagnosis. Calcification can occur, particularly in neuroblastoma; the presence of calcium does not help in distinguishing benign from malignant lesions.

A neurofibroma arising in a nerve root can be dumb-bell shaped, part being inside and part outside the spinal canal. In such cases, the intervertebral foramen may be enlarged. CT can be helpful in determining the extent of the mass and associated vertebral abnormalities and can distinguish the mass from an aortic aneurysm or other vascular lesion if an intravenous contrast agent is given. CT after injection of myelographic contrast medium may be useful in demonstrating intraspinal extension.

Anterior or Lateral Thoracic Meningocele

A thoracic meningocele represents anomalous herniation of the spinal meninges through an intervertebral foramen or a defect in the vertebral body. It results in a soft tissue mass visible on chest radiographs. In most patients, this abnormality is associated with neurofibromatosis; most are detected in adults. It is said that meningocele is the most common cause of a posterior mediastinal mass in patients with neurofibromatosis.

Meningoceles are described as lateral or anterior, depending on their relationship to the spine. They are slightly more common on the right. Findings that suggest the diagnosis include rib or vertebral anomalies at the same level or an association with scoliosis. The mass is often visible at the apex of the scoliotic curve. CT after intraspinal contrast medium injection shows filling of the meningocele and is diagnostic (Fig. 4–25).

Neuroenteric Cyst

This rare cyst is composed of both neural and gastrointestinal elements and frequently is attached to both the meninges and gastrointestinal tract. They appear as homogeneous posterior mediastinal masses but rarely contain air because of communication with abdominal viscera. As with meningocele, they are frequently associated with vertebral anomalies or scoliosis. They rarely fill with myelographic contrast medium. As opposed to meningocele, they frequently cause pain and are generally diagnosed at a young age.

Diseases of the Thoracic Spine

Tumors (either benign or malignant), infectious spondylitis, or vertebral fracture with associated hemorrhage can produce a paravertebral mass. Frequently, the abnormality is bilateral and fusiform, allowing it to be distinguished from solitary masses such as a neurogenic tumor. Associated abnormalities of the vertebral bodies or discs assist in diagnosis and should be sought. Preservation of discs in association with vertebral body destruction suggests neoplasm or tuberculosis; disc destruction suggests infection other than tuberculosis.

Extramedullary Hematopoiesis

Extramedullary hematopoiesis can result in a paravertebral mass in patients with severe anemia (usually congenital hemolytic anemias or thalassemia). These masses are of unknown origin but perhaps arise from lymph nodes, veins, or an extension of rib marrow. Masses can be multiple and bilateral and are most commonly associated with the lower thoracic spine. They have no specific CT characteristics.

Fluid Collections

Occasionally, posterior pleural fluid collections can simulate a paravertebral medias-

tinal mass. Mediastinal extension of a pancreatic pseudocyst through the aortic or esophageal hiatus can occur but is rare.

Vascular Abnormalities

Posteriorly located aortic aneurysms can occupy this part of the mediastinum. Also, azygos and hemiazygos vein dilatation will produce abnormalities in this region. Dilated azygos or hemiazygos veins, because they are visible on a number of contiguous slices, are easily distinguished from a focal mass.

DIFFUSE MEDIASTINAL ABNORMALITIES

Mediastinitis

Mediastinal infections can be acute or chronic. Acute mediastinitis results from bacterial infection, has a rapid onset and acute symptoms, and is sometimes fatal. Chronic mediastinitis is usually granulomatous in origin and often is asymptomatic, coming to attention only because of a radiographic abnormality. Chronic sclerosing mediastinitis unassociated with infection is rare but results in similar findings.

Acute Mediastinitis

This usually results from esophageal perforation or the spread of infection from

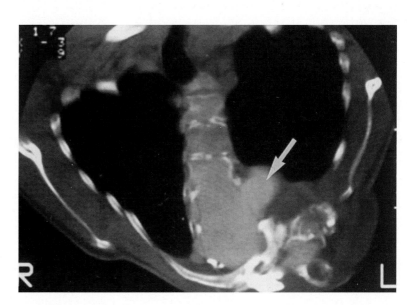

Figure 4–25. Lateral thoracic meningocele. In a patient with neurofibromatosis and scoliosis, a meningocele *(arrow)* is associated with a large foraminal defect. Myelographic contrast material opacifies the meningocele. (From Putman CE, Ravin CE [eds]. Textbook of Diagnostic Imaging, 2nd ed. Philadelphia, WB Saunders, 1994.)

adjacent tissue spaces, including the pharynx, lungs, pleura, and lymph nodes. The primary symptoms are substernal chest pain and fever. CT shows mediastinal widening and replacement of normal fat by fluid attenuation and can detect the presence of gas bubbles (Fig. 4–26). Prognosis is particularly poor in patients with esophageal perforation.

Granulomatous Mediastinitis

In patients with histoplasmosis, tuberculosis, and sarcoidosis, chronic mediastinal lymph node enlargement and associated fibrosis can result in so-called granulomatous mediastinitis. In these patients, the large nodes and associated fibrous tissue form a mediastinal mass that can compress the superior vena cava, pulmonary arteries or veins, bronchi, and esophagus (see Figs. 4–3 through 4–15).

The node enlargement tends to be asymmetric except in patients with sarcoidosis. Fibrosis can replace normally visible mediastinal fat. Calcification of the nodes can be seen in some patients, indicating the benign nature of the disease process. Compression of the main bronchi (usually the left) or pulmonary arteries (usually the right) can sometimes be recognized.

Sclerosing Mediastinitis

In some patients, a similar mediastinal fibrosis is unassociated with obvious granulomatous disease. In a few, this is associated with a similar fibrosis elsewhere (retroperitoneal fibrosis). Symptoms and radiographic findings are similar to granulomatous mediastinitis, but calcification does not occur.

Mediastinal Hemorrhage

Mediastinal hemorrhage usually results from trauma such as venous or arterial laceration, from aortic rupture or dissection, or as a result of anticoagulation therapy. Superior mediastinal widening is usually present, associated with blurring of normal mediastinal contours. Blood can dissect extrapleurally over the lung apex, resulting in a so-called apical cap. In some patients, blood will also be present in the left pleural space. CT is rarely of value in diagnosing the site of bleeding unless a dissection is present.

HEART AND PERICARDIUM

CT is not used much in clinical practice for the evaluation of cardiac abnormalities, but some knowledge of cardiac anatomy on CT is necessary for the proper interpretation of scans and the identification of paracardiac abnormalities or masses and the effect they have on the heart. Only occasionally are incidental cardiac abnormalities detected on CT. CT, on the other hand, is excellent for evaluating pericardial abnormalities.

Cardiac Pathology

Although CT can show a number of abnormalities in patients with ischemic heart dis-

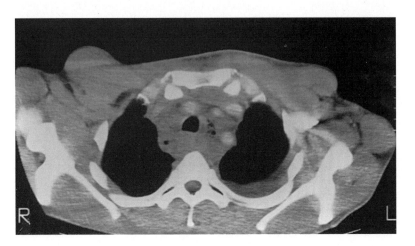

Figure 4–26. Acute mediastinitis. A patient with a retropharyngeal abscess developed secondary mediastinitis. There is mediastinal widening, increased attenuation of mediastinal fat as a result of abscess or inflammation, and small bubbles of air.

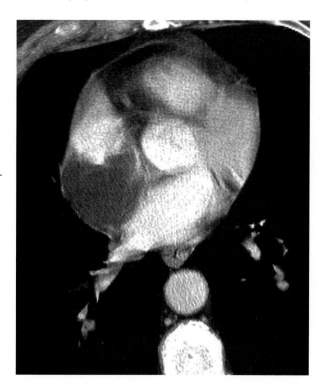

Figure 4–27. Right atrial lipoma. A low attenuation mass partially filling the posterior right atrium and compressing the anterior left atrium was detected incidentally on CT. The patient had no cardiac symptoms.

ease or other cardiac abnormalities, it does not usually play a significant role in the clinical evaluation of patients with cardiac pathology. Echocardiography, magnetic resonance imaging, and angiography are more commonly used.

In patients with an acute myocardial infarction, after the bolus injection of contrast medium, infarcted myocardium can show less opacification than normal myocardium and, to some degree, infarct size can be quantitated. Ventricular thrombus can also be shown in patients with an acute myocardial infarction.

In patients with prior infarct, CT can be valuable in showing ventricular aneurysms and associated thrombus. In patients who have had coronary artery bypass grafts, graft patency can be determined with an accuracy of about 90%, by performing dynamic sequential bolus-enhanced CT. However, significant stenoses of patent grafts are difficult to see.

Intracardiac tumors can be shown with contrast medium–enhanced CT (Figs. 4–27 and 4–28) but are rare and usually evaluated using other techniques. Myocardial wall thickening can be seen in some patients with myocardiopathy.

CT is very sensitive in detecting great vessel (aortic), valve, and annular calcification.

Coronary Artery Calcification

Coronary artery calcification can be clearly identified on CT scans at and below the level of the aortic root. In recent studies, the presence and extent of coronary artery calcification has been correlated with the likelihood of clinically significant coronary artery disease.

The left main coronary artery is about 1 cm in length; it arises from the aorta at about 4 o'clock and gives rise to the left anterior descending coronary artery extending anteriorly and inferiorly and the circumflex coronary artery extending posteriorly and inferiorly. Left main coronary calcification is said to be present if calcium is seen proximal to its point of bifurcation into the left anterior descending and circumflex arteries. The right coronary artery arises from the anterior aorta (at about 11 o'clock) slightly caudad to the left main artery and extends anteriorly and inferiorly in the atrioventricular groove. Left anterior descending artery calcification almost always predominates.

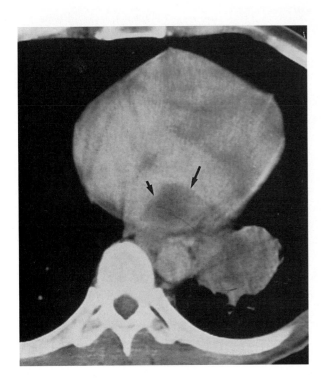

Figure 4–28. Left atrial metastasis. In a patient with renal cell carcinoma and a left hilar mass, a mass within the opacified left atrium represents a large metastasis *(arrows)*.

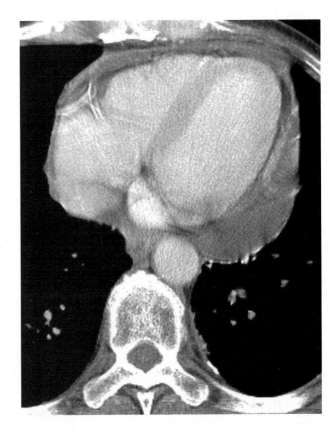

Figure 4–29. Pericardial effusion from metastatic lung cancer. Fluid accumulates first in the dependent portions of the pericardium, posterior to the left ventricle. In this patient, most fluid collection has accumulated in this region.

Pericardial Abnormalities

Pericardial Effusion, Thickening, and Fibrosis

Pericardial effusion results in thickening of the normal pericardial stripe. When fluid begins to accumulate, it accumulates first in the dependent portions of the pericardium, typically posterior to the left ventricle (Fig. 4–29; see also Figs. 4–3 through 4–8). As the effusion increases in size, it is visible lateral and anterior to the right atrium and ventricle and, when large, as a concentric opacity surrounding the heart. Large effusions can also extend into the superior pericardial recess in the mediastinum. The presence of tamponade, associated with pericardial effusion, may be more directly related to the speed at which the fluid accumulates, and the distensibility of the pericardium, rather than the size of the effusion alone.

Pericardial thickening or fibrosis, usually as a result of inflammation, can produce a similar thickening of the pericardial stripe. With contrast medium infusion, the thickened pericardium may be seen to enhance, thus distinguishing it from effusion. Also, pericardial thickening may be denser than fluid collections that also may be present, even without contrast medium infusion. Thickening may be smooth or focal and nodular. Calcification can occur, particularly as a result of tuberculosis, purulent pericarditis, or hemopericardium.

In the presence of symptoms of constrictive pericarditis, the CT appearance of a normal pericardium rules out the diagnosis, whereas a thickened pericardium allows a presumptive diagnosis of constriction to be made. In the presence of pericardial metastases, CT can show an effusion, or nodular masses may be visible, particularly after contrast medium infusion.

PARACARDIAC MASSES

Compression of the atria or right ventricle can be seen in the presence of a paracardiac mass, but left ventricular compression is uncommon because of the thickness of its wall and the relatively high pressure of its contents.

Anterior Cardiophrenic Angle Masses

Although a number of the mediastinal masses already described can occur at the level of the anterior cardiophrenic angle, the differential diagnosis of lesions occurring in this location includes several additional entities. These include pericardial cyst, large epicardiac fat pad, Morgagni's hernia, and enlargement of paracardiac lymph nodes (discussed earlier).

Pericardial Cyst

Most commonly, pericardial cysts touch the diaphragm, 60% in the anterior right cardiophrenic angle and 30% in the left cardiophrenic angle; 10% occur higher in the mediastinum. Most patients are asymptomatic. The cysts typically appear as smooth, round, homogeneous masses. They range up to 15 cm in diameter. As with other mediastinal cysts, their attenuation may be that of water or soft tissue.

Fat Pad

Deposition of fat in either cardiophrenic angle is not uncommon, particularly in obese patients, and can simulate a mass on plain radiographs. CT, of course, is diagnostic.

Morgagni Hernia

Hernias of abdominal contents through the anteromedial diaphragmatic foramen of Morgagni can result in a cardiophrenic angle mass; 90% of these occur on the right. Hernia contents are usually omentum or liver, but they can contain bowel. When the hernia contains fat, CT can confirm its benign nature but does not allow its differentiation from a fat pad. When it contains liver, CT may allow diagnosis by showing hepatic vessels or bile ducts. If bowel is present in the hernia sac, gas is usually visible.

Suggested Reading

Ahn JM, Lee KS, Goo JM, et al. Predicting the histology of anterior mediastinal masses: comparison of chest radiography on CT. J Thorac Imaging 1996; 265–271.

Aronberg DJ, Peterson RR, Glazer HS, Sagel SS. Superior diaphragmatic lymph nodes: CT assessment. J Comput Assist Tomogr 1986; 10:937–941.

Bashist B, Ellis K, Gold RP. Computed tomography of intrathoracic goiters. AJR 1983; 140:455–460.

Buy JN, Ghossain MA, Poirson F, et al. Computed tomography of mediastinal lymph nodes in non–small cell lung cancer: a new approach based on the lymphatic pathway of tumor spread. J Comput Assist Tomogr 1988; 12:545–552.

Dales RE, Stark RM, Raman S. Computed tomography to stage lung cancer: approaching a controversy using meta-analysis. Am Rev Respir Dis 1990; 141:1096–1101.

Daly BD, Faling LJ, Bite G, et al. Mediastinal lymph node evaluation by computed tomography in lung cancer: an analysis of 345 patients grouped by TNM staging, tumor size, and tumor location. J Thorac Cardiovasc Surg 1987; 94:664–672.

Freundlich IM, McGavran MH. Abnormalities of the thymus. J Thorac Imaging 1996; 11:58–65.

Glazer GM, Gross BH, Quint LE, et al. Normal mediastinal lymph nodes: number and size according to American Thoracic Society mapping. AJR 1985; 144:261–265.

Glazer GM, Orringer MB, Gross BH, Quint LE. The mediastinum in non-small cell lung cancer: CT-surgical correlation. AJR 1984; 142:1101–1105.

Glazer HS, Aronberg DJ, Sagel SS. Pitfalls in CT recognition of mediastinal lymphadenopathy. AJR 1985; 144:267–274.

Glazer HS, Aronberg DJ, Sagel SS, Friedman PJ. CT demonstration of calcified mediastinal lymph nodes: a guide to the new ATS classification. AJR 1986; 147:17–20.

Glazer HS, Kaiser LR, Anderson DJ, et al. Indeterminate mediastinal invasion in bronchogenic carcinoma: CT evaluation. Radiology 1989; 173:37–42.

Hopper KD, Diehl LF, Cole BA, et al. The significance of necrotic mediastinal lymph nodes on CT in patients with newly diagnosed Hodgkin disease. AJR 1990; 155:267–270.

Hopper KD, Diehl LF, Lesar M, et al. Hodgkin disease: clinical utility of CT in initial staging and treatment. Radiology 169:17–22, 1988.

Im J-G, Song KS, Kang HS, et al. Mediastinal tuberculous lymphadenitis: CT manifestations. Radiology 1987; 164:115–119.

Kiyono K, Sone S, Sakai F, et al. The number and size of normal mediastinal lymph nodes: a postmortem study. AJR 1988; 150:771–776.

Kuhlman JE, Deutsch JH, Fishman EK, Siegelman SS. CT features of thoracic mycobacterial disease. Radiographics 1990; 10:413–431.

Levitt RG, Husband JE, Glazer HS. CT of primary germ-cell tumors of the mediastinum. AJR 1984; 142:73–78.

McLoud TC, Bourgouin PM, Greenberg RW, et al. Bronchogenic carcinoma: analysis of staging in the mediastinum with CT by correlative lymph node mapping and sampling. Radiology 1992; 182:319–323.

Müller NL, Webb WR, Gamsu G. Paratracheal lymphadenopathy: radiographic findings and correlation with CT. Radiology 1985; 156:761–765.

Müller NL, Webb WR, Gamsu G. Subcarinal lymph node enlargement: radiographic findings and CT correlation. AJR 1985; 145:15–19.

Pastores SM, Naidich DP, Aranda CP, et al. Intrathoracic adenopathy associated with pulmonary tuberculosis in patients with human immunodeficiency virus infection. Chest 1993; 103:1433–1437.

Platt JF, Glazer GM, Gross BH, et al. CT evaluation of mediastinal lymph nodes in lung cancer: influence of the lobar site of the primary neoplasm. AJR 1987; 149:683–686.

Pugatch RD, Faling LJ, Robbins AH, Spira R. CT diagnosis of benign mediastinal abnormalities. AJR 1980; 134:685–694.

Quint LE, Glazer GM, Orringer MB, et al. Mediastinal lymph node detection and sizing at CT and autopsy. AJR 1986; 147:469–472.

Staples CA, Müller NL, Miller RR, et al. Mediastinal nodes in bronchogenic carcinoma: comparison between CT and mediastinoscopy. Radiology 1988; 167:367–372.

5

The Pulmonary Hila

W. Richard Webb, M.D.

The pulmonary hila are difficult to evaluate on plain radiographs because they have extremely complex and somewhat variable silhouettes. It is often hard to decide if a hilum is normal or abnormal and, if it is abnormal, what the abnormal finding represents.

CT is very helpful in the diagnosis of endobronchial lesions, hilar and parahilar masses, and hilar vascular lesions. The sensitivity and specificity of CT in diagnosing a hilar mass or adenopathy in patients with lung cancer average between 80% and 90% and are highest when bolus contrast medium enhancement is used.

TECHNIQUE

As with the different parts of the mediastinum described in Chapter 2, it takes about 10 contiguous 7-mm slices, 7 contiguous 10-mm slices, or 14 contiguous 5-mm slices to image the hila. If spiral CT is used, the hila are adequately assessed using 7-mm collimation and a pitch of 1, with continuous infusion of contrast medium.

With a conventional CT scanner, it is best to think of the hilar examination as a separate and distinct part of the chest CT study. Unless this is done, the technique may not be optimal. Although scans 8 to 10 mm thick are routinely used when chest CT is performed with a conventional scanner, it is a good idea to image the hila with 5-mm collimation, because this provides a better

look at the bronchi. Contrast medium is given by bolus injection with scans obtained dynamically at successive levels (i.e., dynamic incremental CT). Although the method of contrast medium infusion and scanning sequence that is used can be varied, it is important to keep in mind that the more rapidly the contrast medium is given, the better the vascular opacification will be, and the easier it is to distinguish normal hilar vessels from masses or enlarged lymph nodes.

When dynamic incremental CT of the hilum is performed, an intravenous bolus injection of approximately 50 mL of contrast medium is administered, with the scanner positioned at the level of the upper lobe bronchus. Midway through the bolus administration, rapid sequential scanning is performed at 5-mm intervals to the level of the inferior hila. If the patient cannot hold his or her breath for the entire sequence (which is typical), the bolus and scanning sequence can be divided as necessary. In patients who cannot hold their breath for more than one or two slices, hilar CT can be done during the slow infusion of the contrast agent.

Scans are viewed with a mean window level of − 700 H and a window width of 1000 H or 1500 H (lung windows) for accurate assessment of hilar contours and bronchial anatomy. Scans are also viewed at a mean window value of 0 to 50 H and a window width of 500 H (soft tissue windows) to obtain additional information about hilar structures and masses, as well as a more accurate assessment of bronchial narrowing. These windows are also necessary to observe vascular opacification, allowing vessels and mass or node enlargement to be distinguished.

DIAGNOSIS OF HILAR MASS OR ADENOPATHY

A detailed understanding of cross-sectional hilar anatomy is necessary to identify hilar abnormalities on CT.

Lobar and segmental bronchi (Fig. 5–1) are consistently seen on CT and reliably identify successive hilar levels. Their recognition is key to interpreting the pulmonary hila. In general, hilar anatomy and contours at the same bronchial levels are relatively constant from one patient to the next. The bronchi should be looked at first, whenever you read a CT scan of the hila.

In some locations, normal hilar contours are consistent enough that a diagnosis of hilar adenopathy or mass can be made on the basis of an abnormality in hilar contour alone, seen using lung windows. In other locations, however, contours can vary according to the size and position of the hilar pulmonary arteries and veins. In these locations, opacification with contrast medium of the pulmonary vessels is essential for accurate diagnosis. Also, in any location, infusion of a contrast agent can be helpful if you are uncertain as to the presence of a mass. It is always wise to perform hilar CT with contrast medium infusion.

A hilar mass or lymph node enlargement may be suggested by a local or generalized alteration in hilar contour; bronchial narrowing, obstruction, or displacement; and thickening or obliteration of the walls of bronchi that normally contact lung. At soft tissue window settings, any nonenhancing hilar structure larger than 5 mm has been considered abnormal by some, but this is not always the case. Normal soft tissue collections larger than this, representing fat and normal nodes, are sometimes visible.

Normal and Abnormal Hilar Anatomy

There are two ways to read hilar CT. The first is to look at each hilum separately, identifying each important structure, and the second is to compare one side to the

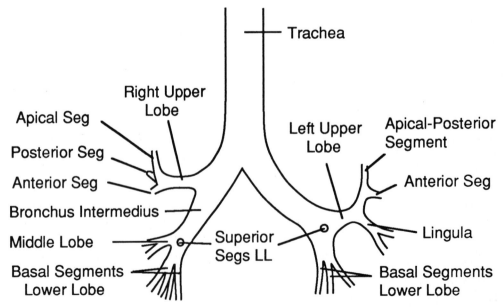

Figure 5–1. Normal bronchial tree. All the bronchi shown are visible on CT in most patients. Those bronchi that appear horizontal (such as those of the right upper lobe) or nearly vertical are usually better seen than those that have an oblique course relative to the plane of scan (such as right middle lobe or lingular bronchi).

TABLE 5–1. **Lobar and Segmental Bronchial Anatomy**

Right Upper Lobe Segments	*Left Upper Lobe Segments*
Apical	Apical-posterior
Posterior	Anterior
Anterior	Superior lingula
	Inferior lingula
Right Middle Lobe Segments	
Medial	
Lateral	
Right Lower Lobe Segments	*Left Lower Lobe Segments*
Superior	Superior
Anterior	Anteromedial
Medial	Lateral
Lateral	Posterior
Posterior	

other at successive scan levels, looking for points of similarity and dissimilarity. In fact, it is wise to do both.

I suggest that as you read the next section, you first learn about right hilar anatomy, skipping what is written about the left hilum. When you finish, and are somewhat oriented, you should start over, reading about both hila, comparing their anatomy, noting what is symmetric and what is not, and learning how the left hilum differs from the right. Also, you should learn to trace each lobar bronchus from its origin to its segmental branches, because this should be done during interpretation of the CT scan.

With one or two exceptions, rather than providing a description of the anatomy of each hilum separately, the normal anatomy for both hila is illustrated as seen on the same scan, at the same time. Although this will seem somewhat complicated at first, it is actually easier and is, in fact, the best way to read hilar CT. Looking at both hila at the same time allows you to compare each hilum to the other. Although the hila are not symmetric structures, they have a number of similarities, and identifying these can be of value. These similarities are emphasized in the following description. To reinforce the normal appearances and their significance, and expected alterations in anatomy occurring because of mass of node enlargement, abnormal findings are discussed at each hilar level described.

Some variation exists among patients in the relative levels of the hila, and, therefore, there is some variation in the levels at which right and left hilar structures are visible on CT. The right-to-left relationships illustrated in Figure 5–1 and described in the following text may or may not be present in individual cases, although variation will usually be minor (1 or 2 cm).

Because recognizing lobar and segmental bronchial anatomy is fundamental to interpreting hilar CT, it is reviewed briefly (Table 5–1). Each of the segments listed is commonly (but not invariably) visible.

Upper Hila

Right Hilum. CT at the level of the distal trachea or carina will show the apical segmental bronchus of the right upper lobe in cross section, surrounded by several vessels of similar size (Fig. 5–2A and B). On either side, mass or lymphadenopathy is easily recognizable. Anything larger than the expected pulmonary vessels is abnormal (Figs. 5–3 and 5–4). Comparing with the opposite side at this level is very helpful.

Left Hilum. The apical-posterior segmental bronchus and associated arteries and veins have a similar appearance to the right side at this level (Fig. 5–2A and B), as does lymph node enlargement (Fig. 5–3).

Right Upper Lobe Bronchus and Left Upper Lobe Segments

Right Hilum. Approximately 1 cm distal to the carina, the right upper lobe bronchus

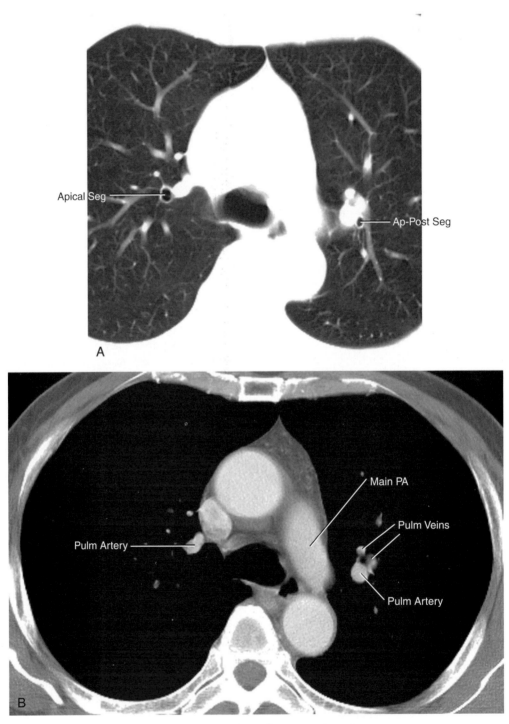

Figure 5–2 *See legend on opposite page*

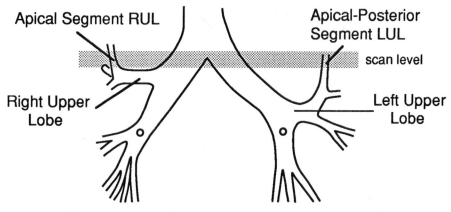

Figure 5–2. Upper hilar level: normal anatomy. CT, with lung *(A)* and soft tissue *(B)* window images at the level of the carina, shows the apical segmental bronchus of the right upper lobe in cross section, with several adjacent vessels of similar size. On the left, the apical posterior segmental bronchus of the left upper lobe and associated arteries and veins have a similar appearance. Note that this same patient is also used to illustrate normal anatomy at lower levels, with lung and soft tissue windows shown together. Generally, the bronchi are identified on the lung window scans and the vessels are identified on the soft tissue window scans.

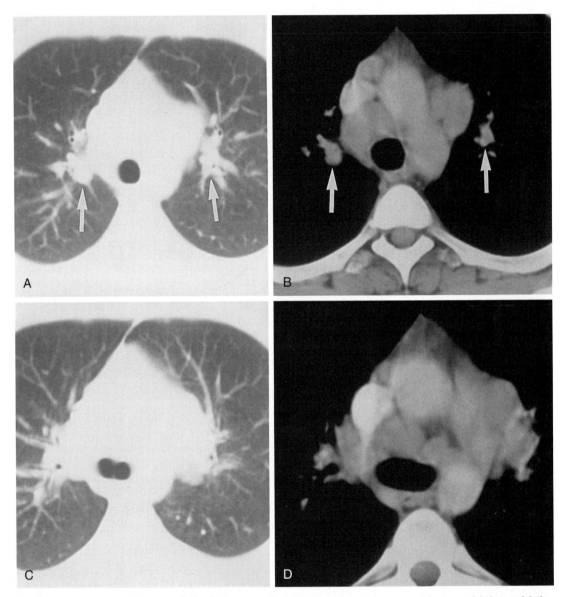

Figure 5–3. Abnormal upper hila (adenopathy). In a patient with sarcoidosis and bilateral hilar adenopathy, contrast medium–enhanced scans at two levels through the upper hila have been photographed with lung *(A, C)* and mediastinal *(B, D)* window settings. *A and B,* This scan level is slightly above that illustrated in Figure 5–2. Note that two small bronchial branches are visible on each side, rather than a single apical or apical-posterior bronchus. Enlarged nodes *(arrows)* adjacent to the bronchi are too large to represent normal vessels and appear unopacified on the mediastinal window scan. *C and D,* At a level 1 cm below *A* and *B,* extensive hilar lobulation is visible, reflecting the adenopathy.

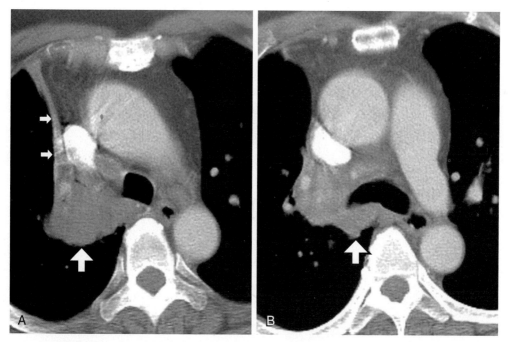

Figure 5–4. Abnormal upper right hilum (bronchogenic carcinoma). *A,* A large mass *(large arrow)* encompasses the region of the apical segmental bronchus of the right upper lobe. A thin linear opacity *(small arrows)* along the right mediastinum reflects collapse of the right upper lobe. *B,* At 7 mm below the level in *A,* the mass results in obstruction of the right upper lobe bronchus. The mass *(arrow)* is also visible posterior to the right main bronchus.

is usually visible along its length, with its anterior and posterior segmental branches both generally seen at the same level (Fig. 5–5). The anterior segment, usually lying in or near the scan plane, is very commonly seen over a length of 2 to 3 cm. The posterior segment bronchus usually angles slightly cephalad, out of the plane of scan, and may not be as well seen. If it is not seen one should look for it on the next highest level. In some normal subjects, the origin of the apical segment can be seen at this level as a round lucency, usually at the point of bifurcation (or, in this case, trifurcation) of the right upper lobe bronchus.

Anterior to the right upper lobe bronchus, the truncus anterior produces an oval opacity of variable size, but often about the same size as the right main bronchus visible at the same level. An upper lobe vein branch (posterior vein), lying in the angle between anterior and posterior segmental branches is present and visible in almost all patients. The posterior wall of the upper lobe bronchus is usually outlined by lung and appears smooth and 2 to 3 mm thick.

Within the anterior right hilum at this level, mass or lymph node enlargement can be identified if a soft tissue opacity larger than the expected size of the truncus anterior is visible (Fig. 5–6). This, of course, could be confirmed by contrast medium injection. Laterally, in the angle between the anterior and posterior segmental bronchi, anything larger than the expected vein is abnormal (see Fig. 5–6). This vein should not be significantly larger than at the level 1 cm above. Posteriorly, thickening of the wall of the upper lobe bronchus or main bronchus (Fig. 5–7; see also Fig. 5–6A) or a focal soft tissue opacity behind it will almost always be abnormal.

Left Hilum. On the left side, at or near this level, the apical-posterior and anterior segmental bronchi of the left upper lobe are usually visible (Fig. 5–5). The apical-posterior segment is seen in cross section as a round lucency, whereas the anterior segment is directed anteriorly, roughly in the plane of scan, at an angle of about 1 o'clock; in some subjects, the anterior segmental

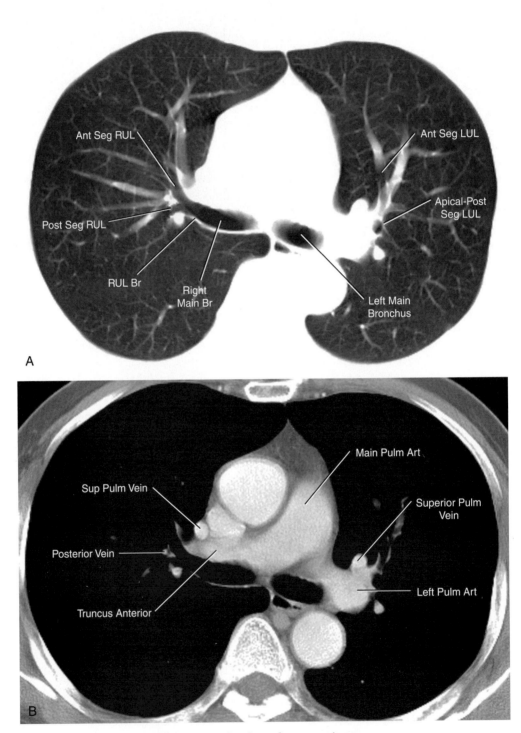

Figure 5–5 *See legend on opposite page*

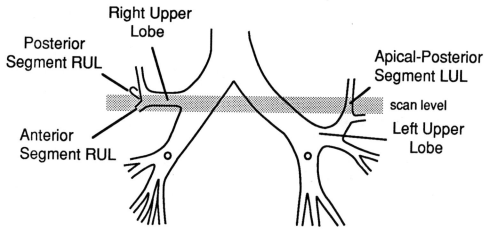

Figure 5–5. Right upper lobe bronchus and left upper lobe segments level: normal anatomy.
The diagram indicates the approximate plane of scan relative to the bronchial tree. *A and B,* Right hilum: The right upper lobe bronchus is visible along its length, along with its anterior and posterior segmental branches. The truncus anterior is anterior to the right upper lobe bronchus. An upper lobe vein branch (posterior vein) lies in the angle between the anterior and posterior segmental branches; the superior pulmonary veins result in some lobulation anterior to the truncus anterior. The posterior wall of the upper lobe bronchus appears smooth and 2 to 3 mm in thickness. Left hilum: On the left side, the apical-posterior and anterior segmental bronchi of the left upper lobe are visible. The apical-posterior segment is seen in cross section as a round lucency, whereas the anterior segment is directed anteriorly. These bronchi lie lateral to the main branch of the left pulmonary artery, which produces a convexity in the posterior hilum, and the superior pulmonary vein, which results in an anterior convexity. The artery supplying the anterior segment of the left upper lobe is seen medial to the anterior segment bronchus.

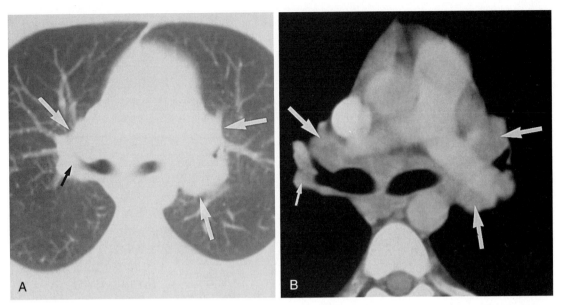

Figure 5–6. Hilar adenopathy. *A and B,* In the patient with sarcoidosis illustrated in Figure 5–3, there is extensive adenopathy *(arrows)* at this level. On the right, nodes are visible as unopacified structures anteriorly and laterally in the angle of the bifurcation of the right upper lobe bronchus into its anterior and posterior segments *(small arrows).* The soft tissue opacity seen in the position of the posterior vein on the right *(small arrow)* is too large to represent a vessel. The posterior wall of the right upper lobe bronchus is thickened; this is best seen at the lung window setting *(A).* On the left side, there are enlarged nodes *(arrows)* in both the anterior and posterior hilum, which are distinguishable from the opacified left pulmonary artery in *B.*

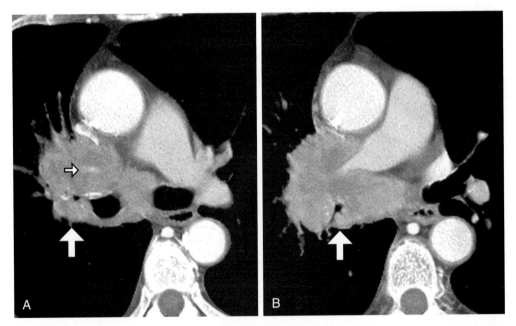

Figure 5–7. Bronchogenic carcinoma with a right hilar mass. *A,* A large carcinoma causes narrowing of the right upper lobe bronchus and obstruction of the anterior and posterior segmental bronchi. The truncus anterior *(small arrow),* anterior to the bronchus, is markedly narrowed and surrounded by tumor. The posterior walls of the right upper lobe bronchus *(large arrow)* and right main bronchus are thickened. *B,* At a lower level, the bronchus intermedius is narrowed and its posterior wall is thickened *(arrow).* The mass also invades the mediastinum, surrounding and narrowing the right pulmonary artery.

bronchus is seen at a lower level. These bronchi lie lateral to the main branch of the left pulmonary artery, which produces a large convexity in the posterior hilum at this level, and the superior pulmonary vein, which results in an anterior convexity. In a number of normal subjects, the artery supplying the anterior segment of the left upper lobe is seen medial to the anterior segment bronchus. Lymphadenopathy can be seen in relation to all these structures, most easily recognized after contrast medium infusion (see Fig. 5–6B).

A small vein is visible lateral to the apical-posterior bronchus in about 40% of individuals. In this location, mass or adenopathy can be recognized when a mass larger than the normal vein is present within the lateral hilum (Fig. 5–8).

Right Bronchus Intermedius

Below the level of the right upper lobe bronchus the bronchus intermedius is visible as an oval lucency at two or three adjacent levels (Fig. 5–9A and C). Its posterior wall is sharply outlined by lung. Anterior and lateral to the bronchus the hilar silhouette may vary in appearance, primarily because

of variations in the sizes and positions of pulmonary veins. A collection of fat and normal-sized nodes, sometimes measuring more than 1 cm in diameter, is commonly seen at the level of the bifurcation of the right pulmonary artery, anterior and lateral to the bronchus intermedius (Fig. 5–10; see also Fig. 5–9). A mass involving the posterior hilum can be readily diagnosed without contrast medium injection, because of thickening of the posterior bronchial wall (Fig. 5–11; see also Fig. 5–7); thickening of the posterior wall of the bronchus intermedius is a common finding in patients with right hilar mass, particularly resulting from lung cancer.

The diagnosis of anterior or lateral hilar masses at this level generally requires contrast medium administration (Fig. 5–12; see also Fig. 5–11). Normal soft tissue and nodes (see Figs. 5–9 and 5–10) should not be mistaken for a hilar mass.

Right Middle Lobe Bronchus and Left Upper Lobe/Lingular Bronchus

Right Middle Lobe Bronchus. On the right, at the level of the lower bronchus intermedius, the middle lobe bronchus

Text continued on page 89

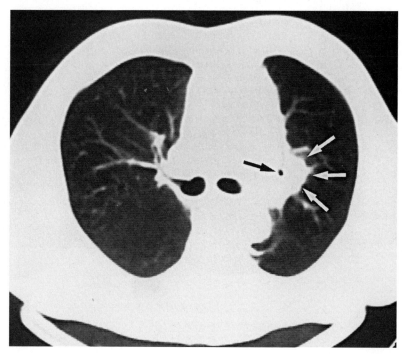

Figure 5–8. Bronchogenic carcinoma with a left hilar mass. A soft tissue mass *(white arrows)* is visible lateral to the left apical posterior segmental bronchus *(black arrow)*. Only a small vein should be seen in this location. (From Webb WR, et al: Computed tomography of the pulmonary hilum in patients with bronchogenic carcinoma. J Comput Assist Tomogr 1983; 7:219—225.)

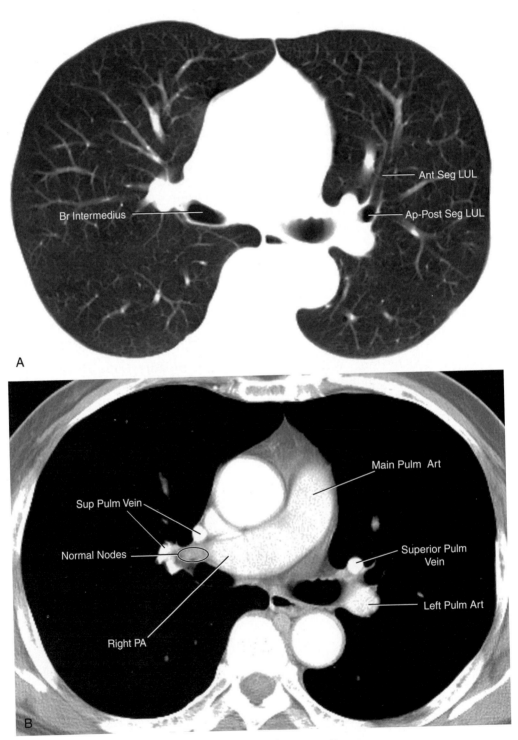

Figure 5–9 *See legend on opposite page*

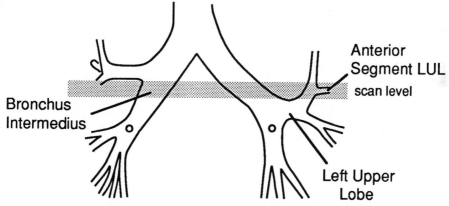

Figure 5–9. Normal bronchus intermedius and left upper lobe bronchus level. *A and B,* The bronchus intermedius is visible as an oval lucency with its posterior wall sharply outlined by lung. Anterior and lateral to the bronchus, the hilum is made up of the interlobar pulmonary artery and superior pulmonary veins. Normal lymph nodes and fat are visible in the anterolateral hilum, between the opacified pulmonary artery and veins. On the left, the anterior and the apical-posterior segmental bronchi of the left upper lobe are visible. The left superior pulmonary vein is anterior and medial to the bronchi, and the descending branch of the left pulmonary artery forms an oval soft tissue opacity posterior and lateral to them.

Illustration continued on following page

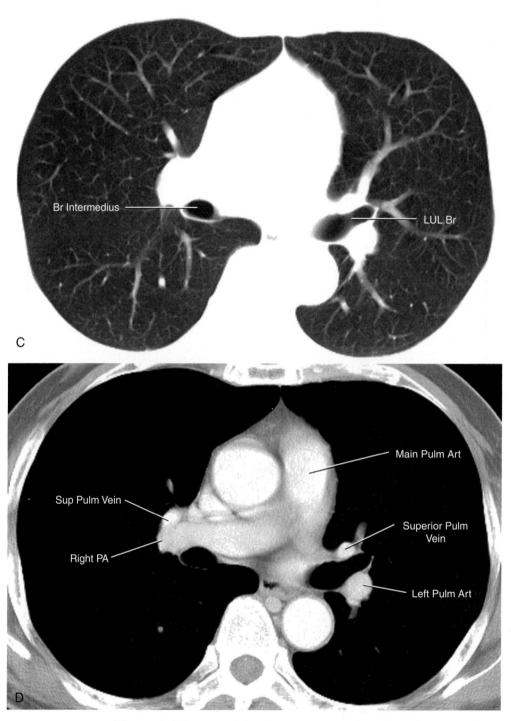

Figure 5–9 *Continued. See legend on opposite page*

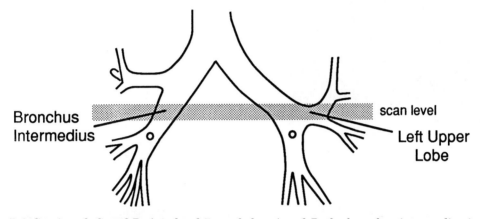

Figure 5–9 *Continued. C and D,* At a level 7 mm below *A* and *B*, the bronchus intermedius is visible as an oval lucency with its posterior wall sharply outlined by lung. The interlobar pulmonary artery and superior pulmonary veins are anterior and lateral to the bronchus. On the left, the upper lobe bronchus is usually seen along its axis, extending anteriorly and laterally from its origin. The left superior pulmonary vein is anterior and medial to the bronchus, and the descending branch of the left pulmonary artery is posterior and lateral to it. The left posterior bronchial wall is outlined by lung at this level.

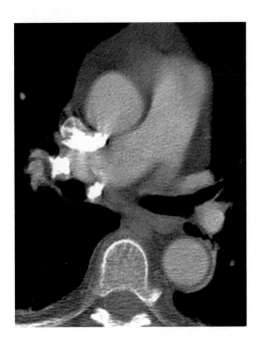

Figure 5–10. Calcified right hilar lymph nodes.
The location of normal lymph nodes in the lateral right hilum at the level of the bronchus intermedius is shown in this patient with lymph node calcification from tuberculosis. These nodes are the same as normal nodes shown in Figure 5–9B. Calcified mediastinal lymph nodes are also visible.

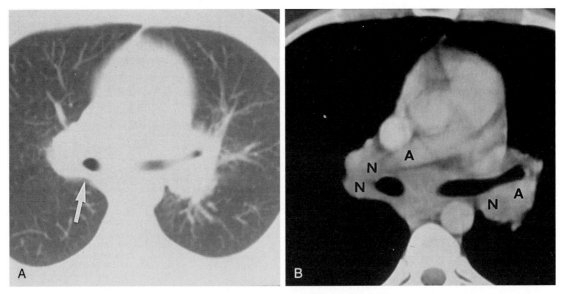

Figure 5–11. Abnormal bronchus intermedius and left upper lobe bronchus level. *A and B,*
In the patient with sarcoidosis, there is lymph node enlargement (N) in the lateral right hilum, distinguishable from the opacified pulmonary artery (A) at a mediastinal window setting. Thickening of the posterior wall of the bronchus intermedius *(arrow)* is also seen. On the left, there are large nodes (N) posterior to the left bronchus and medial to the pulmonary artery (A). These nodes obscure the posterior wall of the left bronchus. Subcarinal node enlargement is also present.

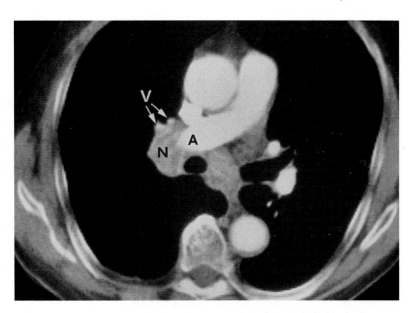

Figure 5–12. Abnormal bronchus intermedius level. In a patient with bronchogenic carcinoma and right hilar adenopathy (N), the soft tissue mass is clearly distinguished from the opacified artery (A). Veins (V) are displaced anteriorly. Note that this mass is much larger than the normal collection of nodes and fat that can be seen in this location (see Fig. 5–9*B*).

arises anteriorly and extends anteriorly, laterally, and inferiorly at angles of 30° to 45° (Fig. 5–13). Because of its obliquity, only a short segment of its lumen is visible at each level on CT, and this appearance should not be misinterpreted as bronchial obstruction. Often the superior segmental bronchus of the lower lobe arises posterolaterally at this level (see Fig. 5–13).

At the level of the origin of the middle lobe bronchus, the superior pulmonary veins lie anterior and medial to the bronchus, whereas the descending (interlobar) branch of the right pulmonary artery lies beside and behind it (see Fig. 5–13). Because of this separation of artery and veins, the lateral hilum at this level (representing the artery) is oval, without prominent lobulations. Any lobulation of significant size suggests hilar adenopathy (Figs. 5–14 and 5–15). Contrast medium injection would be confirmatory.

Left Upper Lobe Bronchus. The appearance of the left hilum at the level of the left upper lobe bronchus is quite similar to that of the right hilum at the level of the middle lobe bronchus; however, the left upper lobe bronchus is usually visible about 1 cm above the right middle lobe bronchus (see Fig. 5–9*C* and *D*).

The left upper lobe bronchus is usually seen along its axis, extending anteriorly and laterally from its origin, at an angle of 10° to 30° (see Fig. 5–9*C* and *D*). The left superior pulmonary veins are anterior and medial to the bronchus at this level, and the descending branch of the left pulmonary artery forms an oval soft tissue opacity posterior and lateral to it. Because only the oval artery occupies the lateral hilum, lobulation of the lateral hilum (more than one convexity) indicates lymphadenopathy (Fig. 5–16; see also Fig. 5–11). The superior segment bronchus of the left lower lobe can arise at this level.

Although lung contacts and sharply outlines the posterior wall of the bronchus intermedius at several levels, the left posterior bronchial wall is usually outlined only at this level, that is, at the level of the left upper lobe bronchus. In approximately 90% of individuals, lung sharply outlines the posterior wall of the left main or upper lobe bronchus, medial to the descending pulmonary artery (Fig. 5–17; see also Fig. 5–11). As on the right, the bronchial wall should measure 2 to 3 mm in thickness. Thickening of this stripe of opacity, or a focal soft tissue opacity behind it, indicates lymph node enlargement or bronchial wall thickening (see Fig. 5–17). In 10% of normal individuals, however, lung does not contact the bronchial wall because the descending pulmonary ar-

Text continued on page 95

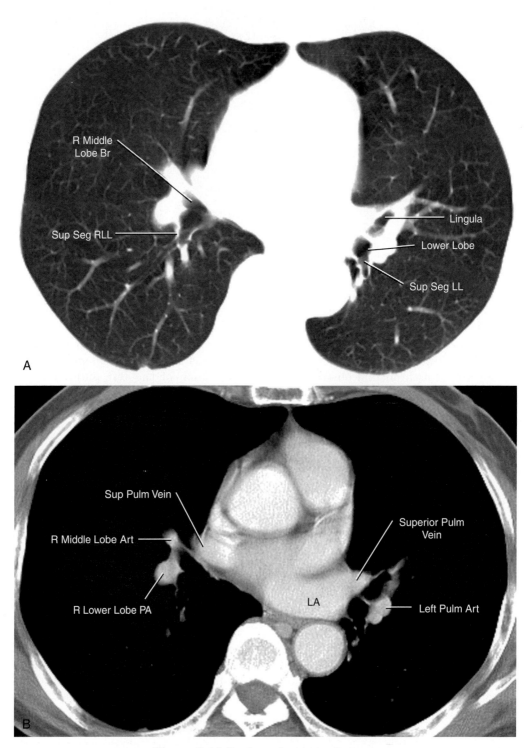

Figure 5–13 *See legend on opposite page*

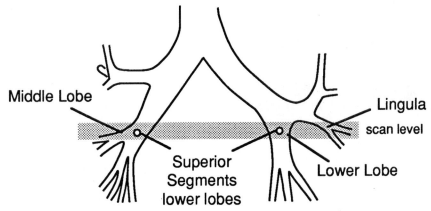

Figure 5–13. Normal right middle lobe and lingular level. *A and B,* Right hilum: The middle lobe bronchus arises anteriorly and extends anteriorly and laterally at an angle of about 45°. Because it is also angled caudad, only a short segment of its lumen is visible. The superior segmental bronchus of the lower lobe arises posterolaterally. The superior pulmonary veins lie anterior and medial to the bronchus, whereas the oval descending (interlobar) branch of the right pulmonary artery lies beside and behind it. The appearance of the right hilum at this level is quite similar to that of the left hilum at the levels of the left upper lobe and lingular bronchi. Left hilum: The lingular bronchus is visible slightly below the level of the upper lobe bronchus. The left lower lobe bronchus and the superior segment branch of the lower lobe is also seen at this level. The descending pulmonary artery appears oval and is located lateral to the bronchi. The appearances of the hila are roughly symmetric.

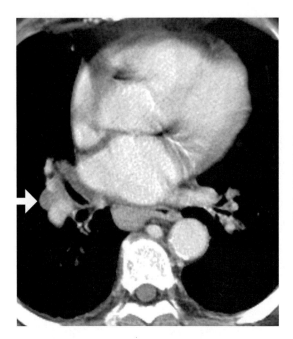

Figure 5–14. Lymphoma with right hilar adenopathy. Enlarged lymph nodes *(arrow)* are visible lateral to the descending right pulmonary artery and middle lobe bronchus. Lymph node enlargement is also visible in the azygoesophageal recess.

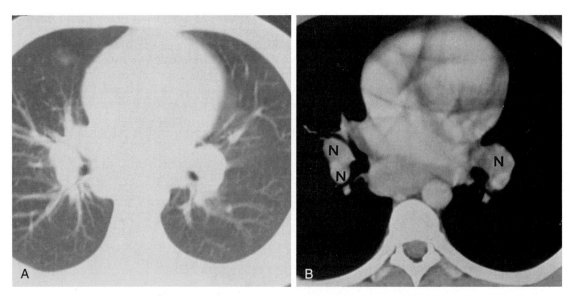

Figure 5–15. Abnormal right middle lobe bronchus level (adenopathy). *A and B,* There is lobulation of the right hilum and adenopathy is visible on mediastinal window scans. On the left, the hilum is enlarged relative to the bronchus and adenopathy is clearly visible on mediastinal windows anterior to the bronchus. N = node.

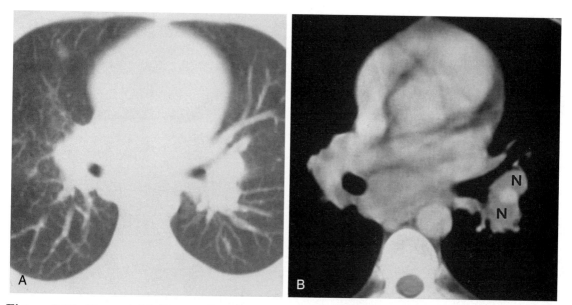

Figure 5–16. Abnormal left upper lobe and lingular bronchus level (adenopathy). *A and B,* On the left, there is lobulation of the hilum. With contrast medium infusion, the enlarged nodes (N) and the pulmonary artery can be distinguished. On the right, the posterior wall of the bronchus intermedius is thickened. Subcarinal lymph node enlargement is also visible.

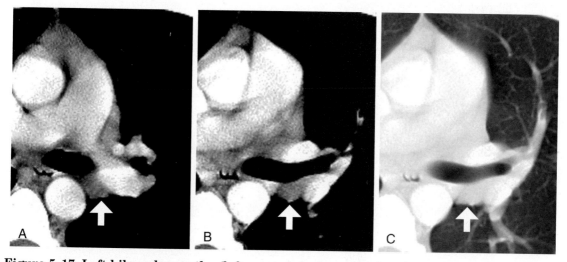

Figure 5–17. Left hilar adenopathy (left upper lobe bronchus level). *A,* Lymph node enlargement *(arrow)* is visible in the posterior hilum, behind the left upper lobe bronchus, and between the aorta and left pulmonary artery. *B and C,* The enlarged lymph node *(arrow)* lies posterior to the bronchus and prevents lung from outlining its posterior wall.

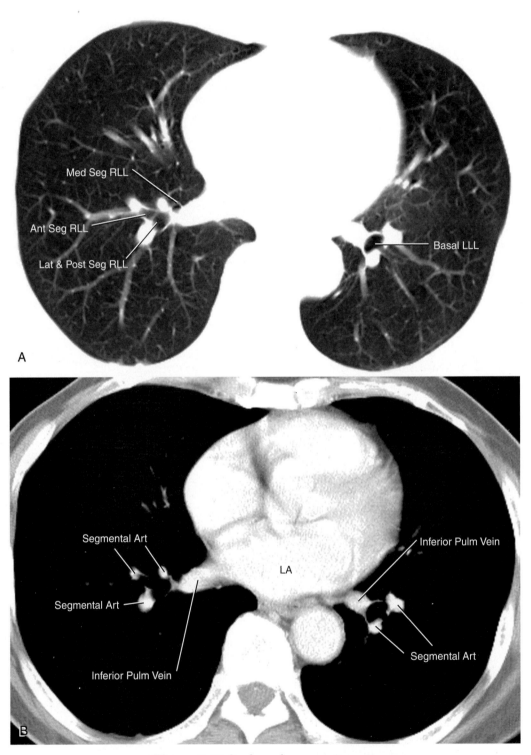

Figure 5–18 *See legend on opposite page*

tery is medially positioned against the aorta. This should not be misinterpreted as abnormal.

Lingular Bronchus. The lingular bronchus is usually visible at a level near the undersurface of the left upper lobe bronchus; its two segments (superior and inferior can sometimes be seen). The pulmonary artery and veins appear the same as at the level of the left upper lobe bronchus (see Fig. 5–13). At this level, significant lobulation of the lateral hilar contour indicates mass or adenopathy (see Fig. 5–16). As can the right upper lobe bronchus, the lingular bronchus can appear as the mirror image of the right middle lobe.

Lower Lobe Bronchi (Basal Segments)

Right and Left Hilum. At this level, the hila are relatively symmetric, and comparing one side to the other can be helpful.

The main lower lobe bronchial trunk on each side (Fig. 5–18), which eventually gives rise to the basal segmental bronchi, branches in a variable fashion. It is common for the lower lobe bronchial trunk on the right to divide into two basal bronchial branches or trunks, at a level above the origins of the basal segmental bronchi.

At the level of the lower lobe bronchial trunk, on either side, the anterior bronchial wall is usually outlined by lung, with pulmonary artery branches being lateral to the bronchus and veins being posterior and medial to the bronchus (see Fig. 5–18A and B). Enlarged lymph nodes can be identified anterior to the bronchus at this level.

The basal segmental branches of the lower lobe bronchi vary in appearance depending on their courses (see Fig. 5–18). On the right, the four segmental branches (medial, anterior, lateral, and posterior) are sometimes visible; on the left, there are three basal segments (anteromedial, lateral, and posterior). However, even on good quality scans it is not unusual for one or more segmental bronchi to be invisible with 1-cm collimation. With thin collimation, the segments are much better seen.

The segmental bronchi are accompanied by pulmonary artery branches that are somewhat larger than the bronchi (see Fig. 5–18). At this level, the inferior pulmonary veins pass behind and medial to the bronchi to enter the left atrium. Hilar masses or lymph node enlargement can be diagnosed on the basis of contour abnormalities or asymmetries between the hila. Soft tissue densities that seem too large to be the pulmonary artery or vein branches should

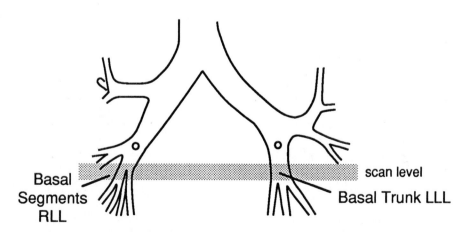

Basal Segments RLL

scan level

Basal Trunk LLL

Figure 5–18. Normal lower lobe bronchi (basal segments). *A and B,* On the right, anterior and medial segmental bronchi are visible, whereas a common trunk is yet to divide into the lateral and posterior branches. The basal segmental bronchi arise in a variable fashion. The inferior pulmonary veins are posterior and medial, and pulmonary artery branches accompany the bronchi. On the left, a single undivided basal lower lobe bronchial trunk is seen.

Illustration continued on following page

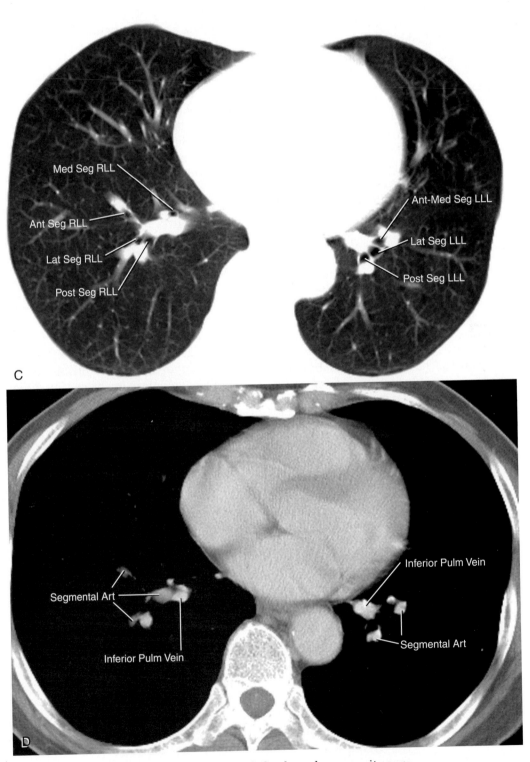

Med Seg RLL

Ant-Med Seg LLL

Ant Seg RLL

Lat Seg LLL

Lat Seg RLL

Post Seg LLL

Post Seg RLL

C

Inferior Pulm Vein

Segmental Art

Inferior Pulm Vein

Segmental Art

D

Figure 5–18 *Continued. See legend on opposite page*

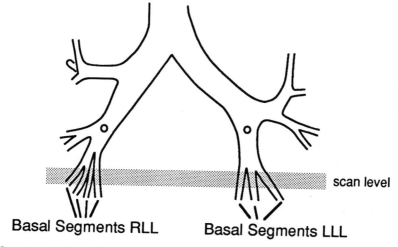

Figure 5–18 *Continued. C and D,* At a level 7 mm below *A* and *B,* the four basal segmental branches of the right lower lobe, the three segmental branches of the left lower lobe, and their associated vessels are all visible.

be regarded with suspicion (Figs. 5–19 through 5–21).

BRONCHIAL ABNORMALITIES

The excellent contrast and spatial resolution of CT allow for good assessment of bronchial lesions, and CT is often performed to guide bronchoscopy in patients who have a suspected hilar or bronchial abnormality. Accurate indicators of bronchial pathology are bronchial wall thickening, an endobronchial mass, and narrowing of the bronchial lumen.

Bronchial wall thickening is most easily assessed on CT in regions where the hilar bronchi lie adjacent to lung: the posterior walls of the right main and both upper lobe bronchi and the posterior wall of the bronchus intermedius. Smooth bronchial wall thickening can be due to inflammation or tumor infiltration (Fig. 5–22; see also Fig. 5–7), whereas a localized or lobulated thickening usually indicates tumor or lymph node enlargement (see Fig. 5–17).

Bronchial narrowing and endobronchial lesions that may be extremely difficult to detect on plain radiographs can be reliably diagnosed on CT (Fig. 5–23). However, it may be difficult to distinguish endobronchial tumor from compression by an exobronchial mass (see Fig. 5–7). Abrupt changes in bronchial caliber on CT usually indicate circumferential tumor infiltration or an endobronchial mass (Fig. 5–24); but it is important to look at adjacent scans to confirm that the apparent bronchial narrowing does not reflect an oblique bronchial course, with the bronchus leaving the plane of scan (as with the right middle lobe bronchus).

In general, scans viewed with a lung window setting are best for identifying normal bronchi and detecting bronchial abnormalities but often overestimate the degree of bronchial narrowing when it is present. Thus, a narrowed but patent bronchus may appear obstructed with this window setting, when 10-mm collimation is used. Also, a normal bronchus, slightly out of the plane of scan, and being volume averaged with adjacent soft tissue, can appear narrowed on lung window scans. Tissue window settings more accurately assess bronchial lumen diameter in the presence of an abnormality but somewhat overestimate luminal

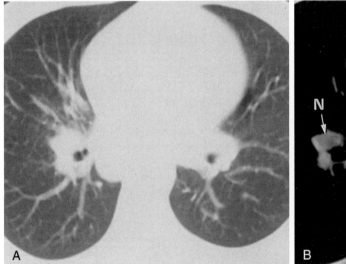
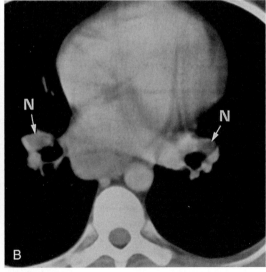

Figure 5–19. Abnormal lower lobe bronchi level (adenopathy). *A and B,* The hila are enlarged bilaterally, and nodes (N) are visible at mediastinal window settings as illustrated at higher levels in this patient with sarcoidosis.

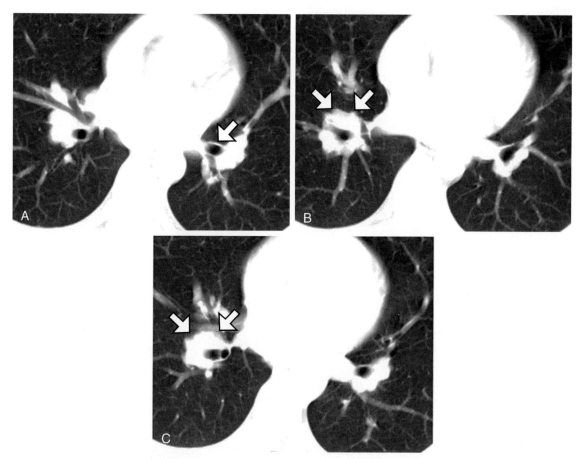

Figure 5–20. Right hilar adenopathy, lower lobe bronchi and basal segments. *A,* Lobulation of the right hilum at the level of the right middle lobe bronchus indicates lymph node enlargement. Note that lung contacts the anterior wall of the left lower lobe bronchial trunk *(arrow),* with arteries and veins being lateral, posterior, and medial to the bronchus. This appearance is normal. *B,* The right lower lobe bronchial trunk has divided into two branches. Soft tissue anterior to these branches represents lymph node enlargement *(arrows).* On the left, the lower lobe bronchial trunk remains outlined by lung anteriorly. *C,* At the level of the basal segments, the right and left sides appear asymmetric. The right bronchial segments are surrounded by soft tissue. Nodes *(arrows)* are anterior to the bronchi.

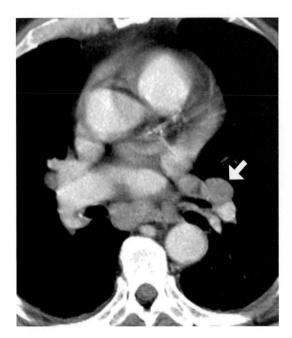

Figure 5–21. Left hilar adenopathy, lower lobe bronchial trunk. In a patient with lymphoma, an enlarged lymph node *(arrow)* is visible anterior to the left lower lobe bronchial trunk.

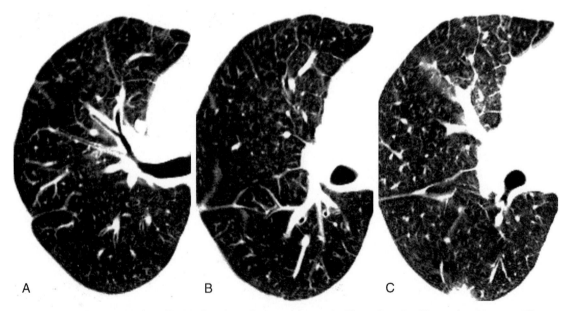

Figure 5–22. Bronchial wall thickening due to tumor infiltration by Kaposi sarcoma. There is thickening of the posterior wall of the right upper lobe bronchus *(A)* and bronchus intermedius *(B and C)*. Interlobular septal thickening is visible in the right lung, as is typical of lymphangitic spread of carcinoma.

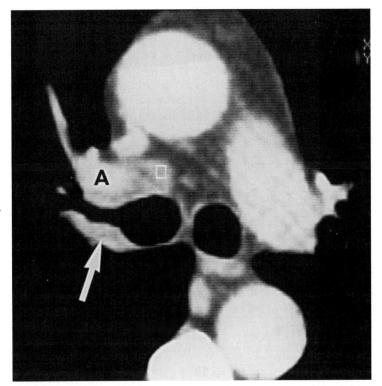

Figure 5–23. Bronchogenic carcinoma, right upper lobe bronchus. There is irregular thickening *(arrow)* of the posterior wall of the right upper lobe bronchus, with narrowing of its lumen, as a result of a carcinoma arising from its posterior wall. The truncus anterior (A) is opacified, as are pulmonary veins.

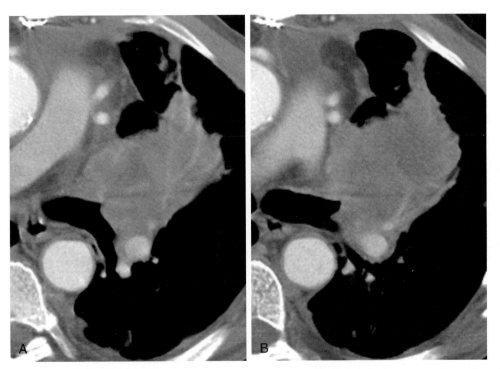

Figure 5–24. Bronchogenic carcinoma, with left upper lobe bronchus obstruction. *A and B,* There is abrupt termination of the left upper lobe bronchus, associated with distal collapse and consolidation of the left upper lobe. This appearance strongly suggests bronchogenic carcinoma.

size. If a bronchial lesion is suspected, both window settings should be used. Thin-collimation scans or high-resolution CT, particularly with spiral acquisition, can be of great value in identifying bronchial abnormalities.

Bronchial abnormalities that are primarily mucosal can be missed using CT because of their small size or minimal thickness. Also, volume averaging at the upper or lower edges of a bronchus can mimic the presence of bronchial obstruction. It is always a good idea to obtain additional views (preferably with thin collimation) of a questionable bronchial lesion before making a definite diagnosis. With spiral CT, scans can be reconstructed at intervals of a few millimeters to optimize visibility of bronchial lesions or confirm that a bronchus is normal.

DIFFERENTIAL DIAGNOSIS OF HILAR AND BRONCHIAL ABNORMALITIES

Lung Cancer

The most common cause of hilar mass or lymph node enlargement is bronchogenic carcinoma. The hilar mass can appear irregular because of local infiltration of the lung parenchyma. In patients with tumors arising centrally (usually squamous cell carcinoma or small cell carcinoma), bronchial abnormalities (narrowing, obstruction) visible on CT are common. In such patients, an endobronchial lesion is commonly visible at bronchoscopy, correlating with the CT abnormality. If the bronchial abnormality involves the carina, resection may be impossible (Fig. 5–25); bronchoscopy rather than CT, however, is most accurate for making this determination.

When the carcinoma arises within the peripheral lung, and the hila are abnormal because of node metastases, the hilar mass or masses may be smoother and more sharply defined than when the hilar mass represents the primary tumor. However, this distinction is not always easily made. Patients with a central mass and bronchial obstruction often show peripheral parenchy-

mal abnormalities. In patients with hilar node metastases, a bronchial abnormality seen at CT usually reflects external compression by the enlarged hilar nodes, but bronchial invasion also may be present. Hilar node metastases are present at surgery in 15% to 40% of patients with lung cancer.

In patients with bronchogenic carcinoma, enlarged hilar nodes visible on CT may not be due to node metastasis. Hyperplastic nodal enlargement often occurs in lung cancer patients, particularly when there is bronchial obstruction and distal pneumonia or atelectasis is present. Conversely, a normal-sized hilar node can harbor microscopic metastases. In the lung cancer staging system, ipsilateral hilar lymph node metastases are termed *N1*.

Other Primary Bronchial Tumors

Other primary bronchial tumors can produce a hilar mass. The most common of these is carcinoid tumor. This malignant tumor arises from the main, lobar, or segmental bronchi in 80% of cases. It tends to be slow growing and locally invasive. A well-defined endobronchial mass is typical, but a large exobronchial, hilar mass is sometimes seen as well. Adenoid cystic carcinoma (cylindroma) can result in a similar appearance. Carcinoid tumors are very vascular and can enhance somewhat after contrast medium infusion. Carcinoid tumors occasionally calcify.

Benign bronchial tumors, such as fibroma, chondroma, or lipoma, usually appear focal and endobronchial on CT, rather than infiltrative and do not commonly produce an exobronchial mass. Obstruction is the primary finding on CT. These tumors are relatively rare.

Lymphoma

Hilar adenopathy is present in 25% of patients with Hodgkin's lymphoma and 10% of patients with non-Hodgkin's lymphoma. Hilar involvement is usually asymmetric. Multiple nodes in the hilum or mediastinum are usually involved. Endobronchial lesions can also be seen, or bronchi may be compressed by enlarged nodes, but this is much less common than with lung cancer. There

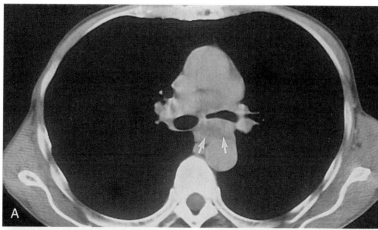

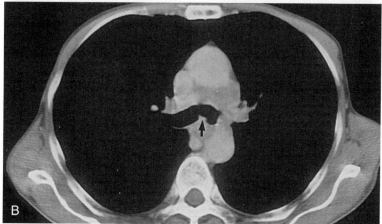

Figure 5–25. Bronchogenic carcinoma, left main bronchus. *A,* Infiltrating tumor is narrowing the left main bronchus and producing a significant mass posterior to the bronchus *(arrows).* This appearance is typical of bronchogenic carcinoma. *B,* At 1 cm cephalad there is thickening of the posterior carina *(arrow),* suggesting infiltration by tumor. This was confirmed at bronchoscopy, making this tumor unresectable.

are no specific features of the hilar abnormality seen in patients with lymphoma that allow a definite diagnosis.

Metastases

Metastases to hilar lymph nodes from an extrathoracic primary tumor are not uncommon. Hilar node metastases may be unilateral or bilateral. Endobronchial metastases can also be seen (Fig. 5–26), without there being hilar node metastases; these may appear to be focal and endobronchial or infiltrative. Head and neck carcinomas, thyroid carcinoma, genitourinary tumors (particularly renal cell and testicular carcinoma), melanoma, and breast carcinomas are most commonly responsible for hilar or endobronchial metastases.

Inflammatory Disease

Unilateral or bilateral hilar lymphadenopathy, and bronchial narrowing, can be seen

in a number of infectious or inflammatory conditions. Primary tuberculosis usually causes unilateral hilar adenopathy. Fungal infections, most notably histoplasmosis and coccidioidomycosis, cause unilateral or bilateral adenopathy. Sarcoidosis causes bilateral and symmetric adenopathy in most patients (see Fig. 5–11).

In patients with prior tuberculosis or histoplasmosis, calcified hilar nodes are commonly seen (see Fig. 5–10). Calcified nodes can erode into a bronchus causing obstruction, so-called broncholithiasis. Because of its ability to diagnose bronchial lesions, and detect calcification, CT can be very helpful in diagnosing this entity.

Mucus

Blobs of mucus may simulate one or more endobronchial lesions on CT; if this diagnosis is suggested, for instance, if you see a focal bronchial lesion when you do not ex-

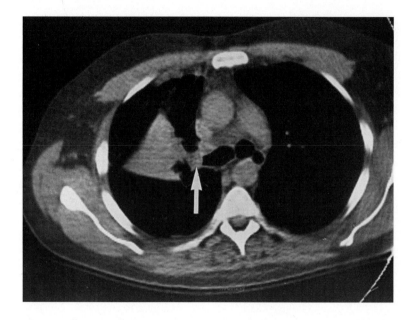

Figure 5–26. Endobronchial metastasis. In a patient with thyroid carcinoma, an endobronchial metastasis appears as a focal endobronchial mass *(arrow)* obstructing the right upper lobe bronchus. Right upper lobe consolidation is associated. (From Webb WR. Computed tomography of the thorax. Radiol Clin N Am 1983; 21:723–739.)

pect one, a repeat scan can be obtained after having the patient cough. The abnormality will disappear. Large mucus plugs can also mimic hilar masses or be seen as a bronchial abnormality on CT.

PULMONARY VASCULAR DISEASE

CT is also useful in differentiating pulmonary vascular disease from hilar adenopathy. Pulmonary hypertension with dilatation of the pulmonary arteries is relatively common and can simulate a hilar mass on plain radiographs (Fig. 5–27). CT can accurately define the size of the pulmonary arteries in patients with arterial dilatation. Rarely, in patients with chronic pulmonary hypertension, pulmonary artery calcification can be seen as a result of atherosclerosis.

Encasement or compression of one of the main pulmonary arteries by tumor in patients with a bronchogenic carcinoma can be diagnosed with CT and can be of value in assessing the extent of surgery that will be required for resection. For example, tu-

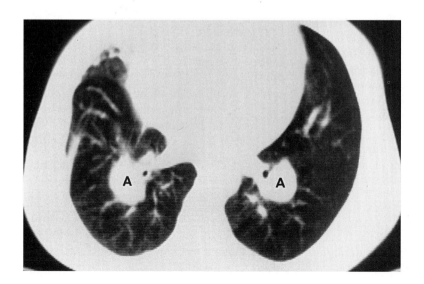

Figure 5–27. Pulmonary artery enlargement. Severe pulmonary hypertension has resulted in enlargement of the descending pulmonary arteries (A). The hila are smoothly enlarged, without lobulation, and the arteries maintain their normal oval shapes. There is some consolidation in the anterior right lung.

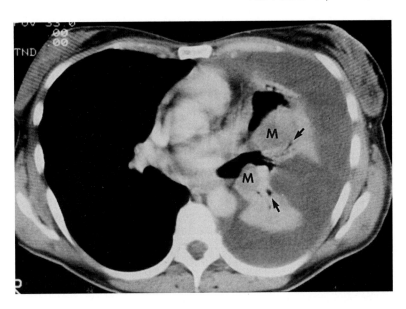

Figure 5–28. Hilar mass with atelectasis. In a patient with left hilar bronchogenic carcinoma, associated with collapse and pleural effusion, the hilar mass can be distinguished from collapsed lung after contrast medium infusion. The mass (M) appears less dense than opacified lung. Air-filled bronchi *(arrows)* delineate consolidated lung. There is also a large pleural effusion.

mor surrounding the left pulmonary artery generally indicates that pneumonectomy rather than lobectomy will be required. However, one must be cautious; narrowing of the pulmonary artery can reflect compression rather than encasement. Adequate assessment requires the use of a bolus of intravenous contrast medium.

Other than pulmonary artery dilatation because of pulmonary hypertension, or pulmonary artery involvement by tumor, pulmonary artery abnormalities are uncommon. Pulmonary artery aneurysms are rarely seen. Pulmonary artery sarcoma is a rare neoplasm resulting in an intravascular mass, which usually results in dilatation of the artery.

The CT diagnosis of pulmonary embolism is discussed in Chapter 3.

MASS VERSUS ATELECTASIS

In patients with a hilar mass and bronchial obstruction, collapse or consolidation of distal lung can obscure the margins of the mass, making it difficult to diagnose. On plain radiographs, the mass can sometimes be detected because of alterations in the shape of the collapsed or consolidated lobe or lobes (i.e., Golden's S sign). Similarly, alterations in the shape of a collapsed lobe can be seen on CT in the presence of a mass.

Also, in some patients, if a bolus of contrast medium is injected, and particularly if dynamic CT is performed, the collapsed lobe can be seen to enhance to a greater degree than the mass (Fig. 5–28). Of additional value in distinguishing mass and lung consolidation are air-filled bronchi as seen on CT. These obviously indicate the presence of lung consolidation. In some patients, in the presence of total obstruction and complete lung collapse, low attenuation, fluid-filled bronchi can be seen within the lung; these are termed *mucus-bronchograms.*

Suggested Reading

Glazer GM, Francis IR, Gebarski K, et al. Dynamic incremental computed tomography in evaluation of the pulmonary hila. J Comput Assist Tomogr 1983; 7:59–64.

Glazer GM, Francis IR, Shirazi KK, et al. Evaluation of the pulmonary hilum: comparison of conventional radiography, 55 degrees posterior oblique tomography, and dynamic computed tomography. J Comput Assist Tomogr 1983; 7:983–989.

Glazer GM, Gross BH, Aisen AM, et al. Imaging of the pulmonary hilum: a prospective comparative study in patients with lung cancer. AJR 1985; 145:245–248.

Im J-G, Song KS, Kang HS, et al. Mediastinal tuberculous lymphadenitis: CT manifestations. Radiology 1987; 164:115–119.

Libshitz HI, McKenna RJ, Mountain CF. Patterns of mediastinal metastases in bronchogenic carcinoma. Chest 1986; 90:229–232.

Müller NL, Webb WR. Radiographic imaging of the pulmonary hila. Invest Radiol 1985; 20:661–671.

Naidich DP, Khouri NF, Scott WJ, et al. Computed tomography of the pulmonary hila: I. Normal anatomy. J Comput Assist Tomogr 1981; 5:459–467.

Naidich DP, Khouri NF, Stitik FP, et al. Computed tomography of the pulmonary hila: II. Abnormal anatomy. J Comput Assist Tomogr 1981; 5:468–475.

Naidich DP, Tarras M, Garay SM, et al. Kaposi sarcoma: CT-radiographic correlation. Chest 1989; 96:723–728.

Park CK, Webb WR, Klein JS. Inferior hilar window. Radiology 1991; 178:163–168.

Webb WR, Gamsu G, Glazer G. Computed tomography of the abnormal pulmonary hilum. J Comput Assist Tomogr 1981; 5:485–490.

Webb WR, Gamsu G, Speckman JM: Computed tomography of the pulmonary hilum in patients with bronchogenic carcinoma. J Comput Assist Tomogr 1983; 7:219–225.

Webb WR, Glazer G, Gamsu G. Computed tomography of the normal pulmonary hilum. J Comput Assist Tomogr 1981; 5:476–484.

Webb WR, Hirji M, Gamsu G. Posterior wall of the bronchus intermedius: radiographic-CT correlation. AJR 1984; 142:907–911.

6

Lung Disease

W. Richard Webb, M.D.

On CT, normal lung varies in appearance depending on the window settings used. With window settings of $-700/1000$ to 1500 H, the lungs appear dark, but not as black as the air visible in the trachea or bronchi. This slight difference in attenuation between lung parenchyma and air should be sought in choosing an appropriate window setting. If the lungs are viewed with too high a window mean, soft tissue structures in the lung (vessels, bronchi, or lung nodules) are difficult to see or underestimated as to their size and also any areas of lucency, such as bullae, may be missed. The lungs, after all, are not simply bags of air, and they should not appear to be. If too low a window mean is used, the size of soft tissue structures in the lung will be overestimated.

NORMAL ANATOMY

Intrapulmonary Fissures and Lobar Anatomy

Major Fissures

Because they are thin and oblique relative to the plane of the scan, the normal major fissures are not usually visible on CT obtained with 7- to 10-mm collimation. However, the position of each major fissure can be inferred from the location of the relatively avascular region of lung 2 to 3 cm

thick (representing the lung on each side of the fissure), which contains no large vessels (Fig. 6–1). Sometimes, an ill-defined band of density is seen in the middle of the avascular area; this band represents volume averaging of the fissure with adjacent lung. In 10% to 20% of patients, the major fissures are visible as a thin line, although low window levels and narrow window widths may be required to see them. On thin-collimation scans or high-resolution CT (HRCT), the major fissures are almost always recognizable as thin white lines.

Within the lower thorax, the major fissures angle anterolaterally from the mediastinum, contacting the anterior third of the hemidiaphragms. They separate the lower lobes posteriorly from the upper lobe on the left and the middle and upper lobes on the right. In the upper thorax, the major fissures angle posterolaterally. Above the aortic arch, they contact the posterior chest wall and terminate.

Minor Fissure

The minor fissure is usually hard to see because it parallels the plane of scan. However, its approximate position can be determined by noting an avascular region in the anterior right lung, corresponding to lung on each side of the fissure (see Fig. 6–1C). This avascular plane is visible on CT in most patients. In some patients, the minor fissure mimics the appearance of the major fissure but is seen anterior to it. On HRCT,

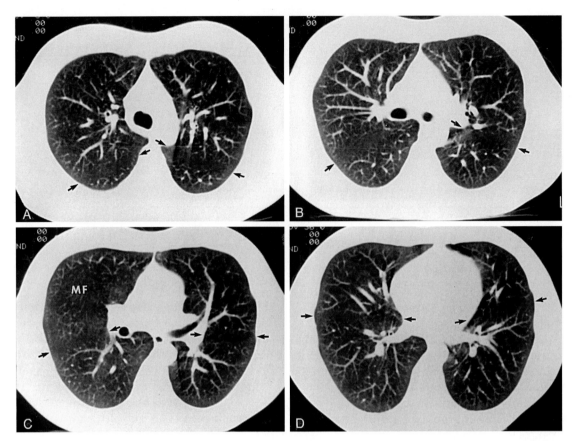

Figure 6–1. Normal fissures. *A,* At the level of the aortic arch, an avascular band *(arrows)* within the posterior lungs marks the locations of the major fissures. They angle posterolaterally. *B,* Several centimeters lower, the major fissures *(arrows)* are more anteriorly positioned. The upper lobes are anterior to the fissures. *C,* The major fissures *(arrows)* remain visible. The location of the minor fissure is indicated by the rounded region (MF), which contains no large vessels. *D,* Near the diaphragm, the major fissures angle anterolaterally *(arrows)*. The middle lobe is located anterior to the right major fissure.

the minor fissure can often be seen as a white line of varying sharpness and thickness, depending on its orientation.

Because the minor fissure often angles caudad, the lower lobe, middle lobe, and upper lobe may all be seen on a single scan (Fig. 6–2). If the minor fissure is concave caudad, it can sometimes be seen in two locations or can appear ring shaped (see Fig. 6–2), with the middle lobe between the fissure lines or in the center of the ring and the upper lobe anterior to the most anterior part of the fissure.

Accessory Fissures

In patients with an azygos lobe, the four layers of the *mesoazygos,* or azygos fissure, are invariably visible above the level of the

intrapulmonary azygos vein. The azygos fissure is C shaped and convex laterally, beginning anteriorly at the right brachiocephalic vein and ending posteriorly at the right anterolateral surface of the vertebral body (see Fig. 6–8; see also Fig. 3–11). Other accessory fissures, most commonly the inferior accessory fissure, are occasionally seen on CT. They are not generally of diagnostic significance.

CONGENITAL LESIONS

Pulmonary Agenesis and Aplasia

Pulmonary agenesis consists of complete absence of lung, bronchi, and vascular supply.

With *pulmonary aplasia*, a rudimentary bronchus is present, ending in a blind pouch, but lung parenchyma and pulmonary vessels are absent (Fig. 6–3).

BRONCHIAL ANOMALIES

Tracheal Bronchus

Tracheal bronchus represents the origin of all or part (usually the apical segment) of the right upper lobe bronchus from the trachea (Fig. 6–4); its incidence may be as high as 1%. The left tracheal bronchus is much less common. Tracheal bronchus is common in cloven-hoofed animals such as the pig, sheep, goat, camel, and giraffe; it may be associated with recurrent infection.

Bronchial Isomerism

Bronchial isomerism refers to bilateral symmetry of the bronchi. It may be isolated or associated with a variety of anomalies.

Bronchial Atresia

Bronchial atresia is characterized by local narrowing or obliteration of a lobar, segmental, or subsegmental bronchus. It is most common in the left upper lobe, followed by the right upper and right middle lobes. Mucus commonly accumulates in dilated bronchi distal to the obstruction, resulting in a tubular, branching, or ovoid mucus plug. Air trapping in the lobe or segment distal to the obstruction occurs because of collateral ventilation. Obstructed distal lung can appear hyperlucent and hypovascular.

BRONCHOGENIC CYST

The appearance of mediastinal bronchogenic cyst has been described. Pulmonary bronchogenic cysts are typically well defined, round or oval, and of fluid or soft tissue attenuation; previously infected cysts can contain air or an air–fluid level. When a cyst contains air, its wall appears very thin, although consolidation of surrounding lung may be present.

ARTERIOVENOUS FISTULA

Pulmonary arteriovenous fistulas can be single (65%) or multiple (35%) and are often

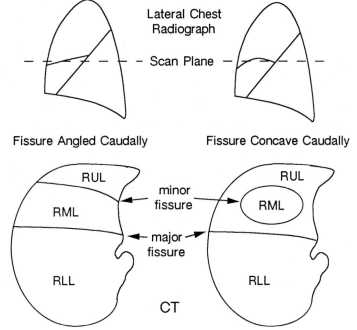

Figure 6–2. Possible appearances of minor fissure. Depending on the orientation of the minor fissure, its appearance and the relationships of the lobes of the right lung can vary. If the minor fissure angles downward, both the middle and upper lobes can be seen on a single scan. If the minor fissure is concave caudad, it may appear ring shaped. RLL = right lower lobe; RML = right middle lobe; RUL = right upper lobe.

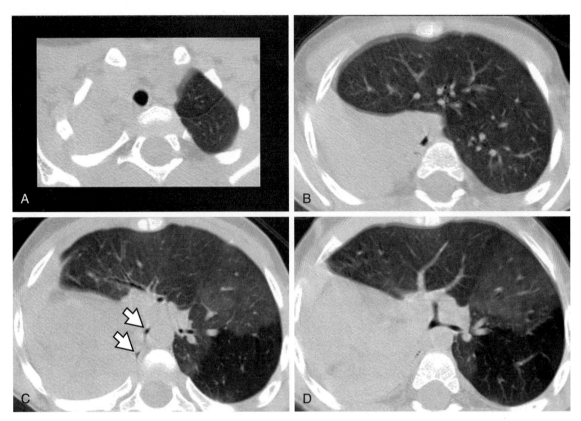

Figure 6–3. Pulmonary aplasia in a child. *A through D,* The right lung is completely absent with mediastinal shift to the right and herniation of the left lung across the midline. The presence of rudimentary bronchi on the right *(arrows, C)* indicates that this represents aplasia rather than agenesis.

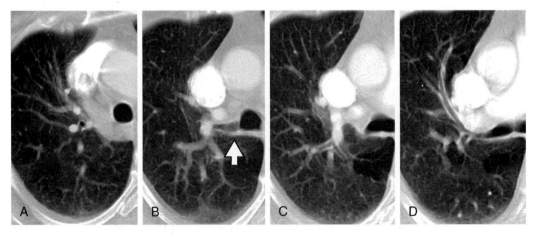

Figure 6–4. Tracheal bronchus. Four images *(A through D)* at contiguous levels in a patient with tracheal bronchus. The tracheal bronchus *(arrow, B)* arises from the lateral tracheal wall *(B)* above the level of the right upper lobe bronchus *(D)*. The tracheal bronchus supplies the apical segment of the right upper lobe. Note that the azygos arch is visible above the tracheal bronchus.

associated with Osler-Weber-Rendu syndrome (65%). On CT, an arteriovenous fistula can appear as (1) a single dilated vascular sac, visible as a smooth, sharply defined, round or oval nodule (most common) or (2) a tangle of dilated tortuous vessels seen as a lobulated or serpiginous mass. In each type, the feeding pulmonary artery branch and draining pulmonary vein are dilated and should be easily seen on CT (Fig. 6–5).

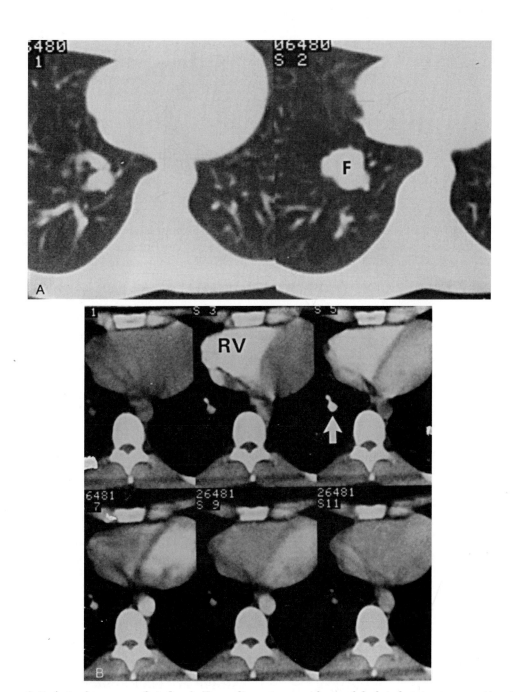

Figure 6–5. Arteriovenous fistula. *A,* Two adjacent scans show a lobulated mass representing the fistula (F) and its large feeding vessels. *B,* After contrast medium injection, the fistula and its feeding vessels opacify rapidly *(arrow),* at the same time as the right ventricle (RV), and the contrast medium then washes out rapidly. (From Godwin JD, Webb WR. Dynamic computed tomography in the evaluation of vascular lung lesions. Radiology 1981; 138:629–635.)

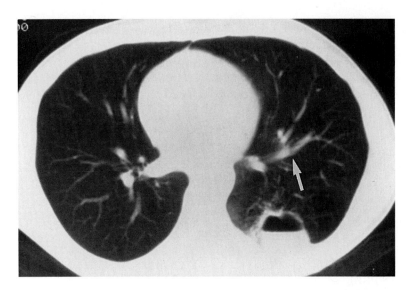

Figure 6–6. Sequestration. An intralobar sequestration presents with an air- and fluid-filled cyst in the left lower lobe. A bronchogenic cyst would have a similar appearance. Note that pulmonary vessels and bronchi *(arrow)* are displaced anteriorly by the sequestration.

In most cases, the fistula will be subpleural. These findings should be sufficient to make a specific diagnosis on scans without contrast medium infusion. Spiral CT without contrast medium infusion is at least as accurate as angiography in detecting arteriovenous fistulas and in showing their vascular architecture.

Although contrast medium is not usually needed for diagnosis, an arteriovenous fistula shows rapid and dense opacification after bolus contrast medium injection, followed by rapid washout of the contrast medium (see Fig. 6–5). As would be expected, opacification occurs at the same time or just after opacification of the right ventricle. Solid tumors can opacify after contrast medium injection, but rapid and dense opacification and washout of contrast medium, typical of an arteriovenous fistula, is not seen with tumors.

SEQUESTRATION

Pulmonary sequestrations can appear cystic or solid on CT. From 70% to 90% are located posteromedially on the left; all have anomalous systemic arterial supply from the thoracic or abdominal aorta. There is no bronchial or pulmonary artery supply to the lesion. In some cases of sequestration, the feeding systemic artery is visible on contrast medium–enhanced CT. Demonstration of this is optimal using spiral CT.

Intralobar Sequestration

Intralobar sequestration is usually diagnosed in adults, and recurrent or chronic infection is common. Venous drainage is usually by means of the pulmonary veins. Intralobar sequestration typically contains air but can be quite variable in appearance. On CT, intralobar sequestration can appear as

1. A region of hyperlucent lung
2. A cystic or multicystic structure (sometimes with air–fluid levels) (Fig. 6–6)
3. Consolidated and collapsed lung
4. A combination of these findings

Areas of lucent lung in association with, or representing part of, an intralobar sequestration are common; these areas are usually due to air trapping. Normal bronchi are not seen in the sequestration; and if the sequestration is aerated, the vascular branching pattern within it may appear abnormal.

Extralobar Sequestration

Extralobar sequestration is usually diagnosed in infants or children, and infection is rare. It almost always appears as a solid mass and rarely contains air. Venous drainage is usually through systemic veins.

HYPOGENETIC LUNG (SCIMITAR) SYNDROME

This rare anomaly, almost always occurring on the right side, is characterized by four features that coexist to varying degrees:

1. Hypoplasia of the lung with abnormal segmental or lobar anatomy
2. Hypoplasia of the ipsilateral pulmonary artery
3. Anomalous pulmonary venous return (the *scimitar vein*) from the right upper lobe or the entire right lung, usually to the vena cava or right atrium
4. Anomalous systemic arterial supply to a portion of the hypoplastic lung, usually the lower lobe

On CT, the hypoplastic lung is recognizable because of dextroposition of the heart and mediastinal shift to the right (Fig. 6–7). The hypoplastic lung may also show abnormal bronchial anatomy, deficient bronchial divisions, or mirror image bronchial or pulmonary artery branching. When the anomalous (scimitar) vein is present, it is clearly visible on CT. Hypoplasia of the pulmonary artery is usually recognizable by the decreased size of vessels in the hypoplastic lung. This entity may be associated with congenital heart disease.

PULMONARY VEIN ANOMALIES AND VEIN VARIX

Anomalous Pulmonary Venous Return

Anomalous pulmonary veins commonly drain into the superior vena cava on the right or an anomalous vertical vein on the left (Fig. 6–8). These can be seen as an isolated anomaly or in association with congenital heart disease.

Pulmonary Vein Varix

A dilated central pulmonary vein, or vein varix, can be congenital or result from elevated left atrial pressure (often with mitral stenosis). It is most common on the right side, corresponding to the inferior pulmonary vein branch in most cases. The dilated segment of vein opacifies after contrast medium infusion. In some cases, a vein varix may be associated with anomalous pulmonary venous return.

FOCAL LUNG LESIONS AND THE SOLITARY PULMONARY NODULE

CT is often used to evaluate focal lung lesions or solitary nodules detected on chest radiographs. It is of value in (1) confirming the presence of a parenchymal lesion, (2) determining its morphology, (3) detecting

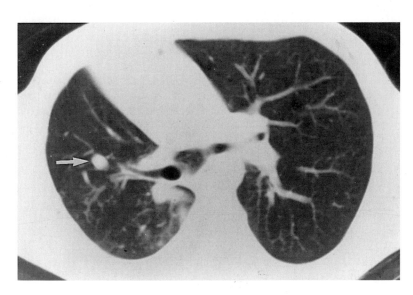

Figure 6–7. Hypogenetic lung syndrome. The right lung is reduced in volume, and the mediastinum is shifted toward the right. The scimitar vein *(arrow)* is visible within the right lung.

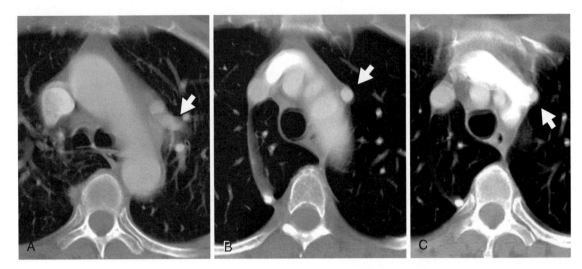

Figure 6–8. Anomalous pulmonary vein drainage. A pulmonary vein branch *(arrow, A)* enters the left mediastinum, draining through an anomalous left vertical vein *(arrow, B),* which drains *(arrow, C)* into the left brachiocephalic vein. An azygos lobe is also present.

the presence of calcium or fat, (4) determining if the lesion opacifies after contrast medium infusion, and (5) planning biopsy.

Morphology of Some Focal Lesions and Lung Nodules

HRCT scans are valuable in defining the morphology of focal pulmonary parenchymal lesions. If spiral CT is available, scanning through the entire nodule with 1-mm collimation (HRCT) and a pitch of 1 is recommended. With a conventional scanner, several contiguous HRCT scans through a lung nodule or mass should be obtained. Lung cancers and several other focal lesions can have characteristic appearances on CT.

Lung Cancer

A definite diagnosis of lung cancer cannot be made on CT. However, HRCT findings that strongly suggest malignancy in a patient with a solitary nodule include

1. An irregular or spiculated edge, usually due to fibrosis surrounding the tumor

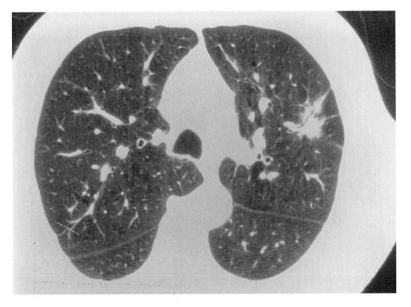

Figure 6–9. Spiculated carcinoma. High-resolution CT in a patient with an upper lobe nodule shows a spiculated mass, very suggestive of carcinoma. Note that the nodule contains an air bronchogram. An adenocarcinoma was found at surgery. Note the sharp definition of the major fissures with high-resolution CT. (From Webb WR. Radiologic evaluation of the solitary pulmonary nodule. AJR 1990; 154:701–708, with permission.)

(90% of nodules with a spiculated edge are malignant) (Fig. 6–9)

2. A lobulated contour (Fig. 6–10)

3. Air-bronchograms (see Fig. 6–9), cystic or "bubbly" air-containing regions within the nodule (seen in 65% of cancers but only 5% of benign lesions)

4. Cavitation (see Fig. 6–10), with a nodular cavity wall or a wall exceeding 15 mm in greatest thickness (90% are cancers)

5. A diameter exceeding 2 cm (95% are cancers)

A spiculated edge and the presence of air-bronchograms or cystic regions are particularly common with adenocarcinomas and bronchioloalveolar carcinoma. Lobulation also suggests the diagnosis of carcinoma but may be seen with other lesions as well, particularly hamartomas.

Both primary lung carcinomas and metastases can cavitate. Typically, a cavitary carcinoma has a thick, irregular, and nodular wall (see Fig. 6–10), but some metastatic tumors, particularly those of squamous cell origin, can be relatively thin walled. A cavitary nodule with a thin wall (<5 mm) is likely (90%) benign.

Hamartoma

HRCT can be valuable in diagnosing pulmonary hamartomas. Using CT with thin colli-mation, about two thirds of hamartomas can be correctly diagnosed because of visible fat (60%), either focal or diffuse (Fig. 6–11), fat and calcification (30%) (Fig. 6–12), or diffuse calcification (10%). Usually fat is easily seen on the scans; CT numbers range between −40 and −120 H.

Rounded Atelectasis

Rounded atelectasis represents focal, collapsed, and often folded lung. It almost always occurs in association with pleural thickening or effusion.

Rounded atelectasis is most common in the posterior, paravertebral regions and may be bilateral in patients with bilateral pleural disease. Areas of rounded atelectasis are usually several centimeters in diameter. Bending or bowing of adjacent bronchi and arteries toward the edge of the area of round atelectasis, because of volume loss or folding of lung, is characteristic (Fig. 6–13) and has been likened to a "comet tail." Air-bronchograms can sometimes be seen within the mass. Rounded atelectasis opacifies densely after contrast medium infusion.

Four findings must be present to make a confident diagnosis of rounded atelectasis on CT; if these are present, follow-up is usually sufficient (see Fig. 6–13). If one of these findings is lacking, you should be cautious

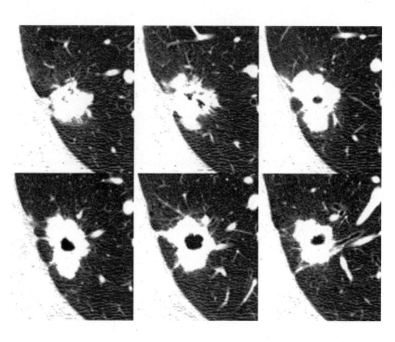

Figure 6–10. Spiculated carcinoma with an irregular cavity. Six scans through a nodule were obtained with spiral technique and 1-mm collimation. The nodule has a lobulated and spiculated margin and contains a thick-walled cavity.

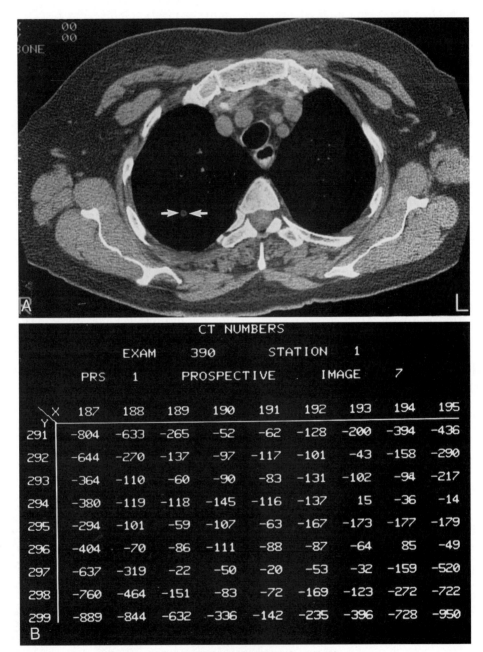

Figure 6–11. Hamartoma with fat density. *A,* High-resolution CT with mediastinal window settings in a patient with a small lung nodule detected on plain films. The nodule *(arrows)* is difficult to see and appears similar in density to subcutaneous fat. *B,* CT numbers are mostly between -40 and -120 H. (From Webb WR. Radiologic evaluation of the solitary pulmonary nodule. AJR 1990; 154:701–708, with permission.)

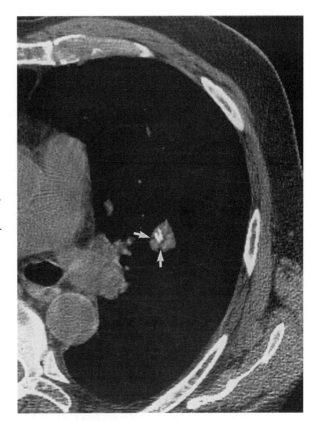

Figure 6–12. Hamartoma with fat and calcium. High-resolution CT shows dense calcification and areas of low density *(arrows)* representing fat.

in making the diagnosis, and biopsy is probably warranted. These four findings are

1. Ipsilateral pleural thickening or effusion
2. Significant contact between the lung lesion and the pleural surface
3. The "comet tail" sign
4. Volume loss in the lobe in which the opacity is seen

Rounded atelectasis is commonly associated with asbestos-related pleural thickening, occurring adjacent to regions of thickened pleura; but often it has an atypical appearance. Areas of atelectasis or focal fibrosis in asbestos-exposed patients can be very irregular, may not have extensive pleural contact, and may not be associated with the "comet tail" sign. Biopsy is often warranted.

Pulmonary Infarction and Septic Embolism

Infarcts can produce a pulmonary nodule. Septic emboli are usually multiple. In either instance, nodules typically

1. Are peripheral or abut a pleural surface
2. Appear round, wedge shaped, or truncated
3. Are often seen to have a pulmonary artery branch leading to them

Using contrast medium–enhanced spiral CT, associated clot may sometimes be identified in the proximal pulmonary artery in patients with pulmonary infarction. In patients with septic embolism, cavitation of lung nodules is common.

The "Halo" Sign and Invasive Pulmonary Aspergillosis

The "halo" sign is said to be present if a soft tissue attenuation nodule is surrounded by a less dense rim or halo of ground-glass opacity (Fig. 6–14). This appearance is typical of invasive aspergillosis occurring in immunosuppressed patients, particularly those with treated leukemia and low white blood cell counts. With invasive aspergillosis, the halo represents hemorrhage surrounding an area of septic infarction; it can

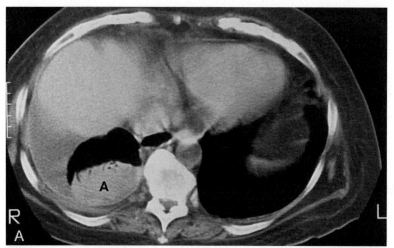

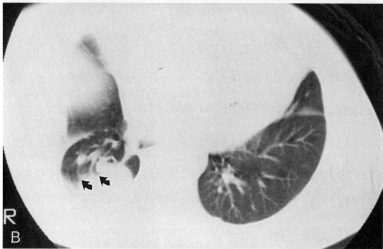

Figure 6–13. Rounded atelectasis. *A,* Adjacent to an area of pleural thickening and effusion, the atelectatic lung (A) shows air bronchograms curving into its edge. The lesion shows extensive pleural contact. *B,* At a lung window setting, the curved vessels and bronchi *(arrows)* entering the atelectatic lung are visible and there is posterior displacement of the major fissure, indicating volume loss.

precede necrosis, cavitation, and the presence of an "air-crescent" sign (Fig. 6–15).

Although suggestive of invasive aspergillosis in the proper clinical setting, the "halo" sign is nonspecific and can be seen with other infections (tuberculosis, legionellosis, nocardiosis, cytomegalovirus infection) and with some tumors (particularly lymphoma and Kaposi's sarcoma). The "air-crescent" sign can also be seen with mycetoma, clot within a cavity, neoplasm arising in a cavity, and echinococcal cyst.

Mycetoma

In patients with a preexisting cyst or cavity, a mycetoma or fungus ball can form as a result of saprophytic infection, usually by *Aspergillus.* On CT, a round or oval mass (the fungus ball) can be seen within the cavity, in a dependent location, and is typi-

cally mobile. Thickening of the cavity wall is common. In patients with a developing mycetoma, the fungus ball can contain multiple air collections. The same appearance can represent semi-invasive aspergillosis, in which the fungus also invades the wall of the cyst or cavity. Hemorrhage and hemoptysis are common associations.

Lung Abscess

A lung abscess can occur with a variety of bacterial, fungal, and parasitic infections. The hallmark of lung abscess is necrosis or cavitation within an area of pneumonia or dense consolidation; the necrotic region can appear quite irregular (see Fig. 6–14). Necrosis is commonly visible on contrast medium–enhanced CT as one or more areas of low attenuation within opacified lung. Cavitation is said to be present if air is visible

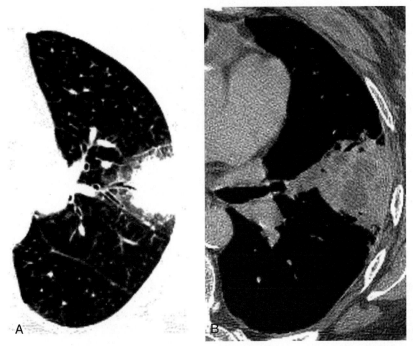

Figure 6–14. Invasive aspergillosis with the halo sign. *A,* In an immunosuppressed patient with leukemia, an ill-defined lung mass is surrounded by a less-dense "halo." This finding is highly suggestive of this diagnosis in a patient with the appropriate history. *B,* Soft tissue window at the same level shows central necrosis.

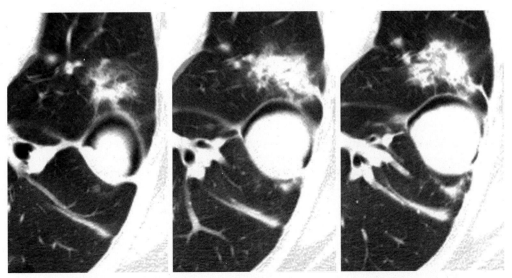

Figure 6–15. Invasive aspergillosis with an air crescent sign. A crescent of air outlines a mass within a cavity. In invasive aspergillosis, the mass represents a ball of infarcted lung and the cavity represents the space the lung used to occupy. This is distinct from aspergilloma, in which an air crescent sign reflects fungus within a preexisting cavity. Focal consolidation is visible anterior to the cavitary lesion, owing to acute infection.

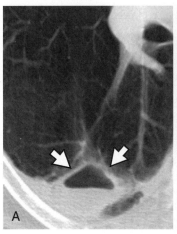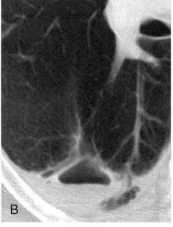

Figure 6–16. Lung abscess. *A and B,* A thin-walled lung abscess *(arrows)* is visible in the posterior lung, containing an air-fluid level.

within the lesion, and often CT is obtained to confirm this diagnosis when the plain radiograph is suggestive. An air-fluid level or levels are commonly present (Fig. 6–16). CT can also be helpful in distinguishing a lung abscess from an empyema. The CT appearances of lung abscess and empyema are contrasted in Chapter 7.

Granulomatous Lesions

Granulomas usually appear rounded and well defined. They may contain calcium (de-

scribed further later). Inflammatory and particularly granulomatous lesions may be associated with small *satellite nodules*— small nodules grouped together or seen in association with a larger nodule or cavity (Fig. 6–17). These are seen in only 1% to 2% of carcinomas.

Lipoid Pneumonia

Chronic aspiration of lipid (animal, vegetable, or mineral) can lead to lipoid pneumo-

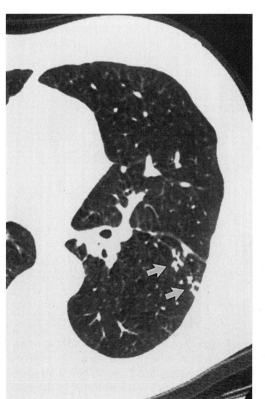

Figure 6–17. Satellite nodules representing atypical mycobacteria. High-resolution CT in a patient with an ill-defined 1-cm nodule visible on a chest radiograph. On high-resolution CT, the "nodule" is seen to consist of a number of smaller, well-defined "satellite" nodules *(arrows),* which suggest a granulomatous process. (From Webb WR. Radiologic evaluation of the solitary pulmonary nodule. AJR 1990; 154:701–708, with permission.)

nia, with fat and variable amount of fibrosis resulting in focal consolidations or masses. In some patients, most typically those with mineral oil aspiration, CT shows low-attenuation consolidation indicative of its lipid content. When fibrosis predominates, the masses are of soft tissue attenuation.

Linear Opacities (Scars or Atelectasis)

Sometimes patients with a solitary nodule on chest radiographs show something on CT that is best categorized as a linear opacity. This may represent scarring from prior infection or infarction or a region of focal atelectasis. Although the cause cannot be determined, these opacities can be distinguished from cancers, which appear round or like a mass. Although their appearance indicates they are likely benign, follow-up is usually appropriate.

Pleural (Fissural) Lesions

Occasionally, a pleural abnormality located in a fissure (e.g., a plaque, loculated effusion, or localized fibrous tumor of the pleura) may be misinterpreted as a lung nodule (see Fig. 7–21). Looking for the fissures on CT, and obtaining HRCT, will sometimes allow you to avoid this mistake. Correlating the CT with the chest radiographs can also be of value.

CT Diagnosis of Calcification in a Lung Nodule

CT can be used to detect calcification in a lung nodule, indicating that the nodule is benign and that resection is not necessary. Twenty-five to 35% of benign nodules appearing uncalcified on radiographs show calcification on HRCT.

Calcification of lung nodules can sometimes be seen using CT with conventional technique (5- to 10-mm collimation). However, thin collimation (1–2 mm) and HRCT technique should be used. Calcium easily diagnosable on thin-section CT is sometimes invisible with 10-mm collimation. Soft tissue window settings are best for detecting calcium.

When using CT to detect "benign" calcification, you must be sure that the calcification is "benign" in appearance; that is, it must be (1) diffuse (see Fig. 6–8), (2) dense and central within the nodule and of significant size, or (3) lamellated. Nodules that show visible calcification will generally have measured CT numbers of about 200 H (Fig. 6–18).

Five to 10% of carcinomas contain some calcium, either as a result of tumor calcification or because the carcinoma has engulfed a preexisting granuloma. Calcification in tumors is typically punctate or stippled or is eccentric within the nodule (Fig. 6–19).

CT Nodule Densitometry

The term *CT nodule densitometry* is used to describe a technique in which measurement of CT numbers is used to detect subtle calcification. Generally, CT numbers of 164 to 200 H are considered to indicate the presence of calcium when using this technique.

Figure 6–18. Diffuse calcification of a granuloma. On high-resolution CT, an apical nodule is diffusely and densely calcified.

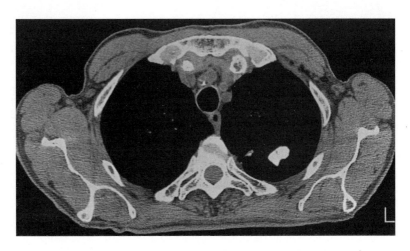

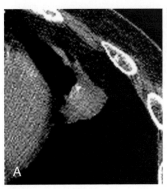

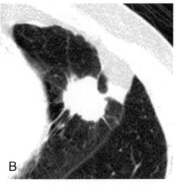

Figure 6–19. Eccentric calcification in adenocarcinoma. *A* and *B,* High-resolution CT in a patient with an adenocarcinoma in the lingula shows a spiculated nodule with eccentric calcification. Eccentric calcification can be seen in carcinomas.

However, because there can be considerable variation in nodule density measurements obtained with different scanners, and for nodules of different sizes, in different locations, and in patients of different body type, an anthropomorphic chest phantom is sometimes used for nodule densitometry (Fig. 6–20). This phantom can simulate the shape, dimensions, and density of thoracic structures in most patients. Cylinders of various

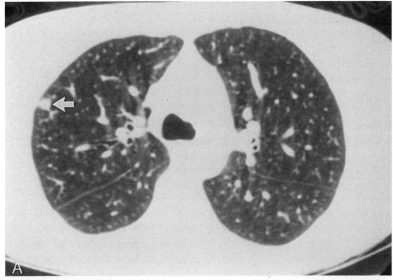

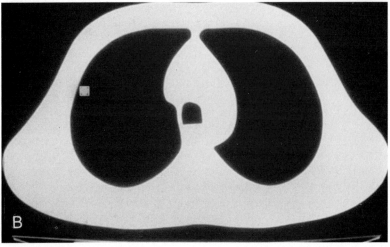

Figure 6–20. CT densitometry using a nodule phantom. *A,* Thin-collimated CT in a patient with a small right lung nodule *(arrow). B,* The CT phantom has been constructed to simulate the same slice level, nodule size, chest wall thickness, and nodule location, and the phantom has been scanned using identical technical factors.

diameters, made of plastic, are used to correspond to the density of a calcified nodule. By comparing the density of a solitary nodule with the density of a similar phantom nodule, a measurement of nodule density independent of equipment-related or patient-related variations can be achieved. Although the use of nodule densitometry and this phantom can increase sensitivity in detecting calcium in benign lesions, its use can also result in some calcium-containing malignancies being called benign.

Nodule Opacification

Lung cancers have been shown to have a greater tendency to enhance after contrast medium infusion than do many benign lesions. Contrast medium enhancement appears to be quite sensitive in detecting cancers, but some benign lesions, such as benign tumors and active granulomatous lesions, also can enhance. In using this technique, an enhancing lesion must be resected; an unenhancing lesion can be observed.

Because the degree of enhancement depends on the amount and rapidity of contrast medium infusion, it is important to use a consistent technique. In one study, 420 mg iodine/kg (usually 75 to 125 mL) was injected at a rate of 2 mL/sec, with HRCT scans through the nodule obtained before the infusion and at 1-minute intervals for 4 minutes following the start of the

CT NUMBERS

EXAM 1799 STATION 1

PRS 1 PROSPECTIVE IMAGE 5

X →	126	127	128	129	130	131	132	133	134
283	-738	-640	-491	-401	-386	-347	-300	-370	-555
284	-648	-489	-294	-177	-126	-64	-24	-147	-430
285	-426	-269	-117	-35	18	82	94	-24	-319
286	-192	-81	5	38	87	141	118	2	-279
287	-118	-23	41	85	161	206	135	-25	-326
288	-187	-77	2	85	184	227	136	-88	-419
289	-354	-183	-55	52	146	186	72	-221	-554
290	-579	-396	-228	-103	3	42	-92	-405	-696
291	-737	-654	-538	-433	-337	-301	-375	-563	-751

C

Figure 6–20 *Continued. C,* CT numbers measured from the nodule include many pixels exceeding 100 H and some that exceed 200 H. *D,* Numbers recorded from the phantom nodule are considerably lower. Thus, the nodule is calcified. (From Webb WR. Radiologic evaluation of the solitary pulmonary nodule. AJR 1990; 154:701–708, with permission.)

CT NUMBERS

EXAM 1799 STATION 1

PRS 1 PROSPECTIVE IMAGE 12

X →	117	118	119	120	121	122	123	124	125
202	-839	-618	-383	-241	-206	-283	-477	-742	-919
203	-627	-279	-61	12	30	-13	-146	-446	-782
204	-399	-64	32	36	38	27	-1	-196	-613
205	-265	13	35	33	31	19	23	-74	-482
206	-241	24	33	33	31	21	36	-52	-461
207	-339	-9	50	42	26	28	43	-113	-549
208	-533	-163	-2	34	37	26	-40	-316	-722
209	-765	-464	-226	-109	-86	-152	-323	-622	-890
210	-921	-799	-623	-499	-473	-562	-714	-880	-972

D

injection. When enhancement of 20 HU or more was used to distinguish malignant from benign lesions, sensitivity was 98% and specificity was 73%. The clinical utility and role of this technique remain to be established.

Use of CT to Guide Biopsy of a Lung Nodule

If CT does not allow a specific diagnosis to be made in a patient with a solitary nodule, and no calcification is visible, a biopsy may be considered necessary for diagnosis. Depending on the clinical situation, several options are available. These include needle lung biopsy, bronchoscopy, and thoracoscopic biopsy. To some degree, CT can be used to help make a choice between these.

Bronchoscopy is most accurate in diagnosing central masses that have an endobronchial component, whereas needle biopsy is best for peripheral lung lesions. For lesions in the central half of the lung, if an endobronchial lesion is seen with CT or a *positive bronchus sign* (bronchial narrowing or obstruction at the site of a nodule, or a bronchus within the mass lesion) is visible, bronchoscopy directed to the proper site is most appropriate. If there is no evidence of an abnormal bronchus at CT, needle biopsy should probably be performed first.

CT can be helpful in planning a needle aspiration biopsy, even if CT is not used for the biopsy itself. First, CT can indicate the depth of the lesion and the needle can be marked accordingly. This is of particular value if only single-plane fluoroscopy is available for the biopsy procedure. Second, CT can help in planning the biopsy approach. If bullae lie in the path of the needle, or the needle must cross a fissure to reach the lesion, the risk of pneumothorax is increased and a different approach might be chosen.

Thoracoscopic biopsy or resection of peripheral lung nodules can be assisted by CT-guided localization techniques, often involving hooked wires or injections of methylene blue.

MULTIPLE LUNG NODULES AND PULMONARY METASTASES

CT is much more sensitive than plain radiographs or conventional tomography in detecting lung nodules. Nodules as small as a few millimeters can be easily detected using CT, even with 10-mm collimation (Fig. 6–21). Spiral CT, because of its ability to acquire data volumetrically, is more sensitive than conventional CT in detecting pulmonary nodules.

Nodules can mimic the appearance of vessels seen in cross section. However, small nodules are usually visible on only one or two adjacent scans, whereas longitudinally oriented vessels can be followed on a number of scans and can be traced to their point

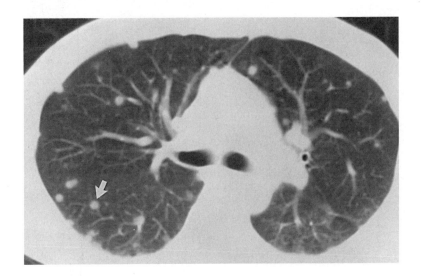

Figure 6–21. Multiple metastases. Multiple small well-defined nodules represent metastases from a renal cell carcinoma. Their peripheral location is typical. A few of these nodules *(arrow)* appear to be related to a pulmonary vessel.

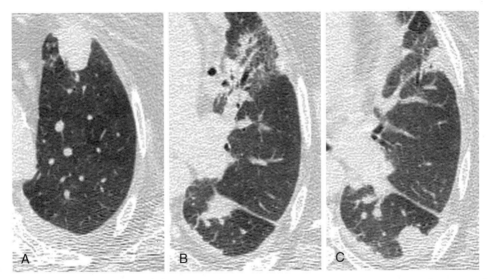

Figure 6–22. Nocardiosis with multiple nodules. Multiple ill-defined nodules reflect nocardial pneumonia in an immunosuppressed patient.

of origin or seen to branch. Contrast medium injection is not usually of value in making this distinction, except in the case of large central nodules, in contiguity with the hilar vessels.

The differential diagnosis of multiple large (>1 cm) pulmonary nodules includes metastases, lymphoma, bronchogenic carcinoma with synchronous primary tumors; bacterial, fungal, and sometimes viral infections (Fig. 6–22); granulomatous diseases; sarcoidosis; Wegener's granulomatosis; rheumatoid nodules; amyloidosis; and septic emboli. In most cases, the CT appearances of large nodules is nonspecific. The differential diagnosis of multiple small nodules (<1 cm) is discussed in the section on HRCT.

Metastases

Nodular metastases can be seen in any part of the lung. However, pulmonary metastases, resulting from tumor embolization, have a predilection for the peripheral lung (see Fig. 6–21) and are commonly visible in a subpleural location. Normal subpleural lymphoid aggregates or granulomas that are a few millimeters in diameter can also have this appearance and in a patient with suspected metastases may be problematic. Because small peripheral densities are too small to sample percutaneously, follow-up CT (at 1–2 months) is often used. Metasta-

ses increase in size. An alternative would be thoracoscopic biopsy. The same rationale is used when small (2–3 mm) intraparenchymal nodules are seen. These small nodules can simply represent granulomas, and follow-up scans are often obtained to evaluate their significance.

In obtaining follow-up CT to assess a small lung nodule for change in size, it is important to obtain scans at exactly the same levels, and with the same window settings as in the original study with which you are comparing it. A small nodule can be missed if the patient breathes differently for two supposedly contiguous scans (the nodule may fall at a level between the two "adjacent" scans) or can appear to be smaller if it is slightly out of the scan plane; the use of spiral CT during a single breath hold helps to avoid these problems. Identifying the pattern of branching vessels within the lung, in the region of the nodule, is an easy way of knowing exactly what level you are looking at. If the same vessels are visible on both the original and follow-up scans, and the nodule looks different, then the nodule is different. If a different branching pattern is visible, an apparent difference in nodule size may not be real. If follow-up scans are viewed at different window settings from the original study, a nodule may appear to be a different size. As stated earlier, low window mean settings make a nodule appear larger.

Pulmonary metastases are typically round and well defined. Some metastases with surrounding hemorrhage can be ill defined or associated with the "halo" sign. Cavitation and calcification can be seen with some metastatic tumors. Pulmonary metastases may be seen to have a connection with a pulmonary artery branch, reflecting their embolic nature (see Fig. 6–21). However, this finding can be present with other causes of pulmonary nodules, such as Wegener's granulomatosis and bland or septic emboli.

Bronchioloalveolar Carcinoma

Approximately 50% of patients with bronchioloalveolar carcinoma present with diffuse or patchy lung consolidation or multiple lung nodules (Fig. 6–23). The presence of visible opacified arteries within the areas of consolidation on contrast medium–enhanced CT (the CT angiogram sign) has been reported to be suggestive of this tumor but can also be seen with other causes of consolidation, such as pneumonia. In patients with bronchioloalveolar carcinoma, the tumor can secrete large amounts of low attenuation fluid, which is partially responsible for lung consolidation and the presence of the CT angiogram sign. Bronchorrhea can also result.

Lymphoma

Pulmonary parenchymal involvement is seen in 10% of patients with Hodgkin's disease at the time of presentation. Direct extension from hilar nodes, focal discrete areas of consolidation, or masslike lesions can be seen. Air-bronchograms or areas of cavitation may be visible within the abnormal regions. In patients with untreated Hodgkin's disease, lung involvement usually does not occur in the absence of radiographically demonstrable mediastinal (and usually ipsilateral hilar) adenopathy.

In patients with non-Hodgkin's lymphoma, pulmonary disease can occur in the absence of lymph node enlargement. This is common in patients with the acquired

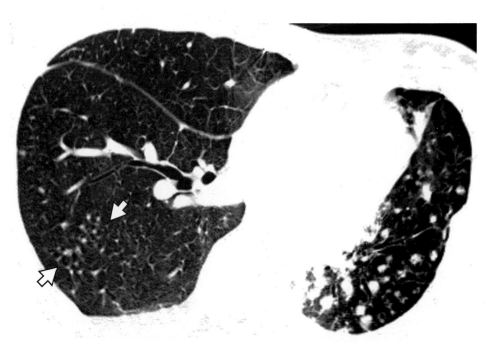

Figure 6–23. Bronchioloalveolar carcinoma with multiple nodules. Multiple nodules are visible in the left lung. A cluster of small nodules *(arrows)* is also visible in the right lung as a result of endobronchial spread of tumor. The left lung is reduced in volume because of prior irradiation.

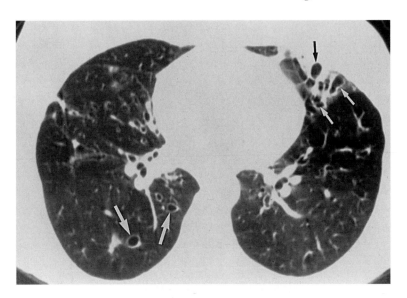

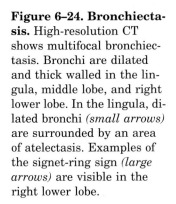

Figure 6–24. Bronchiectasis. High-resolution CT shows multifocal bronchiectasis. Bronchi are dilated and thick walled in the lingula, middle lobe, and right lower lobe. In the lingula, dilated bronchi *(small arrows)* are surrounded by an area of atelectasis. Examples of the signet-ring sign *(large arrows)* are visible in the right lower lobe.

immunodeficiency syndrome. Large ill-defined nodules can be seen.

BRONCHIECTASIS AND BRONCHIAL ABNORMALITIES

Conventional CT is of limited value in diagnosing bronchiectasis, because tubular or cylindrical bronchiectasis is easily missed using this technique. However, HRCT is more accurate than conventional CT and has replaced bronchography. In patients with suspected bronchiectasis, HRCT scans are usually obtained at 1-cm intervals from the lung apices to bases, to show the extent of disease throughout both lungs.

In patients with bronchiectasis, the dilated and thick-walled bronchi are usually visible on several adjacent scans (Fig. 6–24). The smaller pulmonary artery branch and, lying adjacent to it, the dilated, ring-shaped bronchus give their combined shadow the appearance of a signet ring. The "signet ring" sign (see Fig. 6–24) is characteristic of bronchiectasis. Bronchiectasis is usually classified as cylindrical, varicose, and cystic, but these designations are of little clinical significance.

Mucus plugs (Fig. 6–25) associated with bronchiectasis, cystic fibrosis, allergic bronchopulmonary aspergillosis, bronchial obstruction, or congenital bronchial atresia

can sometimes produce nodular opacities that are difficult to diagnose on chest radiographs. On CT, their relation to the bronchial tree, their often branching shape, and their associated bronchiectasis are diagnostic.

In patients with bronchiolitis obliterans (i.e., constrictive bronchiolitis or the Swyer-James syndrome), in addition to findings of bronchiectasis, areas of pulmonary hyperlucency can also be seen on CT, probably as a result of decreased perfusion within areas of lung that are poorly ventilated. This occurrence that gives the lung a patchy inhomogeneous appearance is termed *mosaic perfusion* and is best shown on HRCT (Fig. 6–26). Typically, vessels within the relatively lucent regions appear smaller than in relatively dense lung regions. Bronchiectasis may also be visible.

ATELECTASIS: TYPES AND PATTERNS

Atelectasis most commonly occurs because of bronchial obstruction (obstructive atelectasis), pleural effusion or other pleural processes that allow the lung to collapse (passive atelectasis), or lung fibrosis (cicatrization atelectasis). These can have different appearances. General signs of volume loss on CT are the same as those on chest

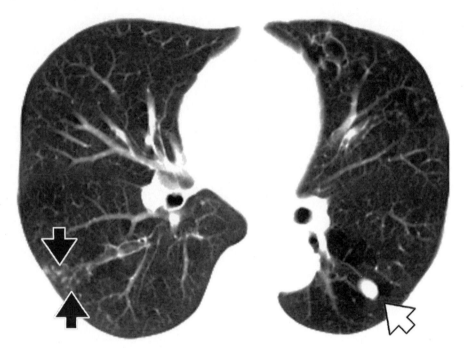

Figure 6–25. Mucus plug with bronchiectasis. In a patient with bilateral bronchiectasis, a nodule visible on chest radiographs *(white arrow)* represents a mucus plug. A dilated bronchus is seen leading to the nodule. Follow-up scans showed no change. A branching appearance in the right lung *(black arrows)* is termed *tree-in-bud* and reflects filling of small airways with infected material or mucus.

radiographs. Mediastinal shift (particularly of the anterior mediastinum) and displacement of fissures are well seen on CT.

Obstructive Atelectasis

Obstructive atelectasis often occurs because of a tumor, and the bronchi should be examined closely. For the most part, the CT findings of obstructive atelectasis are what would be expected from our experience with plain films. Typically, the affected lobe is partially or completely consolidated (Fig. 6–27). Air-bronchograms may be visible (see Fig. 6–27), but typically they are not. Mucus-bronchograms (low-density fluid or mucus within obstructed bronchi) can sometimes be seen on CT. The air- or mucus-filled bronchi can be dilated in the presence of atelectasis, simulating bronchiectasis. If contrast medium infusion is used, opacified vessels are often visible within the consolidated lobe. If little volume loss if present, the term *obstructive pneumonitis* is often used instead (Fig. 6–28).

On CT, atelectasis can be diagnosed when

displacement of fissures is seen. As on plain films, typical patterns of collapse can be identified (Figs. 6–29 and 6–30).

Right Upper Lobe Collapse

The major fissure rotates anteriorly and medially as the upper lobe progressively flattens against the mediastinum (see Figs. 6–27 and 6–29). The fissure can be bowed anteriorly. In the presence of a hilar mass, an appearance similar to Golden's S sign as seen on plain radiographs is visible. In some patients, the lobe assumes a triangular shape (see Fig. 6–27).

Left Upper Lobe Collapse

As on the right, the major fissure rotates anteromedially. However, above the hilum, the superior segment of the lower lobe may displace part of the upper lobe away from the mediastinum, giving the posterior margin of the collapsed lobe a V shape (see Fig. 6–29). A similar appearance is sometimes seen on the right.

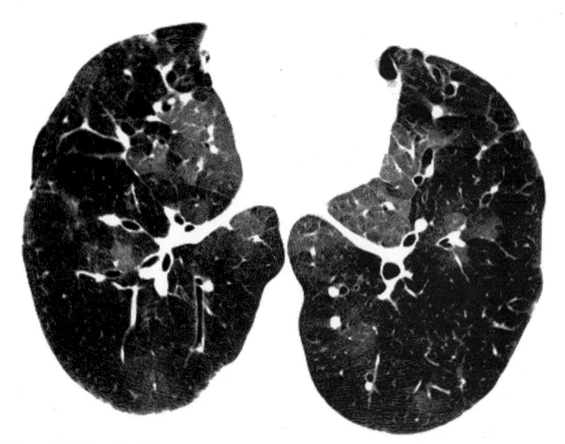

Figure 6–26. Bronchiolitis obliterans with mosaic perfusion. In a patient with bronchiolitis obliterans resulting from a bone marrow transplantation and graft-versus-host reaction, the lung has a patchy appearance on a high-resolution CT. Differences in lung density reflect differences in lung perfusion secondary to abnormal ventilation related to airway obstruction. Note that vessels look larger in the dense lung regions than in the lucent lung regions; this is an important clue to the presence of mosaic perfusion.

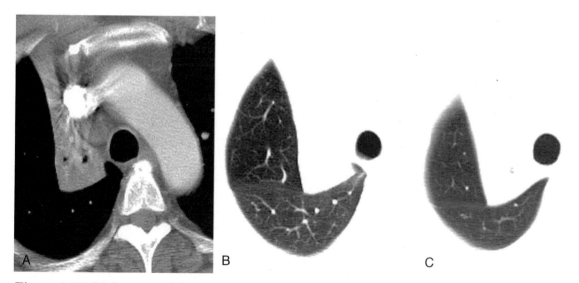

Figure 6–27. Right upper lobe collapse. In a patient with carcinoma obstructing the right upper lobe bronchus, both air bronchograms and opacified vessels are visible *(A)*. The collapsed upper lobe has a triangular shape *(B and C)*. The middle lobe borders the lateral aspect of the collapsed lobe, whereas the lower lobe is posterior to it.

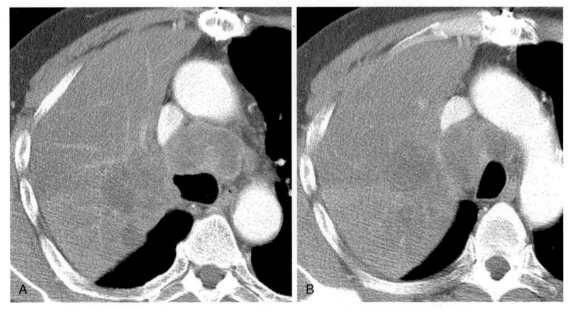

Figure 6–28. Lung carcinoma with obstructive pneumonia. *A and B,* The right upper lobe is consolidated, but no volume loss is present. No air bronchograms are seen, but opacified vessels are visible. Large low-density, necrotic mediastinal lymph nodes are also present.

Middle Lobe Collapse

As the middle lobe loses volume, the minor fissure, which normally is difficult to see because it lies in the plane of scan, rotates downward and medially and becomes visible on CT. The collapsed lobe assumes a triangular shape, with one side of the triangle abutting the mediastinum (see Fig. 6–30). The upper lobe can be seen anterolaterally, bordering the collapsed lobe, with the lower lobe bordering it posterolaterally. These aerated lobes usually separate the collapsed middle lobe from the lateral chest wall.

Lower Lobe Collapse

On either side, the major fissure rotates posteromedially (see Fig. 6–30). The collapsed lobe contacts the posterior mediastinum and posteromedial chest wall and

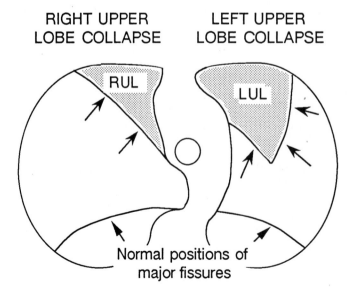

Figure 6–29. Typical patterns of upper lobe collapse.

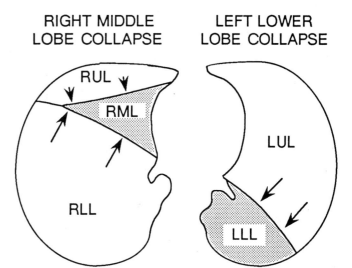

RIGHT MIDDLE
LOBE COLLAPSE

LEFT LOWER
LOBE COLLAPSE

RUL

RML

LUL

RLL

LLL

Figure 6–30. Typical patterns of middle and lower lobe collapse.

maintains contact with the medial diaphragm.

Passive Atelectasis

In the presence of pleural effusion, lung tends to retract or collapse toward the hilum, and fluid entering the fissures allows the lobes to separate (see Fig. 7–5). With the injection of contrast material, the lung opacifies and is clearly distinguishable from surrounding fluid. Air-bronchograms may be seen within the collapsed lobes. Rounded atelectasis is a form of passive atelectasis.

Cicatrization Atelectasis

Cicatrization atelectasis occurs in the presence of pulmonary fibrosis and may be associated with tuberculosis, radiation, or chronic bronchiectasis. In this condition, there is no evidence of bronchial obstruction. Rather, air-bronchograms and bronchial dilatation (bronchiectasis) are usually visible within the area of collapse. The volume loss is often severe.

DIFFUSE INFILTRATIVE LUNG DISEASE

The term *diffuse infiltrative lung disease* is used to describe a variety of conditions, both air space and interstitial, manifested by a generalized parenchymal abnormality. Included in this category are such disparate diseases as diffuse pneumonia, pulmonary edema, and chronic interstitial abnormalities.

CT is not generally used to evaluate patients with acute diffuse lung consolidation or acute interstitial disease visible on chest radiographs, because in most cases the diagnosis of such diseases is clinical. Common causes would be acute pneumonia, pulmonary edema, and adult respiratory distress syndrome.

In some patients with an acute abnormality, however, CT may be done to look for associated findings such as pleural effusion, bronchial obstruction or associated mass, adenopathy, or cavitation, which might be valuable in diagnosis. CT and, particularly, HRCT have been reported to be of some value in the diagnosis of acute lung disease in immunosuppressed patients, especially those with the acquired immunodeficiency syndrome.

HRCT Diagnosis of Diffuse Lung Disease

HRCT is commonly used to evaluate diffuse infiltrative lung diseases, particularly when chronic or progressive, and when the diagnosis is in question. Generally, HRCT is used (1) to detect lung disease in patients with symptoms of respiratory distress or abnormal pulmonary function tests who have normal chest radiographs (approximately

10% of patients with infiltrative lung disease have normal chest radiographs); (2) to characterize lung disease as to its morphologic pattern (e.g., is there honeycombing?), and perhaps make a specific diagnosis; (3) to assess disease activity, and (4) to localize areas of abnormality in patients who are having a lung biopsy. HRCT is more sensitive than plain radiographs (94% vs. 80%), more specific than plain radiographs (96% vs. 82%), and more accurate in making a diagnosis (by more than 10%).

HRCT scans are usually obtained at 1- to 2-cm intervals, because this technique is intended to "sample" lung anatomy at different levels. Scans are usually obtained during full inspiration in the supine position. Prone scans may also be obtained to avoid misdiagnosis when posterior atelectasis develops with the patient lying supine. Some dependent lung collapse is often seen on HRCT, and having scans in both positions allows us to differentiate this finding from true pathologic processes.

HRCT Findings in Normal Subjects

Secondary pulmonary lobules are polygonal and vary in size, usually measuring 1 to 3 cm in diameter. They are marginated by interlobular septa, containing veins and lymphatics (Fig. 6–31). In the center of the lobule are pulmonary artery and bronchiolar branches. On HRCT, normal interlobular septa are sometimes visible as very thin, straight lines of uniform thickness, 1 to 2 cm in length, but usually, only a few well-defined septa are visible in normal subjects.

Branching vessels seen in relation to the septa represent veins. A linear, branching, or dotlike density seen within the secondary lobule, or within a centimeter of the pleural surface, represents the centrilobular artery branch. The centrilobular bronchiole is not normally visible. The visible artery in the center of the lobule does not extend to the pleural surface in the absence of atelectasis.

In normal subjects, the pleural surfaces, fissures, and the margins of central vessels and bronchi appear smooth and sharply defined.

HRCT Findings in Abnormal Subjects

Thickened Interlobular Septa

Thickening of interlobular septa can be seen in patients with a variety of interstitial lung diseases (Fig. 6–32). Within the central lung, thickened septa can outline lobules that appear hexagonal or polygonal and contain a visible, central arterial branch. In the peripheral lung, thickened septa often extend to the pleural surface. Thickening of longer septa, several centimeters in length, which marginate more than one lobule can also be seen. Septal thickening can appear smooth, nodular, or irregular in different diseases (see later).

Often, thickened septa in the peripheral lung reflect generalized interstitial thickening and are also associated with (1) thickening of fissures due to subpleural interstitial thickening, (2) prominent centrilobular structures due to thickening of the sheath

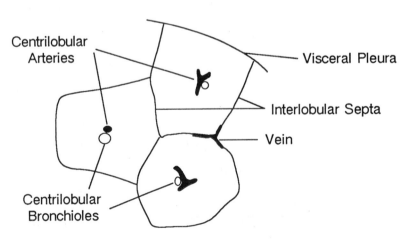

Centrilobular Arteries

Visceral Pleura

Interlobular Septa

Vein

Centrilobular Bronchioles

Figure 6–31. Normal pulmonary lobules.

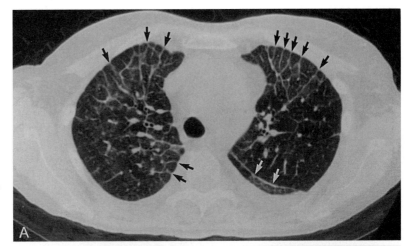

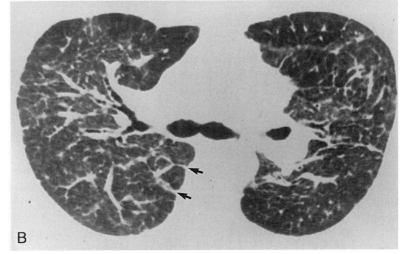

Figure 6–32. Thickening of interlobular septa. *A,* In a patient with lymphangitic spread of carcinoma, high-resolution CT shows evidence of septal thickening *(black arrows)* characteristic of this disease. Apparent thickening of the left major fissure *(white arrows)* represents subpleural interstitial thickening. Notice that the pleural surface appears irregular where it is contacted by the thick septa. *B,* In a patient with sarcoidosis and pulmonary fibrosis, irregular septal thickening *(black arrows)* is visible throughout the lung. The edges of vessels and bronchi appear quite irregular.

of connective tissue that surrounds them, and (3) thickening of the interstitium surrounding central vessels and bronchi (i.e., peribronchial cuffing).

Common causes of interlobular septal thickening as the predominant HRCT finding include

1. Lymphangitic spread of carcinoma (smooth or nodular septal thickening)
2. Interstitial pulmonary edema (smooth)
3. Alveolar proteinosis (smooth, in association with ground-glass opacity)
4. Sarcoidosis (nodular when granulomas present; irregular in fibrotic or end-stage disease)

Pulmonary Fibrosis

Fibrosis results in an irregular reticular pattern on HRCT. *Intralobular interstitial thickening* is a common finding in early fibrosis and appears as a fine reticulation. Fibrosis associated with areas of lung destruction and the disorganization of lung architecture is termed *honeycombing*. Honeycombing results in a coarser reticular pattern or cystic appearance on HRCT, which is characteristic (Fig. 6–33); cystic spaces are several millimeters to several centimeters in diameter, are often peripheral and subpleural, are characterized by thick, clearly definable walls, and tend to occur in groups or layers, with adjacent cysts sharing walls. *Traction bronchiectasis,* dilatation of bronchi in regions of fibrosis, is another common finding. Also, intralobular bronchioles may be visible on HRCT in patients with honeycombing because of a combination of traction bronchiolectasis and thickening of the peribronchiolar interstitium.

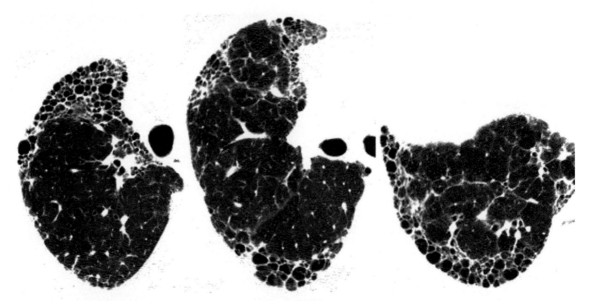

Figure 6–33. Pulmonary fibrosis and honeycombing in rheumatoid arthritis. High-resolution CT of the right lung at three levels shows characteristic small thick-walled cysts (honeycomb cysts), most evident peripherally. This appearance is diagnostic of fibrosis.

Conglomerate masses of fibrous tissue can be seen in the upper lobes of patients with sarcoidosis or silicosis.

Common causes of fibrosis and honeycombing as the predominant HRCT finding include

1. Idiopathic pulmonary fibrosis (60%–70% of cases)
2. Autoimmune diseases, particularly rheumatoid arthritis and scleroderma
3. Asbestosis, in association with pleural thickening
4. End-stage hypersensitivity pneumonitis
5. Drug-related fibrosis
6. End-stage sarcoidosis (a few percent of patients)

Nodules

Small nodules (a few millimeters to 1 cm in diameter) can be detected on HRCT in patients with granulomatous diseases such as sarcoidosis and miliary tuberculosis, in patients with metastatic tumor, and in patients with small airways disease. Three distributions of lung nodules can be identified on HRCT (Fig. 6–34); recognition of one of these three is invaluable in differential diagnosis.

Perilymphatic nodules predominate in relation to (1) the pleural surfaces (particularly the fissures), (2) large vessels and bronchi, (3) interlobular septa, and (4) the centrilobular regions, and they are typically patchy in distribution. They are most common in sarcoidosis (Fig. 6–35; see also Fig. 6–34), silicosis, and lymphangitic carcinoma.

Random nodules also involve the pleural surfaces but have a diffuse and uniform distribution, with a random distribution in relation to structures of the secondary lobule. They are most typical of miliary tuberculosis and hematogenous metastases.

Centrilobular nodules usually spare the pleural surfaces and are centrilobular in distribution (Fig. 6–36). They tend to occur in relation to small vessels, with the most peripheral nodules being 5 to 10 mm from the pleural surface. They usually reflect diseases occurring in relation to small airways and are common with endobronchial spread of infection (e.g., tuberculosis), endobronchial spread of tumor (e.g., bronchioloalveolar carcinoma), hypersensitivity pneumonitis, bronchiolitis obliterans organizing pneumonia, and diseases causing or associated with bronchiectasis.

Centrilobular nodules are sometimes as-

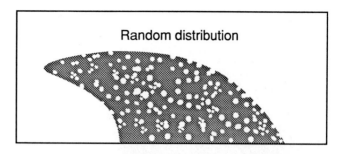

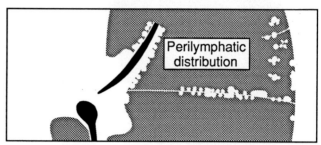

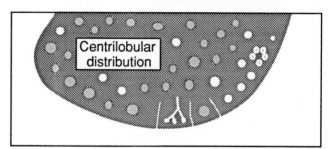

Figure 6–34. Distributions of lung nodules.

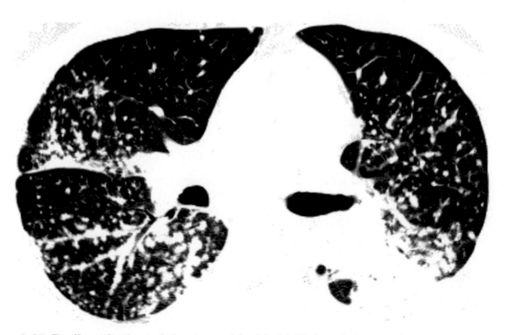

Figure 6–35. Perilymphatic nodules (sarcoidosis). Multiple nodules are visible adjacent to the major fissure and central bronchi and vessels. This pattern is characteristic of sarcoidosis. Note the patchy distribution, with some lung regions being involved, whereas others appear normal. A conglomerate mass of nodules is visible on the left.

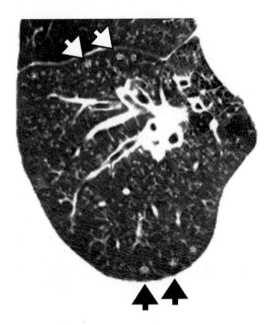

Figure 6–36. Centrilobular nodules in a patient with bronchiectasis and bronchiolar infection. Small ill-defined nodules are visible in the lower lobe. The most peripheral nodules *(arrows)* are 5 to 10 mm from the fissure or the pleural surfaces. Bronchiectasis is also visible.

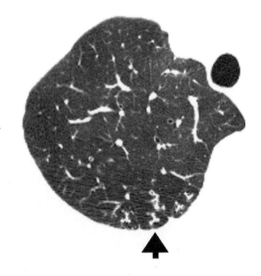

Figure 6–37. "Tree-in-bud" associated with *Mycobacterium avium-intracellulare* complex (MAC) infection. Ill-defined branching structures in the posterior lung *(arrow)* represent dilated bronchioles filled with infected material. These are too large to represent vessels. Endobronchial spread of tuberculosis could have a similar appearance.

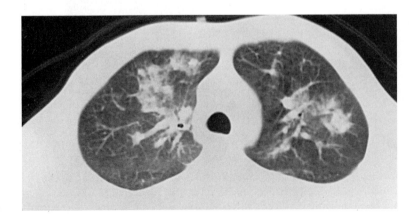

Figure 6–38. Patchy consolidation from pneumonia. Small nodular densities on the edges of larger areas of consolidation represent so-called air-space nodules.

sociated with a finding termed *tree-in-bud*, because that is what it looks like (Fig. 6–37; see also Fig. 6–25). Tree-in-bud reflects mucus or pus in dilated centrilobular bronchioles. The presence of this finding almost always indicates infection, such as caused by endobronchial spread of tuberculosis or *Mycobacterium avium-intracellulare* complex, cystic fibrosis, or bronchiectasis.

In attempting to make the diagnosis of one of these three patterns of multiple nodules, it is easiest to first determine the presence or absence of nodules in relation to the pleural surfaces and particularly along the fissures. If pleural nodules are absent, the distribution is centrilobular; if they are present, then the distribution of lung nodules determines the pattern present. Patchy nodules indicate a perilymphatic distribution; a diffuse and uniform distribution indicates a random pattern. The following algorithm can be used to correctly categorize more than 95% of the cases you see.

Consolidation

HRCT findings of air space consolidation are similar to those seen on plain radiographs, with obscuration of pulmonary vessels and air-bronchograms being the most characteristic findings (Fig. 6–38). Centrilobular nodules, as described earlier, measuring 0.5 to 1 cm in diameter, can also be seen on HRCT in patients with air space diseases (e.g., endobronchial spread of tuberculosis).

Common causes of lung consolidation evaluated using HRCT include tuberculosis, bronchiolitis obliterans obstructing pneumonia, bronchioloalveolar carcinoma, and chronic eosinophilic pneumonia.

Ground-Glass Opacity

In some patients with minimal interstitial disease, alveolitis, alveolar wall thickening, or minimal air space consolidation, a hazy

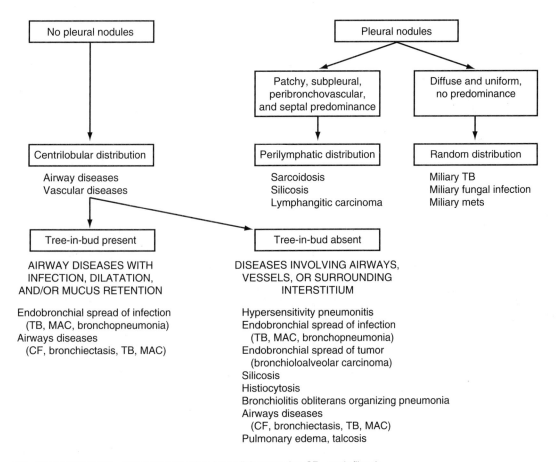

TB = tuberculosis; MAC = *Mycobacterium avium-intracellulare* complex; CF = cystic fibrosis

increase in lung density can be observed on HRCT, which typically has a patchy distribution (Fig. 6–39); this is termed ground-glass opacity. Ground-glass opacity is differentiated from consolidation in that areas of increased opacity do not obscure underlying pulmonary vessels. In about 80% of patients, this appearance correlates with some type of active lung disease.

Ground-glass opacity is nonspecific and can be seen with a variety of diseases (e.g., *Pneumocystis carinii* or viral pneumonia, edema, hypersensitivity pneumonitis, desquamative interstitial pneumonitis, idiopathic pulmonary fibrosis, bronchiolitis obliterans obstructing pneumonia, alveolar proteinosis), but, in most patients, the disease is treatable and the diagnosis should be pursued. However, if ground-glass opacity is seen only in lung regions also showing findings of fibrosis (e.g., honeycombing or traction bronchiectasis), it is likely that this finding represents fibrosis rather than active disease.

Lung Cysts

Lung cysts are thin-walled, air-filled spaces; this term is usually used to describe the air-filled spaces seen in patients with histiocytosis or lymphangiomyomatosis and the pneumatoceles seen in patients with *Pneu-*

mocystis carinii pneumonia. They should be differentiated from the lucencies seen in patients with emphysema.

HRCT Appearances in Specific Diseases: The Top 10

Although more than 200 diseases can result in a diffuse pulmonary abnormality, knowledge of a relatively few allows you to correctly diagnose most cases you see. More than 90% of patients with diffuse lung disease have one of about 10 diseases.

Metastatic Carcinoma

Although lymphangitic spread and hematogenous spread of carcinoma produce somewhat different patterns, overlap is common, and many patients will show some features of both.

In a patient with the appropriate history of malignancy and progressive dyspnea, the HRCT appearance of lymphangitic spread is diagnostic. Often, the plain radiograph will be normal or equivocal in this setting. *Lymphangitic spread of carcinoma* is characterized by

1. Interlobular septal thickening, smooth or nodular (see Fig. 6–32A; see also Fig. 5–22)

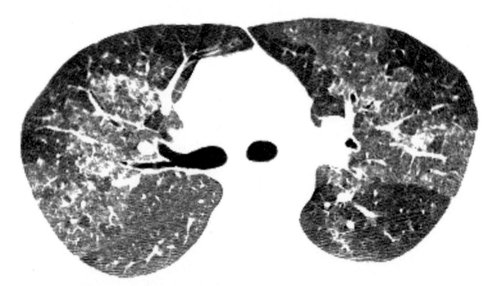

Figure 6–39. "Ground-glass" opacity. Patchy ground-glass opacity in this patient reflects sarcoidosis. Ground-glass opacity is said to be present when areas of increased lung opacity do not obscure vessels.

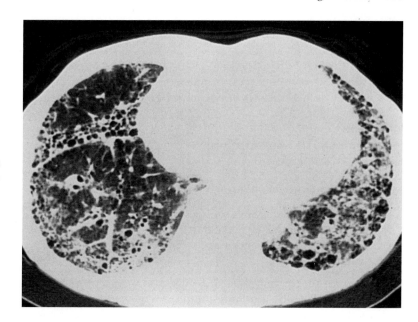

Figure 6–40. Idiopathic pulmonary fibrosis. There is extensive subpleural honeycombing.

2. Peribronchial interstitial thickening (peribronchial cuffing)
3. Thickening of fissures (smooth or nodular)
4. A patchy or unilateral distribution (in many cases)
5. Lymph node enlargement (in some cases)

Hematogenous spread of tumor can be characterized by

1. A random distribution of small nodules, sometimes with a peripheral predominance (see Figs. 6–21 and 6–34)
2. Involvement of fissures and the pleural surfaces
3. A bilateral distribution
4. Presence of large nodules

Idiopathic Pulmonary Fibrosis

Idiopathic pulmonary fibrosis accounts for two thirds of cases of diffuse pulmonary fibrosis with honeycombing. Progressive dyspnea is present. The prognosis is poor. Patients with this disorder typically show

1. Intralobular interstitial thickening
2. Honeycombing (Fig. 6–40)
3. Traction bronchiectasis and bronchiolectasis
4. A predominance in subpleural, posterior, and basal lung regions
5. Ground-glass opacity can be present

in some patients; it suggests active disease when it is a predominant finding.

Collagen Vascular Disease

Rheumatoid lung disease, scleroderma, and other collagen diseases result in findings identical to those of idiopathic pulmonary fibrosis (see Fig. 6–33).

Sarcoidosis

Sarcoidosis can have a highly diagnostic appearance in some patients. Patients may be relatively asymptomatic. HRCT findings in patients with active and end-stage disease differ. Typical findings in patients with active sarcoid are

1. Perilymphatic nodules, 1 to 10 mm (particularly subpleural and peribronchial) (see Figs. 6–34 and 6–35); calcification can occur.
2. A patchy distribution, often asymmetric
3. Upper lobe predominance
4. Hilar and mediastinal node enlargement (helpful in diagnosis, but not always present); calcification can be present.
5. Ground-glass opacity (uncommon) (see Fig. 6–39), reflecting the presence of very small granulomas

HRCT findings in patients with end-stage sarcoidosis and fibrosis include

1. Irregular septal thickening (see Fig. 6–32B)
2. Architectural distortion
3. Parahilar conglomerate masses containing crowded, ectatic bronchi, often involving the upper lobe
4. Honeycombing (a few percent)
5. Hilar and mediastinal node enlargement (not always present)

Silicosis and Coal Workers' Pneumoconiosis

Findings can be similar to those of sarcoidosis, but significant differences are recognizable. Findings include

1. Perilymphatic nodules, 1 to 10 mm (particularly centrilobular and subpleural), with calcification in some
2. Symmetric distribution
3. Posterior lung predominance
4. Upper lobe predominance
5. Conglomerate masses of nodules or fibrosis in the upper lobes
6. Hilar and mediastinal node enlargement; egg-shell calcification may be present.

Tuberculosis

Tuberculosis has different appearances depending on the form of disease. The features of primary tuberculosis resemble those of pneumonia, and HRCT is not commonly used for diagnosis. In patients with disseminated tuberculosis, HRCT findings depend on the mode of spread:

Endobronchial Spread

1. Centrilobular nodules (see Fig. 6–34)
2. Tree-in-bud
3. Focal areas of consolidation
4. Bronchial wall thickening or bronchiectasis
5. Usually patchy or focal

Miliary Spread

1. Random nodules, 1 to 5 mm (see Fig. 6–34)
2. Usually diffuse

Pulmonary Alveolar Proteinosis

Pulmonary alveolar proteinosis is characterized by filling of the alveolar spaces by a proteinaceous material, rich in lipid. A majority of cases are idiopathic, but some are associated with exposure to dusts (particularly silica), hematologic or lymphatic malignancies, or chemotherapy. Nocardial or mycobacterial superinfection may occur. HRCT findings can be diagnostic and include

1. Patchy or geographic ground-glass opacity
2. Smooth interlobular septal thickening in regions of ground-glass opacity

Hypersensitivity Pneumonitis

Hypersensitivity pneumonitis is an allergic lung disease resulting from exposure to one of a number of organic dusts (e.g., farmer's lung). In the acute and subacute stages, alveolitis, interstitial infiltrates, and ill-defined granulomas are present. In the chronic stage, fibrosis and honeycombing occur. In the subacute stage, HRCT typically shows

1. Patchy or geographic ground-glass opacity (Fig. 6–41)
2. Poorly defined centrilobular nodules of ground-glass opacity

Bronchiolitis Obliterans Organizing Pneumonia

This entity can be idiopathic or result from infections, toxic exposures, drug reactions, or autoimmune diseases. It typically results in progressive dyspnea and low-grade fever. Organizing pneumonia is the predominant feature, and the idiopathic form of this disease is also called cryptogenic organizing pneumonia. HRCT features are nonspecific and include

1. Patchy or nodular consolidation
2. Patchy or nodular ground-glass opacity (Fig. 6–42)
3. A peripheral or peribronchial distribution

Eosinophilic Pneumonia

Chronic eosinophilic pneumonia is idiopathic and characterized by filling of alveoli

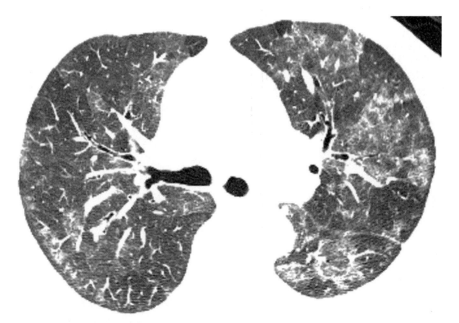

Figure 6–41. "Ground-glass" opacity in hypersensitivity pneumonitis. Multiple patchy areas of increased lung attenuation are typical of ground-glass opacity. Note that vessels remain visible within the abnormal lung regions. Ill-defined centrilobular nodules of ground-glass opacity are also visible. This appearance is typical of hypersensitivity pneumonitis.

by a mixed inflammatory infiltrate consisting primarily of eosinophils. Blood eosinophilia is usually present. Patients present with fever, cough, and shortness of breath of months' duration. HRCT features are nonspecific and similar to those of bronchio-litis obliterans obstructing pneumonia, including

1. Patchy consolidation or, less often, ground-glass opacity
2. A peripheral distribution

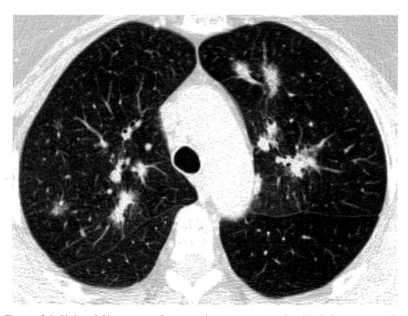

Figure 6–42. Bronchiolitis obliterans obstructing pneumonia. Nodular areas of consolidation in relation to bronchi are common in patients with this disorder.

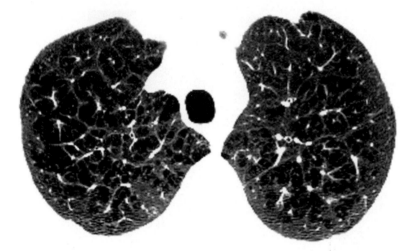

Figure 6–43. Centrilobular emphysema. On high-resolution CT, multiple spotty areas of cystic lucency without visible walls are typical of centrilobular emphysema.

Histiocytosis

Histiocytosis (Langerhans' histiocytosis or eosinophilic granuloma) is associated with centrilobular nodules early in the disease and cystic lesions late in the disease. Nodules and cysts can coexist. It occurs in both men and women, and its features include

1. Centrilobular nodules, which may be cavitary
2. Thin-walled irregular lung cysts
3. Normal-appearing intervening lung
4. Upper lobe predominance
5. Sparing of costophrenic angles

Lymphangiomyomatosis

HRCT demonstrates thin-walled cysts, with intervening lung appearing normal. When seen in a patient with a characteristic history (i.e., a woman with dyspnea, spontaneous pneumothorax, and chylous pleural effusions), the findings are diagnostic. Lymphangiomyomatosis occurs only in women of child-bearing age, but an identical abnormality can occur in patients with tuberous sclerosis, almost entirely in women. Its features include

1. Thin-walled, usually rounded lung cysts

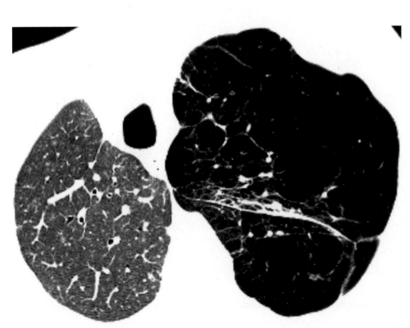

Figure 6–44. Panlobular emphysema. Panlobular emphysema in a patient with a right lung transplant. The native left lung, involved by emphysema, is too lucent and vessels are abnormally small.

2. Normal-appearing intervening lung
3. A diffuse distribution, without sparing of the lung bases
4. Lymph node enlargement or pleural effusion

EMPHYSEMA

On conventional CT, emphysema can sometimes be diagnosed if areas of low attenuation are visible; a paucity of vessels, or draping of vessels around bullae, may also be seen. However, emphysema is most accurately depicted using HRCT. On HRCT, emphysema results in areas of very low attenuation that can be easily contrasted with surrounding normal lung parenchyma if sufficiently low window means (< -700 HU) are used. Emphysema is usually distinguishable from honeycombing or cystic lung disease because in most cases the lucent areas lack visible walls (Fig. 6–43). Emphysema can be diagnosed using HRCT in symptomatic patients when chest films and pulmonary function tests are normal. On HRCT, emphysema may be classified as centrilobular, panlobular, paraseptal, and bullous.

Centrilobular emphysema is most common, usually associated with smoking, and is typically most severe in the upper lobes (see Fig. 6–43). Sometimes it appears "centrilobular" on HRCT, but the presence of "spotty" lucencies is diagnostic.

Panlobular emphysema is much less common and is often related to α_1-antitrypsin deficiency. It is diffuse or most severe at the lung bases and is manifested by an overall decrease in lung attenuation and in the size of pulmonary vessels (Fig. 6–44). Early panlobular emphysema can be very subtle.

Paraseptal emphysema is common. It involves the subpleural lung adjacent to the chest wall and mediastinum. Emphysematous spaces several centimeters in diameter are typical, and their walls are easily seen (Fig. 6–45). It can occur as an isolated abnormality in young patients or be associated with centrilobular emphysema.

Bullous emphysema is said to be present when bullae predominate. It is most often

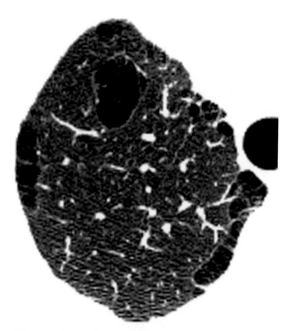

Figure 6–45. Paraseptal emphysema. Subpleural emphysema is present.

associated with paraseptal emphysema. Large bullae can be seen, particularly in young men. Bullae sometimes contain fluid as well as air, which may indicate infection.

Suggested Reading

Aberle DR, Hansell DM, Brown K, Tashkin DP. Lymphangiomyomatosis: CT, chest radiographic, and functional correlations. Radiology 1990; 176:381–387.

Akira M, Yamamoto S, Yokoyama K, et al. Asbestosis: high-resolution CT–pathologic correlation. Radiology 1990; 176:389–394.

Balakrishnan J, Meziane MA, Siegelman SS, Fishman EK. Pulmonary infarction: CT appearance with pathologic correlation. J Comput Assist Tomogr 1989; 13:941–945.

Bhalla M, Turcios N, Aponte V, et al. Cystic fibrosis: scoring system with thin-section CT. Radiology 1991; 179:783–788.

Brauner MW, Grenier P, Mompoint D, et al. Pulmonary sarcoidosis: evaluation with high-resolution CT. Radiology 1989; 172:467–471.

Davis SD. CT evaluation for pulmonary metastases in patients with extrathoracic malignancy. Radiology 1991; 180:1–12.

Engeler CE, Tashjian JH, Trenkner SW, Walsh JW.

Ground-glass opacity of the lung parenchyma: a guide to analysis with high-resolution CT. AJR 1993; 160:249–251.

Foster WL, Gimenez EI, Roubidoux MA, et al. The emphysemas: radiologic-pathologic correlations. RadioGraphics 1993; 13:311–328.

Glazer HS, Anderson DJ, DiCroce JJ, et al. Anatomy of the major fissure: evaluation with standard and thin-section CT. Radiology 1991; 180:839–844.

Grenier P, Maurice F, Musset D, et al. Bronchiectasis: assessment by thin-section CT. Radiology 1986; 161:95–99.

Gruden JF, Webb WR, Warnock M. Centrilobular opacities in the lung on high-resolution CT: diagnostic considerations and pathologic correlation. AJR 1994; 162:569–574.

Hansell DM, Moskovic E. High-resolution computed tomography in extrinsic allergic alveolitis. Clin Radiol 1991; 43:8–12.

Hruban RH, Meziane MA, Zerhouni EA, et al. Radiologic-pathologic correlation of the CT halo sign in invasive pulmonary aspergillosis. J Comput Assist Tomogr 1987; 11:534–536.

Ikezoe J, Murayama S, Godwin JD, et al. Bronchopulmonary sequestration: CT assessment. Radiology 1990; 176:375–379.

Im JG, Han MC, Yu EJ, et al. Lobar bronchioloalveolar carcinoma: "angiogram sign" on CT scans. Radiology 1990; 176:749–753.

Im JG, Itoh H, Shim YS, et al. Pulmonary tuberculosis: CT findings—early active disease and sequential change with antituberculous therapy. Radiology 1993; 186:653–660.

Kuhlman JE, Kavuru M, Fishman EK, Siegelman SS. *Pneumocystis carinii* pneumonia: spectrum of parenchymal CT findings. Radiology 1990; 175:711–714.

Kuhlman JE, Reyes BL, Hruban RH, et al. Abnormal air-filled spaces in the lung. RadioGraphics 1993; 13:47–75.

Lee KS, Kim YH, Kim WS, et al. Endobronchial tuberculosis: CT features. J Comput Assist Tomogr 1991; 15:424–428.

Lewis ER, Caskey CI, Fishman EK. Lymphoma of the lung: CT findings in 31 patients. AJR 1991; 156:711–714.

Mahoney MC, Shipley RT, Cocoran HL, Dickson BA. CT demonstration of calcification in carcinoma of the lung. AJR 1990; 154:255–258.

Mayo JR. High resolution computed tomography: technical aspects. Radiol Clin North Am 1991; 29:1043–1049.

Mayo JR, Webb WR, Gould R, et al. High-resolution CT of the lungs: an optimal approach. Radiology 1987; 163:507–510.

McGuinness G, Naidich DP, Jagirdar J, et al. High resolution CT findings in miliary lung disease. J Comput Assist Tomogr 1992; 16:384–390.

McHugh K, Blaquiere RM. CT features of rounded atelectasis. AJR 1989; 153:257–260.

Moore AD, Godwin JD, Dietrich PA, et al. Swyer-James syndrome: CT findings in eight patients. AJR 1992; 158:1211–1215.

Moore AD, Godwin JD, Müller NL, et al. Pulmonary histiocytosis X: comparison of radiographic and CT findings. Radiology 1989; 172:249–254.

Müller NL, Miller RR. Computed tomography of chronic diffuse infiltrative lung disease: I. Am Rev Respir Dis 1990; 142:1206–1215.

Müller NL, Miller RR. Computed tomography of chronic diffuse infiltrative lung disease: II. Am Rev Respir Dis 1990; 142:1440–1448.

Müller NL, Miller RR, Webb WR, et al. Fibrosing alveolitis: CT-pathologic correlation. Radiology 1986; 160:585–588.

Munk PL, Müller NL, Miller RR, Ostrow DN. Pulmonary lymphangitic carcinomatosis: CT and pathologic findings. Radiology 1988; 166:705–709.

Naidich DP. High-resolution computed tomography of cystic lung disease. Semin Roentgenol 1991; 26:151–174.

Naidich DP, Ettinger N, Leitman BS, McCauley DI. CT of lobar collapse. Semin Roentgenol 1984; 19:222–235.

Naidich DP, Garay SM. Radiographic evaluation of focal lung disease. Clin Chest Med 1991; 12:77–95.

Naidich DP, McCauley DI, Khouri NF, et al. Computed tomography of bronchiectasis. J Comput Assist Tomogr 1982; 6:437–44.

Osborne D, Vock P, Godwin JD, Silverman PM. CT identification of bronchopulmonary segments: 50 normal subjects. AJR 1984; 142:47–52.

Primack SL, Hartman TE, Hansell DM, Müller NL. End-stage lung disease: CT findings in 61 patients. Radiology 1993; 189:681–686.

Proto AV, Ball JB. Computed tomography of the major and minor fissures. AJR 1983; 140:439–448.

Remy J, Remy-Jardin M, Giraud F, Wattinne L. Angioarchitecture of pulmonary arteriovenous malformations: clinical utility of three-dimensional helical CT. Radiology 1994; 191:657–664.

Remy-Jardin M, Giraud F, Remy J, et al. Importance of ground-glass attenuation in chronic diffuse infiltrative lung disease: pathologic-CT correlation. Radiology 1993; 189:693–698.

Remy-Jardin M, Remy J, Cortet B, et al. Lung changes in rheumatoid arthritis: CT findings. Radiology 1994; 193:375–382.

Siegelman SS, Khouri NF, Leo FP, et al. Solitary pulmonary nodules: CT assessment. Radiology 1986; 160:307–312.

Siegelman SS, Khouri NF, Scott WW, et al. Pulmonary hamartoma: CT findings. Radiology 1986; 160:313–317.

Skeens JL, Fuhrman CR, Yousem SA. Bronchiolitis obliterans in heart-lung transplantation patients: radiologic findings in 11 patients. AJR 1989; 153:253–256.

Stern EJ, Frank MS. CT of the lung in patients with pulmonary emphysema: diagnosis, quantification, and correlation with pathologic and physiologic findings. AJR 1994; 162:791–798.

Stern EJ, Webb WR. Dynamic imaging of lung morphology with ultrafast high-resolution computed tomography. J Thorac Imaging 1993; 8:273–282.

Stern EJ, Webb WR, Weinacker A, Müller NL. Idiopathic giant bullous emphysema (vanishing lung syndrome): imaging findings in nine patients. AJR 1994; 162:279–282.

Swensen SJ, Harms GF, Morin RL, Myers JL. CT evaluation of solitary pulmonary nodules: value of 185-H reference phantom. AJR 1991; 156:925–929.

Swensen SJ, Brown LR, Colby TV, Weaver AL, Midthun DE. Lung nodule enhancement at CT: Prospective findings. Radiology 1996; 201:447.

Templeton PA, Zerhouni EA. High-resolution computed tomography of focal lung disease. Semin Roentgenol 1991; 26:143–150.

Webb WR. Radiologic evaluation of the solitary pulmonary nodule. AJR 1990; 154:701–708.

Webb WR. High-resolution computed tomography of the lung: normal and abnormal anatomy. Semin Roentgenol 1991; 26:110–117.

Webb WR: High-resolution CT of the lung parenchyma. Radiol Clin North Am 1989; 27:1085–1097.

Webb WR. High-resolution computed tomography of obstructive lung disease. Radiol Clin North Am 1994; 32:745–757.

Webb WR, Müller NL, Naidich DP. High Resolution CT of the Lung. New York, Lippincott-Raven, 1996.

Zerhouni EA, Stitik FP, Siegelman SS, et al. CT of the pulmonary nodule: a cooperative study. Radiology 1986; 160:319–327.

Zwirewich CV, Vedal S, Miller RR, Müller NL. Solitary pulmonary nodule: high-resolution CT and radiologic-pathologic correlation. Radiology 1991; 179:469–476.

7

Pleura, Chest Wall, and Diaphragm

W. Richard Webb, M.D.

CT plays an important role in the diagnosis of pleural and chest wall abnormalities. The cross-sectional format and excellent density resolution of CT often provide anatomic information that cannot be obtained using conventional radiographs.

TECHNICAL CONSIDERATIONS

In general, the pleura and chest wall are well evaluated using standard thoracic CT techniques with 7- to 10-mm collimation. High-resolution CT (HRCT) techniques can demonstrate the anatomy of the lung/pleura/chest wall interface better than can conventional CT; this is occasionally of value. CT after contrast medium infusion is helpful in showing pleural thickening and in allowing its differentiation from pleural fluid. Soft tissue window settings are most suitable for evaluating pleural abnormalities, the chest wall, and the diaphragm.

One must keep in mind that the diaphragm and posterior pleural space extend well below the lung bases, and scans inferior to the diaphragmatic domes must be obtained to evaluate these structures completely. Scanning with the patient in the prone position may be of assistance in evaluating pleural diseases; free pleural effusions shift to the dependent portion of the pleural space when the patient is moved from the supine position to the prone or decubitus position, whereas loculated effusions or fibrosis shows little or no change. Also, the movement of an effusion helps reveal underlying pulmonary parenchymal or pleural lesions that are otherwise obscured.

PLEURA

Anatomy

Because of the oblique orientation of the lateral ribs, usually only a short segment of each rib is visible on a single CT scan; each progressively more anterior rib represents the one arising at a higher thoracic level (Fig. 7–1). Thus, at any given level, the fifth rib, for example, is anterior to the sixth, and the fourth is anterior to the fifth. At the level of the lung apex, the first rib can be identified by its anterior position and by its articulation with the manubrium immediately below the level of the clavicle.

In some patients, a bony spur projects inferiorly from the undersurface of the first rib at its junction with the manubrium. In cross section, this bony spur can appear to be surrounded by lung and can mimic a lung nodule. This appearance is usually bilateral and symmetric, providing a clue as to its true nature. As would be expected, it often appears calcified.

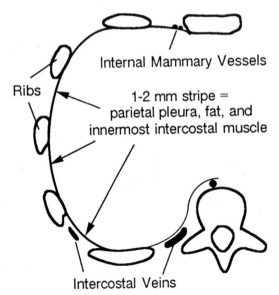

Ribs

Internal Mammary Vessels

1-2 mm stripe = parietal pleura, fat, and innermost intercostal muscle

Intercostal Veins

Figure 7–1. Normal pleura. A 1- to 2-mm line of opacity at the pleural surface primarily represents the innermost intercostal muscle, combined with the two pleural layers and the endothoracic fascia. In the paravertebral region, this stripe is much thinner or invisible.

Costal Pleura

On conventional CT or HRCT in normal subjects, a 1- to 2-mm thick opaque stripe is commonly seen in the intercostal spaces, between adjacent rib segments (see Fig. 7–1). This stripe primarily represents the innermost intercostal muscle. In the paravertebral regions, the innermost intercostal muscle is absent and a much thinner line (or no line at all) is visible at the pleural surface. The visceral and parietal pleura lie internal to ribs and innermost intercostal muscles and are separated from them by a layer of extrapleural fat, but they are not normally visible on CT.

Intrapulmonary Fissures

Intrapulmonary fissures were described in Chapter 6 (see Fig. 6–1). Normal collections of fat extending into the inferior aspects of the major fissures at the diaphragmatic surface can simulate fissural pleural thickening or effusion. These will be low in attenuation at mediastinal window settings.

Inferior Pulmonary Ligament

On each side, below the inferior pulmonary vein, the parietal and visceral pleural layers join, forming a fold that extends inferiorly along the mediastinal surface of the lung and ends at the level of the diaphragm. This fold, the *inferior pulmonary ligament,* anchors the lower lobe. On CT images viewed at lung window settings, it appears as, or is related to, a small triangular opacity 1 cm or less in size with its apex pointing laterally into the lung and its base against the mediastinum. On each side, it usually lies adjacent to the esophagus (Fig. 7–2). Pleural effusion or pneumothoraces can be limited and marginated by the inferior pulmonary ligament.

A very similar opacity can be seen on the right, lateral to the inferior vena cava (and thus anterior to the inferior pulmonary ligament), extending inferiorly to the diaphragm, and then laterally for several centimeters along the diaphragmatic surface (see Fig. 7–2). This represents the right phrenic nerve and its pleural reflection. Its only significance is that it is commonly seen and is just as commonly confusing.

Pleural Abnormalities

Pleural Thickening and Look-Alikes

Pleural thickening is visible on CT as a soft tissue curvilinear stripe, passing internal to the ribs and innermost intercostal muscles. Anytime the pleura is visible on CT, it is thickened. Thickened pleura is best seen after contrast medium infusion.

In the presence of pleural thickening, the extrapleural fat layer is often thickened as well and the visible pleura is often seen to be separated from the ribs and intercostal muscles by this fat layer. In the paravertebral regions or adjacent to the mediastinum, a distinct opaque stripe is visible in the presence of pleural thickening.

A small *pleural effusion* can mimic the appearance of pleural thickening; however, effusion is usually dependent in location and crescentic. Thickened pleura can often be distinguished from small pleural fluid collections by contrast medium infusion; thickened pleura enhances whereas fluid does not.

Normal *extrapleural fat pads*, a few millimeters thick, can sometimes be seen internal to ribs, particularly in the lower postero-

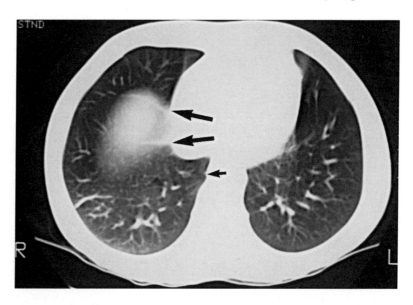

Figure 7–2. Inferior pulmonary ligament and right phrenic nerve. A small triangular opacity *(small arrow)* adjacent to the esophagus represents the right inferior pulmonary ligament. Longer linear densities near the surface of the right diaphragm *(large arrows)* represent pleural reflections adjacent to the phrenic nerves.

lateral thorax, and may not be easily distinguishable from pleural thickening or fluid. However, normal fat pads appear low in attenuation and are often symmetric, whereas pleural abnormalities generally are not. Identifying these fat pads as low in attenuation is easiest on HRCT.

The *subcostalis muscles* are sometimes visible posteriorly in the lower thorax, as a 1- to 2-mm thick stripe internal to one or more ribs. In contrast to pleural thickening, these muscles are smooth, uniform in thickness, and symmetric bilaterally.

Segments of *intercostal veins* are commonly visible in the paravertebral regions and can mimic focal pleural thickening. Continuity of these opacities with the azygos or hemiazygos veins can sometimes allow them to be correctly identified.

Pleural Effusion

Pleural fluid collections are generally crescentic, elliptical, or lenticular (Fig. 7–3). A crescentic and dependent fluid collection is likely free, rather than loculated, but a

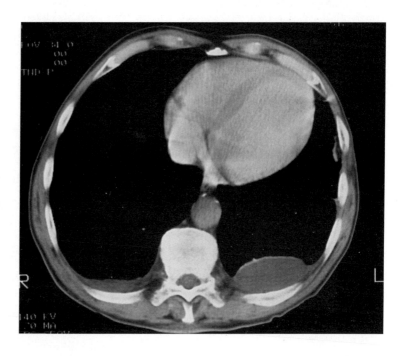

Figure 7–3. Pleural fluid. A crescentic fluid collection on the right is internal to the visible rib segment. On the left, the fluid collection is lenticular but tapers laterally.

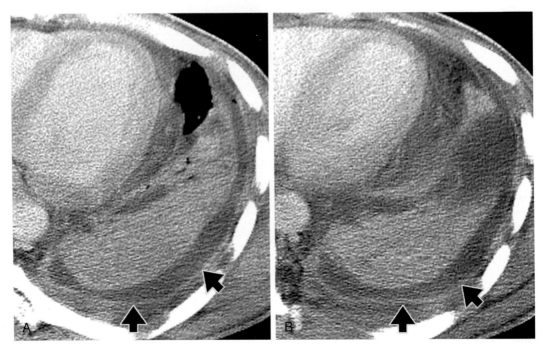

Figure 7–4. Pleural effusion with pleural thickening. In this patient with empyema, the parietal pleura is thickened (i.e., it is visible) *(arrows)*. The left lower lobe is consolidated. No visceral pleural thickening is visible.

definite diagnosis of free pleural fluid requires that a shift in effusion be demonstrated in association with a shift in patient position. Large effusions often extend into the major fissures, displacing the lower lobes medially and posteriorly. Elliptical or crescentic effusions, and effusions that are nondependent, are likely loculated.

Characterization of Pleural Fluid: Exudates and Transudates

Most effusions appear to be near to water in attenuation. CT numbers cannot be used to predict the specific gravity of the fluid or its cause. One exception, however, is acute or subacute hemothorax. Hemothorax can sometimes appear inhomogeneous, with some areas—particularly dependent regions—having an attenuation value higher than that of water. The presence of pleural thickening is usually of more value in predicting the nature of the effusion.

In patients with effusion, the presence of pleural thickening on contrast medium–enhanced CT (Fig. 7–4) indicates that the effusion is an *exudate* (a high-protein effusion associated with pleural disease) rather than a *transudate* (a low-protein effusion associated with alteration in systemic factors governing formation of pleural fluid) (Table 7–1). By definition, the pleura is considered thickened if it is visible on contrast medium–enhanced (or nonenhanced) CT. Transudates are never associated with pleural thickening (except in the rare case of a patient with preexisting pleural disease who subsequently develops an unrelated transudate).

On the other hand, the absence of pleural

TABLE 7–1. **Common Causes of Exudates and Transudates**

Exudates	Transudates
Parapneumonic effusion	Congestive heart failure
Empyema	Liver disease
Malignancy	Renal disease
Collagen vascular disease	Overhydration
Pulmonary embolism	Low serum protein
Abdominal disease	
Hemothorax	
Chylothorax	

thickening on contrast medium–enhanced CT is less helpful—in this case, the effusion can be an exudate or a transudate (Fig. 7–5). Only about 60% of exudates are associated with visible pleural thickening. However, the absence of pleural thickening on a contrast medium–enhanced scan rules out empyema; empyema is always associated with parietal pleural thickening on contrast medium–enhanced CT.

Diagnosis of Paradiaphragmatic Fluid Collections

The visceral pleura covers the surface of the lung, and its inferior extent is defined by the inferior extent of lung in the costophrenic angles. The parietal pleura is contiguous with the chest wall and diaphragm and extends well below the level of the lung bases, in the costophrenic angles. Thus, pleural fluid collections in the costophrenic angles can be seen below the lung base and can mimic collections of fluid in the peritoneal cavity.

The parallel curvilinear configuration of the pleural and peritoneal cavities at the level of the perihepatic and perisplenic recesses allows fluid in either cavity to appear as an arcuate or semilunar opacity displacing liver or spleen away from the adjacent chest wall. The relationship of the fluid collection to the ipsilateral diaphragmatic crus (see later) helps to determine its location. Pleural fluid collections in the posterior costophrenic angle lie posterior to the diaphragm and cause lateral displacement of the crus. Peritoneal fluid collections are anterior to the diaphragm and lateral to the crus, displacing it medially.

Pleural fluid can also be distinguished from ascites by the clarity of the interface of the fluid with the liver and spleen (Fig. 7–6). With pleural fluid the interface is hazy, whereas with ascites it is sharp. In patients with both pleural and peritoneal fluid, the diaphragm can often be seen as a uniform, curvilinear structure of muscle attenuation with relatively low-attenuation fluid both anteriorly and posteriorly or medially and laterally (see Fig. 7–6). Fluid seen posterior to the liver is within the pleural space; the peritoneal space does not extend into this region (this is the "bare area" of the liver).

A large pleural effusion will allow the lower lobe to float anteriorly and lose volume. The posterior edge of the lower lobe, when surrounded by fluid both anteriorly and posteriorly, can appear to represent the diaphragm (a "pseudodiaphragm"), with pleural fluid posteriorly and ascites anteriorly (Fig. 7–7). Sequential scans at more cephalad levels, however, generally will

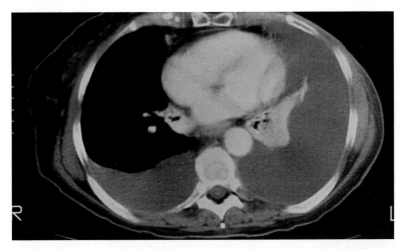

Figure 7–5. Pleural effusion without pleural thickening. Large bilateral effusions appear lower in attenuation than contrast medium–enhanced left lower lobe and heart. There is no evidence of pleural thickening; the thin line seen at the pleural surface represents the normal 1- to 2-mm intercostal stripe (i.e., it does not pass internal to the ribs). This appearance can be associated with either exudate or transudate, but it effectively rules out empyema. These effusions were malignant.

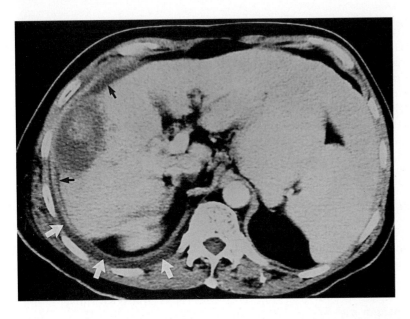

Figure 7–6. Pleural effusion and ascites. In this patient with a liver abscess both pleural effusion and ascites are present. The effusion *(white arrows)* is posterior to the diaphragm. The ascites *(black arrows)* is medial to the diaphragm, and a sharp interface with the liver is evident. Note that the diaphragm is visible as a white stripe with fluid on each side. No ascites is visible posterior to the liver.

allow the correct interpretation to be made. Typically, the arcuate opacity of the atelectatic lower lobe becomes thicker superiorly, is contiguous with the remainder of the lower lobe, and often contains air-bronchograms.

Fissural Fluid

A focal or loculated collection of pleural fluid in a major or minor fissure can have a confusing appearance on CT scans and can be misinterpreted as representing a parenchymal mass. However, careful analysis of contiguous images usually will confirm the re-

lationship of the mass to the plane of the fissure. If the abnormality also is of fluid attenuation, the diagnosis becomes more likely. The edges of the fluid collection may be seen to taper, conforming to the fissure, forming a "beak" (Fig. 7–8). Correlation of CT scans with the plain radiographs can help, particularly for fluid localized in the minor fissure.

Parapneumonic Effusions

Pleural fluid can accumulate in patients with pneumonia, even when the pleural space is uninfected. This is termed a *para-*

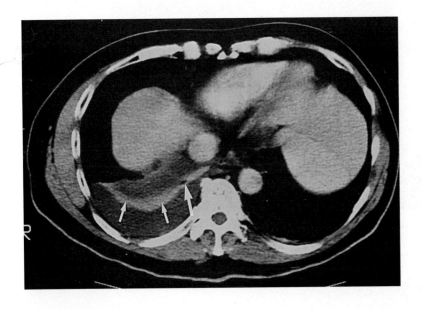

Figure 7–7. Subpulmonic effusion with a "pseudodiaphragm." In a patient with a large right pleural effusion, the collapsed posterior lower lobe *(small arrows)* simulates the diaphragm. However, an air-bronchogram *(large arrow)* within this opacity and contiguity with the lower lobe at more cephalad levels indicate its true nature.

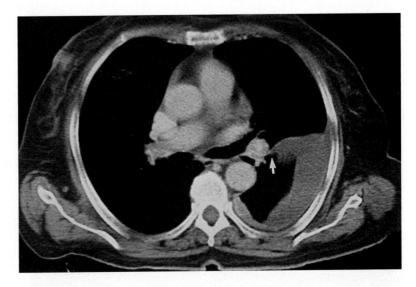

Figure 7–8. Fluid in a fissure. In this patient, fluid extends into the left major fissure. The fluid tapers medially *(arrow),* forming a "beak."

pneumonic effusion and results from increased permeability of the visceral pleura associated with the pneumonia. The effusion is usually an exudate. Distinguishing pleural effusion from adjacent consolidated lung may be difficult unless contrast medium is injected, resulting in lung opacification; the pleural fluid remains low in attenuation. Parietal pleural thickening is present in about half of patients, whereas visceral pleural thickening is seen in one fourth. Because loculation is not present, the effusion is crescentic and dependent.

Empyema

Empyema is diagnosed if pleural fluid contains infectious organisms on smear or culture. Classically, an empyema is associated with the "split-pleura" sign. This sign is said to be present when the thickened visceral and parietal pleural layers are split apart by, and surround, the empyema (Figs. 7–9 and 7–10); these pleural layers are generally of similar thickness. However, this sign is not always present. Although empyema is always associated with parietal pleural thickening on contrast medium–enhanced CT, visceral pleural thickening (and thus the "split-pleura" sign) is only present in half (see Fig. 7–4).

Empyemas can be free or loculated and crescentic (Fig. 7–11; see also Fig. 7–4), rounded, elliptical, or lenticular (see Figs. 7–9 and 7–10). In patients having a dependent and crescentic effusion, associated with pleural thickening, simple parapneumonic effusion and empyema cannot be distinguished. Loculated effusions are typically elliptical or lenticular and often nondependent; loculation is not usually present in parapneumonic effusion.

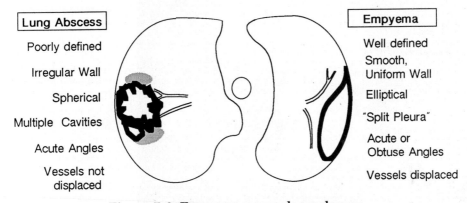

Figure 7–9. Empyema versus lung abscess.

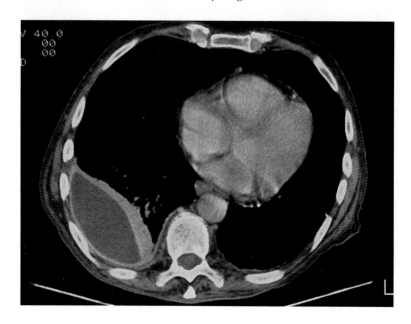

Figure 7–10. Empyema. An empyema is lenticular and well defined. After contrast medium injection, the thickened visceral and parietal pleura and the "split pleura sign" are visible.

The presence of air within the empyema almost always indicates bronchopleural fistula (see Fig. 7–11), although a gas-forming organism can also result in this appearance. This is usually an indication for tube drainage.

Extension of an empyema to involve the chest wall is termed *empyema necessitatis.* Two thirds of cases result from tuberculosis, but other responsible organisms include *Ac-* *tinomyces* and *Nocardia.* CT findings include low-attenuation fluid collections within the chest wall.

Differentiation of Empyema from Lung Abscess

Distinguishing empyema from lung abscess is sometimes important in patients who are clinically infected; empyema is often treated

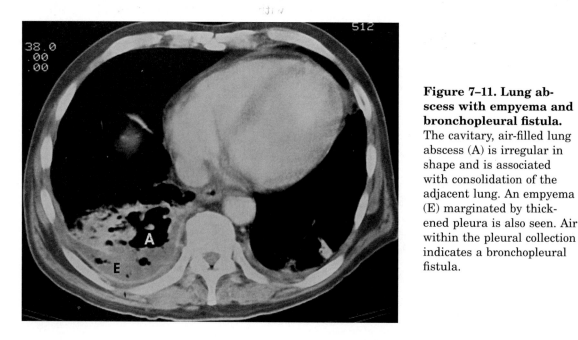

Figure 7–11. Lung abscess with empyema and bronchopleural fistula. The cavitary, air-filled lung abscess (A) is irregular in shape and is associated with consolidation of the adjacent lung. An empyema (E) marginated by thickened pleura is also seen. Air within the pleural collection indicates a bronchopleural fistula.

using tube drainage whereas lung abscess generally is not. CT can be helpful in making this distinction, particularly when contrast medium is infused.

The outer edge of an empyema is sharply demarcated from adjacent lung, and on contrast medium–enhanced scans the empyema wall appears regular in thickness. When a bronchopleural fistula is present and air is contained within the empyema cavity, or when air is introduced into the empyema at thoracentesis, its inner margin usually appears smooth.

In contrast, lung abscesses are irregularly shaped and often contain multiple areas of low-attenuation necrosis or loculated collections of air and fluid. On contrast medium–enhanced scans, the abscess wall will generally opacify relative to fluid in the abscess cavity. The inner surfaces of an abscess are often irregular and ragged, and their outer edges may be poorly defined because of adjacent pulmonary parenchymal consolidation.

At their point of contact with the chest wall, empyemas can show acute or obtuse angles (see Figs. 7–9 and 7–10), whereas abscesses typically have acute angles. Empyemas also tend to compress and displace lung and vessels, acting as a space-occupying mass, whereas lung abscesses destroy lung without displacing it (usually).

Organizing Empyema (Pleural Peel)

In patients with chronic empyema, especially tuberculous in origin, ingrowth of fibroblasts can result in pleural fibrosis and the development of chronic pleural thickening. CT may show a thickened pleural peel (Fig. 7–12). The presence of decreased volume of the affected hemithorax is a very important finding (see Fig. 7–12). Calcification, which typically is focal in its early stages (Fig. 7–13), may become extensive (Figs. 7–14 and 7–15). Frequently, a thickened layer of extrapleural fat is also visible separating the parietal pleura and the ribs (see Fig. 7–14) (this layer is considerably thicker than the fat pads, which can be seen normally). Treatment requires pleural stripping.

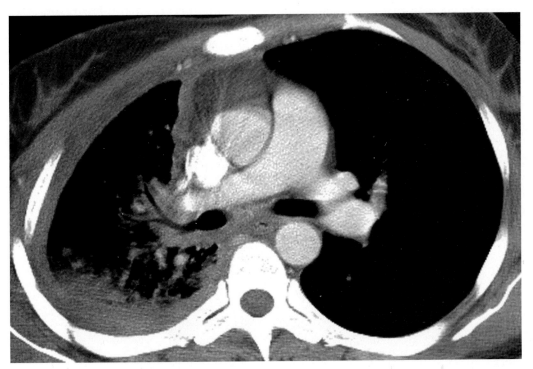

Figure 7–12. Pleural peel. A patient with prior empyema shows extensive smooth thickening of the pleura. Note that the hemithorax is reduced in volume. This is typical of pleural fibrosis.

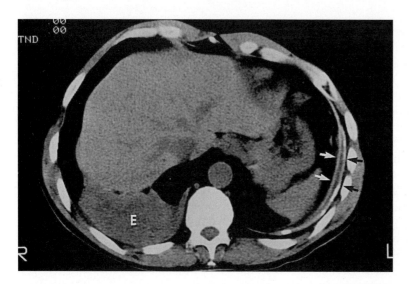

Figure 7–13. Acute and chronic empyemas. On the right side, a fluid collection (E) posterior to the liver is in the pleural space; it represents an acute empyema. On the left, pleural thickening *(arrows)* with areas of calcification reflects a healed tuberculous empyema. The "split pleura" sign is present.

Dense pleural thickening, even with calcification, does not indicate that the pleural disease is inactive. Loculated fluid collections resulting from active infection (see Fig. 7–15) may be seen on CT within the thickened pleura.

Thoracostomy Tubes

Infected pleural fluid collections often become loculated and can be difficult to drain. CT is sometimes indicated to evaluate thoracostomy tube position when the tube is functioning poorly. Malpositioned chest tubes can lie within a fissure, within a locu-

lated fluid collection (while other collections remain undrained), or outside the empyema.

Asbestos-Related Pleural Disease

Asbestos-related pleural thickening has a typical appearance on CT. Early pleural thickening is discontinuous with the intervening pleura appearing normal; focal areas of pleural thickening are termed *pleural plaques* (Fig. 7–16). The pleural disease is typically bilateral. Calcification is common. Diffuse pleural thickening, which is probably the result of prior asbestos-related

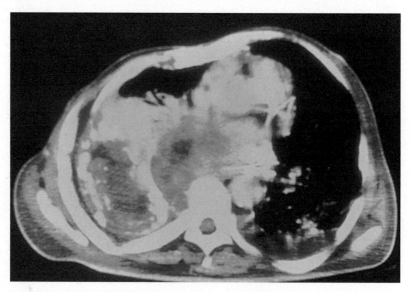

Figure 7–14. Calcified pleural thickening associated with tuberculosis. Densely calcified pleura is evident in a patient with prior tuberculosis. A fat layer separates the calcified pleura from the ribs.

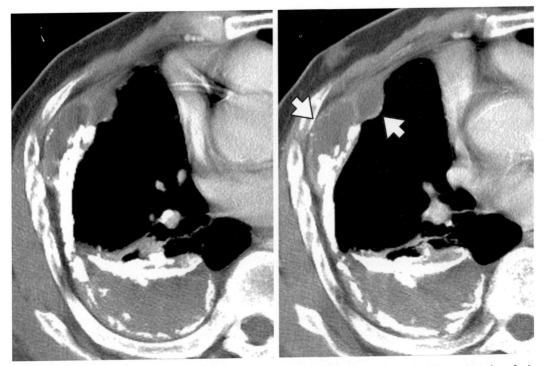

Figure 7–15. Calcified pleural thickening associated with tuberculosis. The parietal and visceral pleura is densely calcified. Residual fluid is evident in the pleural space, and loculated collections anteriorly *(arrows)* reflect active infection.

Figure 7–16. Asbestos-related pleural plaques. Typical calcified pleural plaques *(arrows)* are visible. They are often internal to ribs.

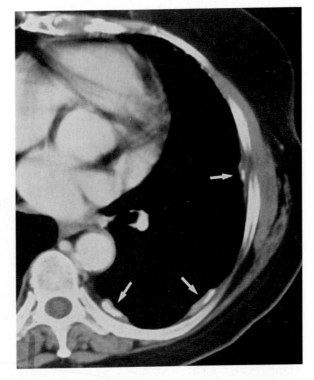

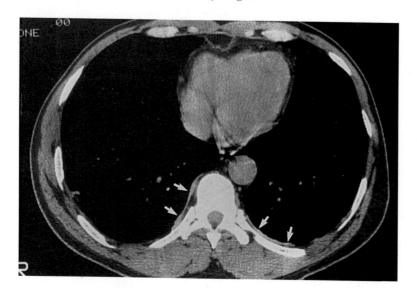

Figure 7–17. Asbestos-related pleural thickening. Linear pleural thickening *(arrows)* can be seen with asbestos exposure or other causes of pleural disease, such as rheumatoid arthritis. The thickened pleura is visible internal to the ribs.

benign pleural effusion, can also be seen (Fig. 7–17). In patients with asbestos-related pleural disease, the pleural thickening, plaques, or calcification typically involve the parietal pleura, but this is difficult to recognize on CT unless the presence of pleural fluid separates the visceral and parietal pleural layers.

The diaphragmatic pleura is commonly involved in patients with asbestos-related pleural disease. However, the diaphragm lies roughly in the plane of the scan, and the detection of uncalcified pleural plaques on the diaphragmatic surface can be difficult. In some patients, diaphragmatic pleu-ral plaques are visible deep in the posterior costophrenic angle, below the lung base; in this location, the pleural disease can be localized to the parietal pleura, because only parietal pleura is present. Pleural plaques along the mediastinum have been considered unusual in patients with asbestos-related pleural disease but are visible on CT scans in about 40% of patients. Paravertebral pleural thickening is also common.

Although it is unusual, pleural thickening can involve a fissure and result in a localized intrapulmonary pleural plaque. These may simulate a lung nodule on CT unless the plane of the fissure is identified.

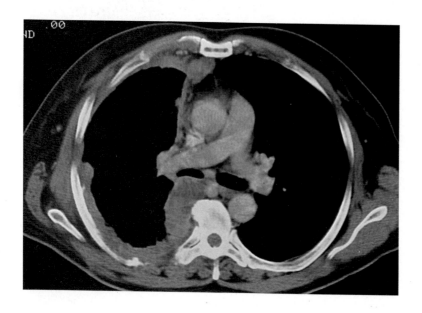

Figure 7–18. Malignant mesothelioma. There is circumferential nodular pleural thickening involving the right hemithorax. The right lung is reduced in volume compared with the left.

Pleural Effusion Associated with Malignancy

In patients with malignancy, pleural effusion can result from tumor involvement of the pleura or lymphatic obstruction in the hila or mediastinum. In both instances, an exudate is typically present. On contrast medium–enhanced CT, pleural thickening is present in a minority of patients.

The term *malignant effusion* means that malignant cells are present in the fluid. It can be present with pleural metastases or malignant mesothelioma. In patients with malignant effusion, pleural thickening may or may not be visible on contrast medium–enhanced CT.

CT findings that are helpful in diagnosing malignant involvement of the pleura are

1. Nodular pleural thickening
2. A pleural thickness of more than 1 cm
3. Thickening that concentrically involves the pleura, encasing the lung
4. Thickening of the mediastinal pleura

Malignant Mesothelioma

Diffuse or malignant mesothelioma is a highly aggressive neoplasm with an extremely poor prognosis. It is characterized morphologically by gross and nodular pleural thickening. However, hemorrhagic pleural effusion is often present and may obscure the underlying pleural thickening, which in early cases can be minimal. Malignant mesothelioma spreads most commonly by local infiltration of the pleura. In most patients, malignant mesothelioma is related to asbestos exposure; and although it is rare in the general population, the incidence in heavily exposed asbestos workers is about 5%.

In patients with malignant mesothelioma, CT can expedite the initial diagnosis and define the extent of tumor. Usually, irregular or nodular pleural thickening is visible (Fig. 7–18), although a new pleural effusion may be the only recognizable finding (Fig. 7–19). Often, pleural thickening is most pro-

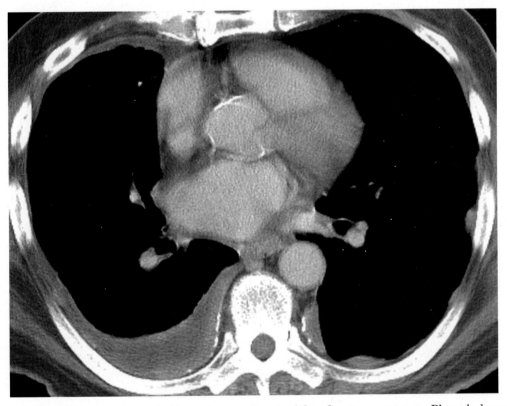

Figure 7–19. Malignant mesothelioma in a patient with asbestos exposure. Pleural plaques on the left and bilateral calcification of the parietal pleura reflect asbestos exposure. A new right pleural effusion indicates the presence of mesothelioma but is nonspecific.

nounced in the inferior thorax. Contrast medium infusion can allow tumor to be distinguished from associated fluid collections. Scans with the patient in the prone or decubitus position can also help in distinguishing underlying mesothelioma from pleural fluid.

Although mesothelioma is visible most frequently along the lateral chest wall, mediastinal pleural thickening or concentric pleural thickening is seen with extensive disease (see Fig. 7–18). The abnormal hemithorax can appear contracted and fixed, with little change in size on inspiration. Thickening of the fissures, particularly the lower part of the major fissures, can reflect tumor infiltration. Malignant mesothelioma typically spreads by local invasion, involving the mediastinum and sometimes the chest wall, but hematogenous pulmonary metastases and distant metastases do occur.

Localized Fibrous Tumor of the Pleura

Localized fibrous tumor of the pleura, previously termed *benign mesothelioma*, is uncommon. It is usually detected incidentally on chest radiographs but can be associated with chest pain, hypoglycemia, and hypertrophic pulmonary osteoarthropathy. About 60% are benign and 40% are malignant.

Localized fibrous tumor usually arises from the visceral pleura and most commonly involves the costal pleural surface (Fig. 7–20); occasionally, it can be seen within a fissure (Fig. 7–21). On CT, these tumors are solitary, smooth, sharply defined, often large lesions, contacting a pleural surface (see Fig. 7–20).

Usually a localized fibrous tumor will appear homogeneous on CT, but necrosis can result in a multicystic appearance with or without contrast medium infusion. Al-

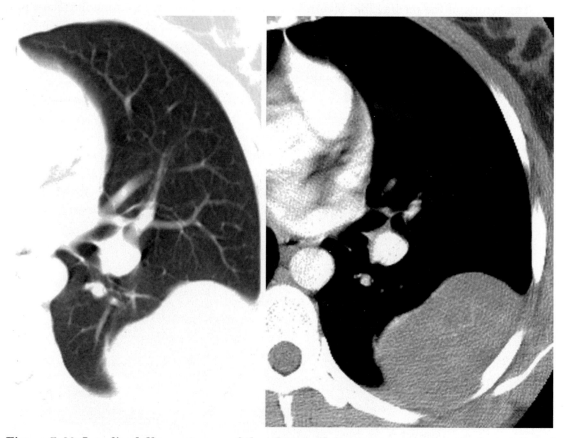

Figure 7–20. Localized fibrous tumor of the pleura. The large homogeneous mass is smooth and sharply defined. Slight "beak"-shaped pleural thickening is seen adjacent to the mass, probably related to a small amount of pleural fluid.

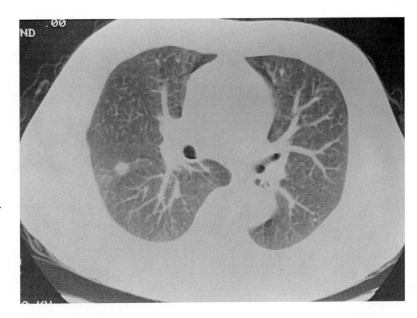

Figure 7–21. Localized fibrous tumor of the pleura. A nodular opacity, mimicking a lung nodule, represents a fibrous tumor arising in the minor fissure.

though it is generally believed that pleural abnormalities result in obtuse angles at the point of contact of the lesion and chest wall, localized fibrous tumors may show acute angles with slightly tapered pleural thickening adjacent to the mass (see Fig. 7–20). This thickening may reflect a small amount of fluid accumulating in the pleural space at the point where the visceral and parietal pleural surfaces are separated by the mass. A similar "beak" or "thorn" sign is often visible on plain radiographs in patients with a benign fissural mesothelioma.

Metastases

Malignant pleural effusion may be unassociated with visible pleural thickening. However, metastases to the pleura can also result in nodular pleural thickening visible on CT; pleural metastases are more easily seen on contrast medium–enhanced scans, being higher in attenuation than the fluid (Figs. 7–22 and 7–23). Usually pleural effusion masks the underlying pleural mass or masses on plain radiographs. Metastatic thymoma can result in pleural nodules unassociated with pleural effusion.

Pleural metastases can diffusely infiltrate the pleura, resulting in an appearance indistinguishable from that of malignant mesothelioma (Fig. 7–24). Extension into the fissures can also be seen.

Lymphoma

Pleural effusions occur in 15% of patients with Hodgkin's disease and usually reflect lymphatic or venous obstruction by mediastinal or hilar tumor, rather than by pleural involvement; effusions in Hodgkin's disease tend to resolve after local mediastinal or hilar radiation. Pericardial effusions, on the other hand, present in 5%, usually indicate direct involvement of the pericardium.

CHEST WALL

Chest Wall Abnormalities

Lung Cancer with Chest Wall Invasion

Direct invasion of the chest wall by a peripheral bronchogenic carcinoma is common. Chest wall invasion by lung cancer does not rule out surgery unless there is invasion of great vessels (i.e., subclavian artery) or vertebral body. In the lung cancer staging system (see Table 4–4), resectable tumors invading chest wall are termed *T3*; unresectable invasive tumors are *T4*. Similarly, Hodgkin's disease can involve structures of the chest wall by direct invasion from the mediastinum or lung in a small percentage of cases. Malignant mesotheli-

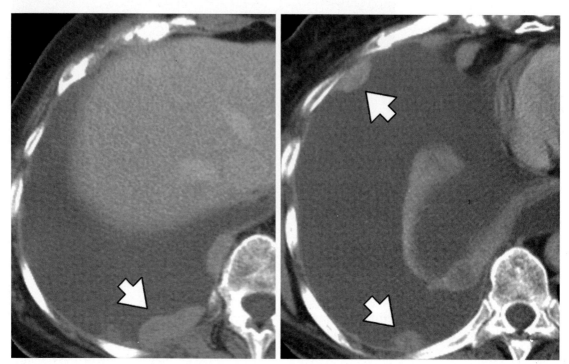

Figure 7–22. Pleural metastases from colon carcinoma. On a contrast medium–enhanced CT scan, focal nodular pleural masses *(arrows)* are visible arising from the parietal pleura. A large pleural effusion is also present.

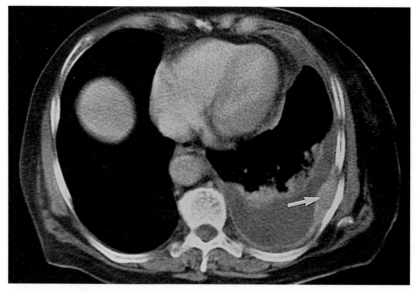

Figure 7–23. Pleural metastasis. Pleural thickening is evident after contrast medium infusion. An enhancing pleural mass *(arrow)* and pleural effusion are visible.

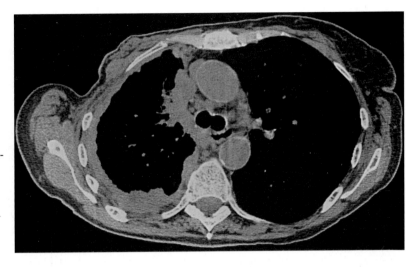

Figure 7–24. Pleural metastasis. Diffuse nodular pleural thickening in a patient with breast cancer simulates mesothelioma.

oma is a less common tumor that also can invade the chest wall.

The CT diagnosis of chest wall invasion can be difficult. A variety of CT findings can indicate chest wall invasion. The most accurate CT findings of chest wall invasion (Fig. 7–25) are

1. Extensive contact between the tumor and chest wall (> 3 cm)

2. Obtuse angles at the point of contact between tumor and pleura

3. A ratio of the length of contact of tumor with chest wall to the tumor's maximum diameter that is greater than 0.7

4. Obliteration of extrapleural fat layers
5. A chest wall mass
6. Bone destruction

Diagnosing chest wall invasion when a tumor simply abuts the pleura should be avoided. Tumors adjacent to the pleura—even when associated with focal pleural thickening and pleural effusion—may not be invasive. In a patient with bronchogenic carcinoma, pleural effusion can occur for a variety of reasons, including obstructive pneumonia and lymphatic or pulmonary venous obstruction by tumor. Only those patients with demonstration of tumor cells in

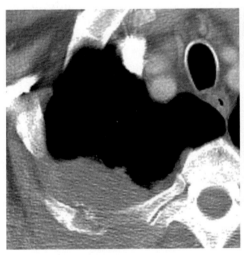 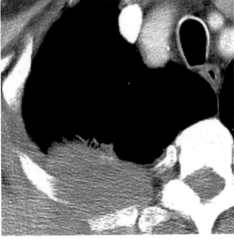

Figure 7–25. Lung carcinoma with chest wall invasion. Findings that suggest or are diagnostic of chest wall invasion in this patient include more than 3 cm of contact between the tumor and chest wall, obtuse angles with the pleura, a ratio of the length of contact of tumor with the chest wall to the tumor's maximum diameter greater than 0.7, obliteration of extrapleural fat layers posteriorly, a chest wall mass, and bone destruction.

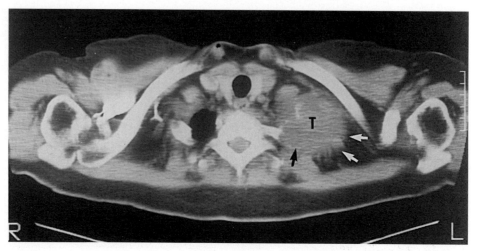

Figure 7–26. Pancoast tumor. A patient with a superior sulcus tumor (T) has rib destruction *(black arrow)* and invasion of fat by tumor *(white arrows).*

the pleural fluid are considered as having unresectable disease.

Superior Sulcus (Pancoast) Tumors

Invasive tumors arising in the superior pulmonary sulcus produce the characteristic clinical findings of Horner's syndrome and shoulder and arm pain; this presentation is termed *Pancoast's syndrome.* In the past, tumors of the superior sulcus carried a very poor prognosis, but combined therapy with radiation followed by resection of the upper lung lobe, chest wall, and adjacent structures has resulted in 5-year survival rates of up to 30%. In patients being considered for this combined therapy, CT scans can provide information on the anatomic extent of tumor spread that is useful in planning both the radiation therapy and the surgical approach to the tumor.

Extension of tumor posteriorly or laterally at the lung apex primarily involves the chest wall (Fig. 7–26). Although such chest wall invasion does not prevent resection, extensive chest wall and bone involvement makes surgical treatment difficult, and the prognosis for patients with extensive chest wall disease is poor. Invasion of tumor posteromedially will involve the ribs or vertebral bodies. This occurs in one third to one half of cases and can usually be seen on CT scans. Anterior and medial extension of tumor can involve the esophagus, trachea, and brachiocephalic vessels. Invasion of

these structures or the vertebral body precludes resection.

AXILLARY SPACE

Anatomy

As usually defined, the axilla is bordered by the fascial coverings of the following muscles: the pectoralis major and pectoralis minor anteriorly; the latissimus dorsi, teres major, and subscapularis posteriorly; the chest wall and serratus anterior medially; and the coracobrachialis and biceps laterally. However, when patients are scanned with their arms above their heads, the axilla is open laterally.

The axilla contains the axillary artery and vein, branches of the brachial plexus, some branches of the intercostal nerves, and a large number of lymph nodes, all surrounded by fat. The axillary vessels and the brachial plexus extend laterally, near the apex of the axilla, close to the pectoralis minor muscle. In general, the axillary vein lies below and anterior to the axillary artery, whereas the brachial plexus is largely above and posterior to the artery. Although these vessels usually can be seen on CT scans, in many normal persons it is impossible to distinguish artery and vein within the axilla, unless the vein is opacification by contrast medium.

Lymphadenopathy or Mass

Axillary lymph nodes, usually up to 1 cm but occasionally 1.5 cm in diameter, can be seen in normal subjects. Lymph nodes larger than 1 cm (least diameter) should be considered suspicious when an abnormality can be suspected on clinical grounds; lymph nodes 2 cm in diameter are considered pathologic regardless of history. Axillary lymphadenopathy is seen most frequently in patients with lymphoma or metastatic carcinoma. Lymph node masses are detected most easily by observing both axillae for symmetry. Enlarged lymph nodes high within the axilla lie beneath the pectoral muscles and may not be palpable, but these nodes can be detected by CT. Axillary masses in relation to nerves of the brachial plexus can also be demonstrated using CT.

BREAST

Soft tissues of the breasts are seen on CT scans of female patients in the supine position. Localized breast masses are occasion-ally visible, but their CT appearance is usually nonspecific. Breast masses detected incidentally on CT images generally should be evaluated by physical examination and mammography.

Breast Carcinoma

CT has not become an established technique for the routine evaluation of patients with breast cancer. However, CT can aid the planning of radiation therapy by providing an accurate measurement of chest wall thickness and by detecting internal mammary lymph node metastases.

Mastectomy

In women who have had a mastectomy, characteristic alterations in chest wall anatomy are seen, depending on the surgical procedure performed. CT is sometimes used to evaluate suspected local tumor recurrence and to guide needle biopsy.

A radical mastectomy consists of complete removal of the breast tissue and pectoralis major and pectoralis minor muscles and extensive axillary lymph node dissection (Fig. 7–27). On CT, although most of the pecto-

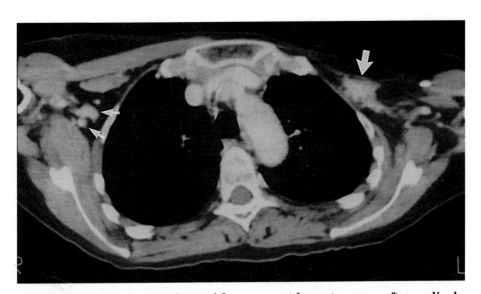

Figure 7–27. Axillary mass in a patient with recurrent breast cancer after radical mastectomy. This patient has been scanned with her arms down. The right axilla is normal, with vessels *(small arrows)* accounting for most of the visible soft tissue. On the left, the pectoralis muscles have been removed. A mass *(large arrow)* is visible in relation to axillary vessels. (From Shea WJ Jr, de Geer G, Webb WR. Chest wall after mastectomy. Part II. CT appearance of tumor recurrence. Radiology 1987; 162:162–164.)

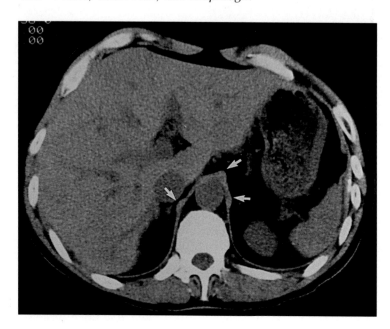

Figure 7–28. Normal diaphragm. The diaphragm is outlined by retroperitoneal fat. Where it contacts the liver and spleen it is not usually visible as a discrete structure. The diaphragmatic crura can appear quite lumpy *(arrows)*. Here they pass anterior to the aorta to form the aortic hiatus.

ralis muscles are absent, residual pectoralis major muscle is sometimes seen at its sternal or costal attachment. This should not be misinterpreted as recurrent tumor.

A typical modified radical mastectomy consists of removal of the breast and pectoralis minor muscle and an axillary lymph node dissection. The precise techniques for this procedure can vary among surgeons, and a discussion with the surgeon concerning the procedure performed is advisable before interpreting the CT scans. In patients who have undergone a modified radical mastectomy, the amount of pectoralis minor muscle remaining is variable. Without careful clinical correlation, it is sometimes difficult to distinguish postsurgical changes from tumor recurrence. This is a particular problem when the patient has difficulty elevating both arms symmetrically for the CT examination. With the arms raised, asymmetry of the pectoralis muscles is accentuated, and the scans are often very difficult to interpret. It is therefore best to obtain scans with the patient's arms at her sides.

A simple mastectomy consists of removal of only breast tissue; the underlying musculature remains intact. Residual breast tissue will remain when segmental or partial mastectomy is performed.

DIAPHRAGM

Anatomy

Because of the transaxial plane of CT, the central portion of the diaphragm does not appear as a distinct structure and its position can only be inferred by the position of the lung base above and upper abdominal organs below. However, as the more peripheral portions of the diaphragm extend caudad toward their sternal and costal attachments, the anterior, posterior, and lateral portions of the diaphragm become visible adjacent to retroperitoneal fat (Fig. 7–28). Where the diaphragm is contiguous with the liver or spleen, it cannot usually be delineated by CT unless thin-collimation CT is used and a subdiaphragmatic fat layer is present.

Diaphragmatic Crura

The right and left diaphragmatic crura are tendinous structures arising inferiorly from the anterior surfaces of the upper lumbar vertebral bodies and intervening discs and continuous with the anterior longitudinal ligament of the spine. The crura ascend anterior to the spine, on each side of the aorta, and then pass medially and anteriorly, joining the muscular diaphragm anterior to the aorta, to form the aortic hiatus (see Fig. 7–28). The right crus, which is larger and longer than the left, arises from the first three lumbar vertebral levels; the left crus arises from the first two lumbar segments.

The diaphragmatic crura can be mistaken for enlarged lymph nodes or masses because of their rounded appearance; paraaortic lymph nodes can indeed be seen in a similar position. However, on contiguous CT scans, the crura merge gradually with the diaphragm at more cephalad levels. The diameter of the crura also will vary with lung volume, increasing in thickness at full inspiration compared with expiration.

Openings in the Diaphragm

The diaphragm is perforated by several openings that allow structures to pass from the thorax to the abdomen. The aortic hiatus is posterior; it is bounded posteriorly by the vertebral body and anteriorly by the crura. Through it pass the aorta, the azygos and hemiazygos veins, the thoracic duct, the intercostal arteries, and the splanchnic nerves. The esophageal hiatus is situated more anteriorly, in the muscular portion of the diaphragm. Through it pass the esophagus, the vagus nerves, and small blood vessels. The foramen of the inferior vena cava pierces the fibrous central tendon of the diaphragm anterior and to the right of the esophageal hiatus.

Of these three structures, the aortic hiatus is defined most easily. On CT scans, the esophageal foramen is visible as an opening at the junction of the esophagus and stomach. The foramen of the inferior vena cava must be inferred from the position of the inferior vena cava. The foramina of Morgagni and of Bochdalek are not visible on CT scans in normal individuals.

Diaphragmatic Abnormalities

Hernias

Abdominal or retroperitoneal contents can herniate into the chest through congenital or acquired areas of weakness in the diaphragm or through traumatic diaphragmatic ruptures. Hernias of the stomach through the esophageal hiatus are the most common.

Hernias through the foramen of Bochdalek were thought to be uncommon in adults; however, CT has shown that small Bochdalek defects may occur in as many as 5% of normal persons. This is the most common type of diaphragmatic hernia in infants. Most are left sided; and although they are often located in the posterolateral diaphragm, they can occur anywhere along the posterior costodiaphragmatic margin (Fig. 7–29). Bochdalek hernias in adults usually contain retroperitoneal fat or, much less commonly, kidney.

Figure 7–29. Bochdalek hernia. In this patient, the hernia (H) consists of a collection of retroperitoneal fat. A small defect in the diaphragm *(arrow)* is visible at this level.

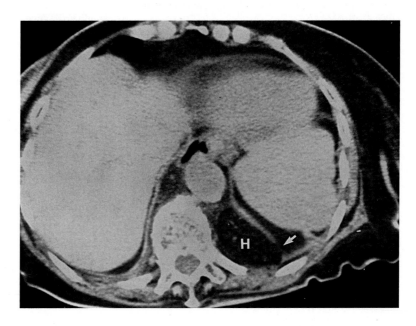

Parasternal hernias through the foramen of Morgagni are relatively rare. Most Morgagni hernias occur on the right and, in contrast to Bochdalek hernias, usually contain an extension of the peritoneal sac. Their contents can include omentum, liver, or bowel.

An understanding of the anatomy of the anterior portion of the diaphragm is essential in correctly diagnosing a Morgagni hernia. The presence of bowel anterior to the heart can suggest the presence of a hernia, but this is not usually the case.

Diaphragmatic rupture can result from penetrating or nonpenetrating trauma to the abdomen or thorax. In nearly all cases, the left hemidiaphragm is affected, with ruptures of the central or posterior diaphragm being the most frequent. Omentum, stomach, small or large intestine, spleen, or kidney may all herniate through the diaphragmatic rent.

Diaphragmatic Eventration

Local eventration of the right hemidiaphragm and superior displacement of the liver can be confused radiographically with a peripheral pulmonary or pleural mass. CT scans after infusion of contrast medium can demonstrate opacification of normal intrahepatic vessels in the apparent mass, allowing its identification. In addition, scans reformatted in the coronal plane can show that the "mass" has the same attenuation as liver.

Suggested Reading

Aberle DR, Gamsu G, Ray CS, Feuerstein IM. Asbestos-related pleural and parenchymal fibrosis: detection with high-resolution CT. Radiology 1988; 166:729–734.

Alexander E, Clark RA, Colley DP, Mitchell SE. CT of malignant pleural mesothelioma. AJR 1981; 137:287–291.

Aquino SL, Webb WR, Gushiken BJ. Pleural exudates and transudates: diagnosis with contrast-enhanced CT. Radiology 1994; 192:803–808.

Dedrick CG, McLoud TC, Shepard JO, Shipley RT. Computed tomography of localized pleural mesothelioma. AJR 1985; 144:275–280.

Friedman AC, Fiel SB, Radecki PD, Lev-Toaff AS. Computed tomography of benign pleural and pulmonary parenchymal abnormalities related to asbestos exposure. Semin Ultrasound CT MR 1990; 11:393–408.

Griffin DJ, Gross BH, McCracken S, Glazer GM. Observations on CT differentiation of pleural and peritoneal fluid. J Comput Assist Tomogr 1984; 8:24–28.

Halvorsen RA, Fedyshin PJ, Korobkin M, et al. Ascites or pleural effusion? CT differentiation: four useful criteria. Radiographics 1986; 6:135–149.

Hulnick DH, Naidich DP, McCauley DI. Pleural tuberculosis evaluated by computed tomography. Radiology 1983; 149:759–765.

Im J-G, Webb WR, Han MC, Park JH. Apical opacity associated with pulmonary tuberculosis: high-resolution CT findings. Radiology 1991; 178:727–731.

Im J-G, Webb WR, Rosen A, Gamsu G: Costal pleura: appearances at high-resolution CT. Radiology 1989; 171:125–131.

Kwong JS, Müller NL, Godwin JD, et al. Thoracic actinomycosis: CT findings in eight patients. Radiology 1992; 183:189–192.

Leung AN, Müller NL, Miller RR. CT in differential diagnosis of diffuse pleural disease. AJR 1990; 154:487–492.

Libshitz HI. Malignant pleural mesothelioma: the role of computed tomography. J Comput Tomogr 1984; 8:15–20.

McLoud TC, Flower CDR. Imaging the pleura: sonography, CT, and MR imaging. AJR 1991; 156:1145–1153.

Mirvis S, Dutcher JP, Haney PJ, et al. CT of malignant pleural mesothelioma. AJR 1983; 140:665–670.

Müller NL. Imaging the pleura. Radiology 1993; 186:297–309.

Naidich DP, Megibow AJ, Hilton S, et al. Computed tomography of the diaphragm: peridiaphragmatic fluid localization. J Comput Assist Tomogr 1983; 7:641–649.

Naidich DP, Megibow AJ, Ross CR, et al. Computed tomography of the diaphragm: normal anatomy and variants. J Comput Assist Tomogr 1983; 7:633–640.

Schmitt WGH, Hübener KH, Rücker HC. Pleural calcification with persistent effusion. Radiology 1983; 149:633–638.

Stark DD, Federle MP, Goodman PC, et al. Differentiating lung abscess and empyema: radiography and computed tomography. AJR 1983; 141:163–167.

Takasugi JE, Godwin JD, Teefey SA. The extrapleural fat in empyema: CT appearance. Br J Radiol 1991; 64:580–583.

Waite RJ, Carbonneau RJ, Balikian JP, et al. Parietal pleural changes in empyema: appearances at CT. Radiology 1990; 175:145–150.

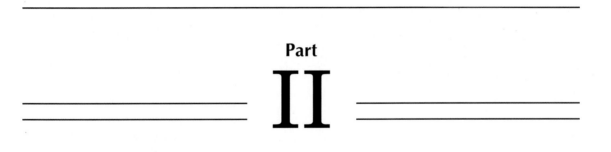

Part II

The Abdomen and Pelvis

8

Introduction to CT of the Abdomen and Pelvis

William E. Brant, M.D.

Helical (spiral) CT has rejuvenated the role of CT of the abdomen, further entrenching CT as one of the primary imaging modalities of the abdomen and pelvis. Helical CT is now the state-of-the-art for abdominal CT. Whereas magnetic resonance imaging of the abdomen continues to improve and plays a greater role in problem solving, CT remains more available, less expensive, and more panoramic for most abdominal applications. Ultrasonography continues to serve as a primary screening modality for diseases of the abdomen and pelvis but is frequently supplemented by CT when disease is found and more comprehensive evaluation is needed.

Evaluation of the abdomen by CT requires greater patient preparation, attention to technique, and individualization than CT evaluation of any other area of the body. The best quality studies are produced when the radiologist is present to evaluate the patient clinically, assess the nature of the imaging problem, and tailor the study to optimize the information the examination provides.

APPROACH

When a patient presents for an abdominal CT scan, the radiologist should assess the clinical problem to be evaluated by taking a brief patient history and reviewing all pertinent previous imaging studies. Medical history of importance to CT examination includes the current indication for the study, contrast agent allergies, cardiac and renal impairments, past abdominal surgeries, history of prior malignancies and radiation therapy, and availability of previous imaging studies. In some cases, such as determining the presence of an abdominal mass, a brief physical examination is helpful. Previous imaging studies are reviewed to ensure that all previously identified abnormalities and questionable findings are appropriately reevaluated.

Decisions to be made to individualize the examination include

1. Contrast medium to be administered: intravenous, oral, rectal, vaginal
2. Intravenous contrast medium administration rates, method of administration, and scan timing
3. Area scanned: anatomic landmarks and scan extent
4. Scan parameters: slice thickness and spacing
5. Technique: helical versus conventional, pitch, maximum breath hold, scan times, reconstruction matrix

The radiologist should review the scan before the patient leaves the CT suite to ensure a superior quality study. Any questionable areas should be reevaluated as needed.

GASTROINTESTINAL CONTRAST AGENTS

Nearly all CT scans of the abdomen require the administration of intraluminal contrast agents to opacify the gastrointestinal tract. The usual agents are radiopaque, consisting of dilute concentrations of barium or iodinated agents. Concentrations of 1% to 3% are optimal for CT, as compared with the 30% to 60% solutions used for fluoroscopy. Barium mixtures and water-soluble iodinated agents are equally effective. A number of commercial preparations are available specifically for CT.

We routinely use dilutions of 3 mL of 60% iodinated oral contrast agent in every 100 mL of water. Our standard bowel preparation for CT includes a clear liquid diet beginning at midnight before the CT examination. The patient ingests only oral contrast agents for the last 4 hours before the examination. Oral contrast agent is given in four doses of 400 mL each; at 10 PM the night before, and at 2 hours, 30 minutes, and immediately before beginning the examination. This dosage regimen will usually opacify the entire bowel including the colon and rectum. Opacification of the upper gastrointestinal tract can be attained rapidly by giving 200-mL doses of oral contrast agents every 10 minutes for 30 to 40 minutes before the CT examination. The same dilution of water-soluble contrast agent can be given as an enema to rapidly opacify the colon. A basic rule of abdominal CT is that no one can receive "too much" oral contrast medium.

Air provides both excellent contrast and bowel distention when used for CT of the gastrointestinal tract. The colon can be insufflated by placement of a Miller air-tip enema tube, such as routinely used for double-contrast barium enemas. The stomach and duodenum can be distended by use of effervescent granules that release carbon dioxide on contact with fluid in the stomach.

INTRAVENOUS CONTRAST AGENTS

Intravenous contrast agents improve the quality of abdominal CT by opacifying blood vessels, increasing the CT density of vascular abdominal organs, and improving image contrast between lesions and normal structures. When properly used, intravenous contrast agents improve the detection of most pathologic processes. Intravenous infusion by controlled mechanical injection through a well-established intravenous line provides more reliable contrast effect than hand injection or drip infusion by gravity. For most abdominal CT scans we use a 150-mL dose of 60% iodinated agent, given at 2.5 mL/sec. Onset of scanning is delayed to allow for circulation of contrast medium into the abdominal vessels. For helical scans, we begin scanning 60 to 70 seconds after initiation of contrast infusion; and for conventional scans, we delay scanning 40 to 50 seconds.

Low-osmolar iodine-based agents are the intravenous contrast media of choice for most abdominal scanning because of their lower rate of adverse reactions. Vomiting and patient motion induced by the "heat" sensation of rapid bolus administration of ionic contrast agents will obviously impair optimal timing of scanning with contrast medium administration. Although cost considerations may force the use of much less expensive ionic contrast agents, the use of low-osmolar agents is considered to be mandatory in the following situations:

1. Prior history of moderate to severe contrast agent reaction, including hypotension, bronchospasm, or required hospitalization

2. History of severe asthma or allergies

3. History of severe heart disease, arrhythmias, congestive heart failure

4. Multiple myeloma or sickle cell anemia

5. Age younger than 1 year

6. Impaired renal function with creatinine value greater than 2 mg/dL

7. CT angiography applications

The goal of contrast medium–enhanced CT scanning of the abdomen is to scan during maximum contrast enhancement and to avoid scanning during the equilibrium phase of contrast enhancement when the contrast concentration within blood vessels is equal to the contrast concentration in the extracellular space. Scanning during maximal enhancement improves the conspicuity of lesions, whereas scanning during equilibrium obscures lesions (Fig. 8–1). Contrast equilibrium is reached in about 2 minutes after the onset of intravenous contrast agent injection.

ADDITIONAL PATIENT PREPARATION

When scanning the female pelvis, particularly when evaluating for pathology of the female organs, the patient is often asked to place a tampon in her vagina. The tampon appears as a cylinder of air density on CT distending the vagina.

Sterile iodinated contrast agents approved for intravenous injection can be injected into indwelling catheters, drainage tubes, sinus tracts, and so on to evaluate extent of disease. Dilution of contrast agent to a 1% to 3% concentration is needed to avoid streak artifact on CT. High-osmolar ionic meglumine-based agents are satisfactory for this application.

SCAN TECHNIQUE

Helical CT

Helical (spiral) CT is performed by moving the patient table at a constant speed through the CT gantry while scanning continuously with an x-ray tube rotating around the patient. A continuous volume of image data is acquired during a single breath hold. This technique dramatically improves the speed of image aquisition, allows scanning during optimal contrast opacification, and eliminates artifacts due to misregistration and variations in patient breathing. The entire liver may be scanned in a single breath hold and the entire abdomen and pelvis in two to three breath holds, all during the first 90 seconds of contrast medium administration. Volume acquisition allows retrospective reconstruction of multiple overlapping slices, improving visualization of small lesions and allowing high-detail three-dimensional CT rendering. The image parameters to be selected for helical CT include the following:

1. *Slice thickness* is selected and fixed before scan acquisition by selecting the collimation setting for the x-ray beam. Most scanners allow choices between 1 and 10 mm. Because volume averaging effects are more pronounced with helical, as compared

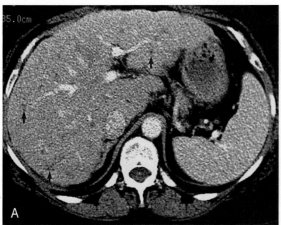 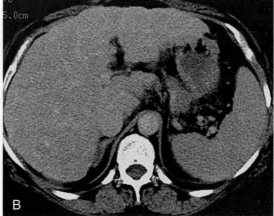

Figure 8–1. Timing of contrast medium administration with CT scanning. Early (arterial phase) *(A)* and later (equilibrium phase) *(B)* CT scans of the liver demonstrate the importance of optimizing the timing of CT scanning with the intravenous bolus administration of contrast agents. Small metastatic nodules *(A, arrows)* from lung carcinoma, seen on the arterial phase scan, cannot be seen on the equilibrium phase scan obtained less than 2 minutes later.

with conventional, CT, most abdomen applications use a slice thickness of 7 or 8 mm. Higher detail scanning, such as for the kidneys or pancreas, frequently use 5-mm thick slices. Slice thickness cannot be altered after scanning is completed.

2. *Slice reconstruction interval* may be selected prospectively (before scanning) or retrospectively (after scanning). Routine survey examinations usually reconstruct slices at intervals equal to slice thickness (i.e., 7-mm thick slices at 7-mm intervals). Better visualization of small lesions can be attained retrospectively by reconstructing overlapping slices (i.e., 7-mm thick slices at 3-mm intervals). CT angiography and three-dimensional CT require many overlapping slices for optimal images (i.e., 5-mm thick slices at 1-mm intervals). Additional slices can be reconstructed after scanning is complete and without additional patient radiation exposure, provided the image "raw data" are still available in the scanner.

3. *Scan time* for helical CT is the time required for the tube to make one 360° rotation. Scan time for modern helical scanners is 1 second or less.

4. *Pitch,* for helical CT, is defined as the ratio of table movement, during one 360° scan, to the slice thickness. With table movement of 7 mm/sec, scan time of 1 second, and slice thickness of 7 mm, pitch is equal to 1. With a table movement of 10.5 mm/sec, scan time of 1 second, and slice thickness of 7 mm, pitch is equal to 1.5. Currently, most abdominal protocols use a pitch of 1 to 1.5. A greater pitch allows scanning of a larger patient volume for any given total scan time, but at the cost of greater image noise and poorer resolution.

5. *Total scanning time and scanned patient volume* is limited primarily by each patient's ability to hold his or her breath. Scan protocols are designed around this limitation. With current helical scanners, the entire liver can be scanned with a 30-second breath hold using 7-mm collimation, a scan time of 1 second, and pitch of 1. This protocol allows a range of 21 cm of patient length to be scanned in a single helical volume acquisition. Patients with shorter breath-holding ability, and longer ranges of coverage, can be scanned by using sequential helical acquisitions separated by a short breathing interval or by increasing the pitch.

6. *Scan delay* refers to time between the initiation of contrast medium injection and the onset of scanning. For helical CT of the liver, a scan delay of 60 to 70 seconds allows, for most patients, optimal contrast opacification of the liver and portal and hepatic veins. The speed of helical scanning allows the liver to be scanned twice, during both early and late (arterial and portal venous) stages of nonequilibrium contrast medium enhancement to optimize lesion detection and characterization.

7. *Field of view and image matrix.* To optimize spatial resolution, the reconstruction field of view must be matched to the cross-sectional area of the patient. Smaller fields of view provide better spatial resolution. The image matrix selected determines the number of pixels (picture elements) that make up the CT image. For abdominal applications, a 512×512 image is usually used. This matrix provides 262,144 pixels in each image.

Some disadvantages of helical CT include vascular flow artifacts and increased volume averaging effects. When intravenously administered contrast agent levels are at their peak in the arterial system, veins usually show no contrast opacification or a confusing mixture of contrast medium with unopacified blood in the veins simulating thrombus (Fig. 8–2). Early scans show the kidneys with only cortical enhancement. Delayed scans may be needed for optimal venous opacification and a total contrast nephrogram effect.

The volume profile for any CT slice obtained by helical technique resembles a triangle with the apex (thinnest portion) at the center of the reconstructed slice and the base (thickest portion) at the periphery of the slice. A 10-mm slice obtained by helical technique has more volume averaging than a 10-mm slice obtained by conventional CT. For this reason, helical CT protocols commonly use narrower slice collimation (i.e., 7 mm rather than 10 mm).

Conventional CT

Conventional (nonhelical) CT obtains image data one slice at a time. The patient holds

Figure 8–2. Poor venous mixing. Early (arterial phase) helical CT scan through the upper abdomen demonstrates limited mixing of contrast medium with unopacified blood in the inferior vena cava *(arrow)*. The appearance of poor contrast medium/venous blood mixing may be indistinguishable from thrombus with the vein. Note the enhancement of only the cortex of the kidneys while the medulla remains unopacified.

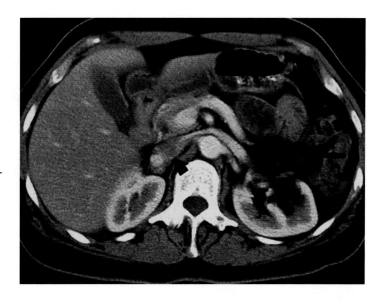

his or her breath, a slice is taken, the patient breathes, the table moves, and the sequence is repeated. This technique requires at least two to three times the total scanning time of helical CT for any given patient scan volume, making optimization of scanning during maximum contrast more difficult. Minor changes in lung volume with each breath hold may make substantial changes in the anatomy scanned, resulting in "skip" areas. More recent scanners can simulate helical scanning by "cluster" technique. Several sequential scans are obtained during a single breath hold. Parameters to be selected for conventional CT include the following:

1. *Slice thickness* for routine conventional CT of the abdomen is 8 to 10 mm.
2. *Slice interval* is routinely equal to slice thickness allowing for contiguous stacked slices (i.e., 10 mm thick at 10-mm intervals).
3. *Scan time* for modern conventional scanning is usually 1 to 2 seconds for each 360° slice. Scan times longer than 2 seconds often result in unacceptable motion artifacts owing to peristalsis, heart motion, vessel pulsation, and patient movement.
4. *Table incrementation time* (interscan delay) is the time required for the patient couch to move from one slice location to the next. The table incrementation time is usually equal to the scan time. Therefore, a single slice may require 4 seconds: 2-second

scan time + 2-second table incrementation time.

5. *Total scanning time and scanned patient volume* is determined by scan time, table incrementation time, and patient breathing time. The total patient volume that can be scanned in any given amount of time is significantly less than with helical technique.
6. *Scan delay* used for conventional technique is usually less than that for helical scanning because of the greater total scan time required to scan any given patient volume. To scan the entire liver during the prime first 2 minutes of contrast medium administration usually requires a scan delay of 30 seconds. The upper liver may be "underenhanced" whereas the lower liver is scanned in equilibrium.
7. *Field of view and image matrix.* As with helical CT, proper technique includes matching the field of view to the cross-sectional area of the patient. An image matrix of 512 × 512 pixels is also standard for conventional CT. When performing interventional procedures, a 256 × 256 matrix is usually adequate and provides a faster image reconstruction time.

CT Angiography

Applications for CT angiography are still being developed. Volumetric CT scanning with helical technique can provide many

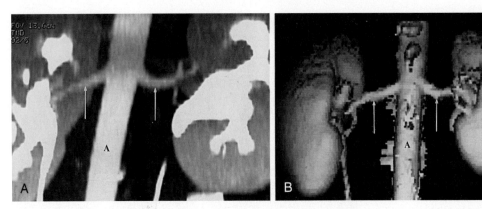

Figure 8–3. CT angiography. CT angiography was performed to demonstrate renal artery (A) anatomy before donation of a kidney for renal transplantation. Maximum intensity projection image *(A)* and shaded surface rendered image *(B)* demonstrate the branching pattern in the renal hilum of single renal arteries *(arrows)* supplying each kidney. This 20-minute CT study provided comprehensive evaluation of the kidneys and their vascular supply and saved the patient the risks of conventional catheter angiography. CT angiography images can be rotated, analyzed, and displayed in multiple projections. A = aorta.

overlapping slices with bright vessel enhancement. Three-dimensional CT angiograms can be constructed by computer from the image reconstructions by using maximum intensity projection or shaded surface display algorithms (Fig. 8–3).

IMAGE PHOTOGRAPHY

Each CT image of the abdomen contains much more information than can be displayed by any one window width and level setting. Routine "soft tissue" windows (win-

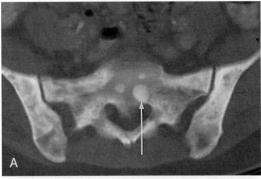

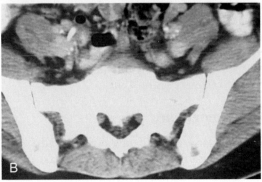

Figure 8–4. Bone windows. Metastatic lesions *(arrow)* from prostate carcinoma to the sacrum and iliac bones are obvious on "bone window" *(A)* but cannot be seen on routine "soft tissue window" *(B)*.

dow width ~400; window level 30–50) define most abdominal anatomy. However, the liver should also be inspected using narrower "liver windows" (window width ~150; window level 70–80) to increase image contrast within the liver and improve visibility of subtle lesions. The lung bases are included on scans through the upper abdomen and should be inspected using "lung windows" (window width 1000–2000; window level 600–700). Lastly, inspection of the bones using "bone windows" (window width ~2000; window level ~600) may yield important clues to pathologic findings within the abdomen (Fig. 8–4).

Suggested Reading

Baron RL. Understanding and optimizing use of contrast material for CT of the liver. AJR 1994; 163:323–331.

Berland LL. Slip-ring and conventional dynamic hepatic CT: contrast material and timing considerations. Radiology 1995; 195:1–8.

Bluemke DA, Chambers TP. Spiral CT angiography: an alternative to conventional angiography. Radiology 1995; 195:317–319.

Dillon EH, van Leeuwen MS, Fernandez A, Mali WPTM. Spiral CT angiography. AJR 1993; 160:1273–1278.

Heiken JP, Brink JA, Vannier MW. Spiral (helical) CT. Radiology 1993; 189:647–656.

Herts BR, Einstein DM, Paushter DM. Spiral CT of the abdomen: artifacts and potential pitfalls. AJR 1993; 161:1185–1190.

Shirkhoda A. Diagnostic pitfalls in abdominal CT. RadioGraphics 1991; 11:969–1002.

Silverman PM, Cooper CJ, Weltman DI, Zeman RK. Helical CT: practical considerations and potential pitfalls. RadioGraphics 1995; 15:25–36.

Stehling MK, Lawrence JA, Weintraub JL, Raptopoulos V. CT angiography: expanded clinical applications. AJR 1994; 163:947–955.

Zeman RK, Fox SH, Silverman PM, et al. Helical (spiral) CT of the abdomen. AJR 1993; 160:719–725.

Zeman RK, Silverman PM, Vieco PT, Costello P. CT angiography. AJR 1995; 165:1079–1088.

Zeman RK, Zeiberg AS, Davros WJ, et al. Routine helical CT of the abdomen: image quality considerations. Radiology 1993; 189:395–400.

9

Peritoneal Cavity, Vessels, and Nodes

William E. Brant, M.D.

PERITONEAL CAVITY

Anatomy

The various recesses and spaces of the peritoneal cavity are easiest to recognize on CT when ascites is present (Fig. 9–1). Identifying the precise compartment that an abnormality is in goes a long way toward identifying the nature of the abnormality and deciding on a plan for intervention. Whereas all the spaces of the peritoneal cavity potentially communicate with one another, diseases, such as abscesses, tend to loculate within one or more specific locations. The right subphrenic space communicates around the liver with the anterior subhepatic and posterior subhepatic (Morison's) space. The left subphrenic space communicates freely with the left subhepatic space. The right and left subphrenic spaces are separated by the falciform ligament and do not communicate directly. The lesser sac is the isolated peritoneal compartment between the stomach and the pancreas (see Fig. 12–1). It communicates with the rest of

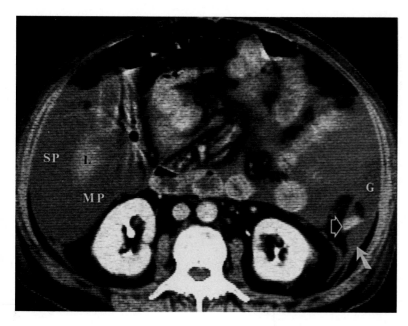

Figure 9–1. Ascites. CT image through the mid abdomen at the level of the tip of the liver (L) demonstrates low-density ascites filling the peritoneal cavity and outlining the peritoneal recesses. The right subphrenic space (SP) is seen to communicate freely with Morison's pouch (MP), the right posterior subhepatic space. The right subphrenic/subhepatic space continues caudad to the pelvis as the right paracolic gutter. The left paracolic gutter (G) is seen to extend three fourths of the way around the descending colon *(open arrow)*, forming a deep recess *(solid arrow)*.

the peritoneal cavity (greater sac) through the foramen of Winslow.

The right subphrenic and subhepatic spaces communicate freely with the pelvic peritoneal cavity by means of the right paracolic gutter. The phrenicocolic ligament prevents free communication between the left subphrenic/subhepatic spaces and the left paracolic gutter. Free fluid, blood, infection, and peritoneal metastases commonly settle in the pelvis because the pelvis is the most dependent portion of the peritoneal cavity, and it communicates with both sides of the abdomen.

The small bowel mesentery suspends the jejunum and ileum and contains branches of the superior mesenteric artery and vein, as well as mesenteric lymph nodes. The mesentery extends like a fan obliquely across the abdomen from the ligament of Treitz in the left upper quadrant to the region of the right sacroiliac joint. Disease originating from above the ligament is directed toward the right lower quadrant. Disease originating from below the ligament has open access to the pelvis.

The greater omentum is a double layer of peritoneum that hangs from the greater curvature of the stomach and descends in front of the abdominal viscera. The greater omentum encloses fat and a few blood vessels. It serves as fertile ground for implantation of peritoneal metastases.

Fluid in the Peritoneal Cavity

Fluid in the peritoneal cavity originates from many different sources and varies greatly in composition. *Ascites* refers to accumulation of serous fluid within the peritoneal cavity and results from cirrhosis, hypoproteinemia, congestive heart failure, or venous obstruction. Exudative ascites is associated with inflammatory processes such as pancreatitis, peritonitis, and bowel perforation. Neoplastic ascites is caused by intraperitoneal tumor. Chylous ascites is due to obstruction or traumatic injury to the thoracic duct or cisterna chyli. Urine and bile may spread through the peritoneal cavity owing to obstruction or injury to the urinary or biliary tracts. *Hemoperitoneum* is an important sign of abdominal injury in blunt trauma.

When the anatomy of the peritoneal cavity is known, recognition of fluid density within its recesses on CT is easy. When free peritoneal fluid is present, bowel loops tend to float to the central abdomen.

Paracentesis is required for precise differentiation of the exact type of fluid present in the peritoneal cavity. However, CT can offer some clues. Serous ascites has an attenuation value near water (-10 to $+15$ H) and tends to accumulate in the greater peritoneal space, sparing the lesser sac. On the other hand, exudative ascites due to pancreatitis tends to preferentially accumulate within the lesser sac. Acute bleeding into the peritoneal cavity has a higher attenuation value, averaging 45 H, and is usually above 30 H. Blood tends to accumulate in greatest amount about the site of hemorrhage. Exudative and neoplastic ascites have intermediate attenuation values that overlap those of both serous ascites and blood.

Loculations of peritoneal fluid due to benign or malignant adhesions may simulate cystic abdominal masses. Tense loculated ascites may accumulate in confined spaces like the lesser sac and compress and displace bowel loops. Loculated ascites, however, tends to conform to the general shape of the space it occupies. Cystic masses make their own space, cause greater displacement of adjacent structures, and have more varied internal consistency.

Pseudomyxoma peritonei is an unusual complication of mucocele of the appendix or of mucinous cystadenocarcinoma manifested by filling of the peritoneal cavity with gelatinous mucin. The mucinous fluid is typically loculated and causes scalloping and mass effect on the liver and adjacent bowel (Fig. 9–2). Septations, mottled densities, and calcification within the fluid may be seen on CT.

Free Air in the Peritoneal Cavity

Free air within the peritoneal cavity is an important sign of perforated viscus but may be surprisingly difficult to recognize on CT. The diagnosis is based on recognizing that the air is outside of the bowel lumen. Images should be routinely examined at "lung

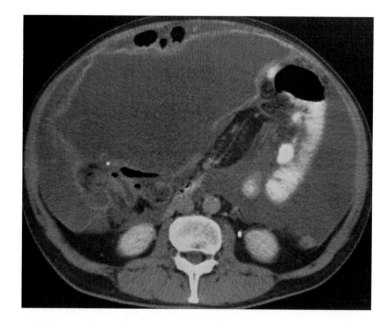

Figure 9–2. Pseudomyxoma peritonei. Gelatinous ascites, from rupture of an appendiceal mucocele, causes septations and loculations of intraperitoneal fluid.

windows" (window level −400 to −600 H; window width 1000–2000 H) for free intra-peritoneal air. Unsuspected pneumothorax may also be detected using this technique on abdominal CT scans obtained because of abdominal trauma. Before ascribing pneu-moperitoneum to bowel perforation, a tho-racic source, such as pneumothorax or me-chanical ventilation, should also be considered.

Tumors in the Peritoneal Cavity

Peritoneal Carcinomatosis. Diffuse met-astatic seeding of the peritoneal cavity oc-curs commonly with abdominopelvic tu-mors. The most common tumors to spread by this method are ovarian carcinoma in females and stomach, pancreas, and colon carcinoma in males. The preferential sites for tumor implantation are the pouch of Douglas, the right paracolic gutter, and the greater omentum. CT findings with perito-neal tumor seeding (Fig. 9–3) are

1. Ascites, frequently loculated
2. Tumor nodules on the parietal perito-neal surface
3. "Omental cake"—thickened nodular greater omentum displacing bowel away from the anterior abdominal wall
4. Tumor nodules in the mesentery
5. Thickening and nodularity of the bowel wall due to serosal tumor implant

Minute implants, which may be painfully obvious and diffuse at surgery, are com-monly missed by CT owing to their small size. The presence of ascites in patients with known abdominopelvic tumor, especially ovarian carcinoma, should be regarded as suspicious for peritoneal seeding. Calcifica-tion of tumor implants may aid in their CT identification.

Peritoneal Mesothelioma. Twenty to 40% of mesotheliomas arise within the abdomen. On CT, mesothelioma causes diffuse irregu-lar thickening of the peritoneal surfaces. Nodules and globular thickening are com-monly evident. Multilocular cystic forms of the tumor also occur. Ascites is present in most cases.

Abscess

CT is commonly performed to search for and destroy abdominal abscesses. Once found, percutaneous aspiration confirms the diag-nosis and provides material for culture. Im-age directed catheter placement is com-monly used for drainage ("pus busting"). Most abscesses occur as complications of ab-dominal trauma, surgery, pancreatitis, or bowel perforation (ruptured appendicitis, diverticulitis). Intraperitoneal abscesses are commonly located in the pelvic cavity and the subphrenic and subhepatic spaces. CT features of abscess (Figs. 9–4 and 9–5) are

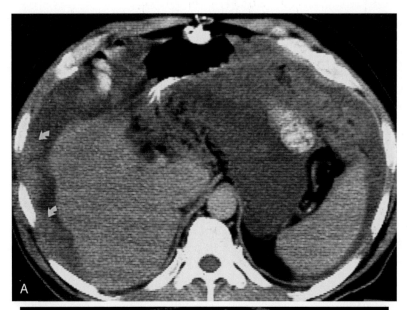

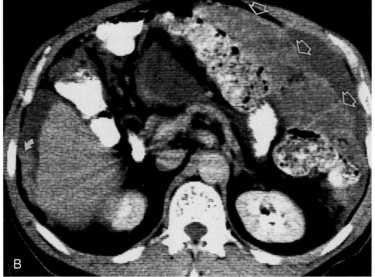

Figure 9–3. Peritoneal implants and omental cake. CT scans through the upper *(A)* and lower *(B)* portions of the liver demonstrate peritoneal metastases due to colon carcinoma. Tumor metastases *(solid arrows)* on the parietal peritoneum are seen as soft tissue density masses projecting into peritoneal fluid. Tumor implants on the greater omentum *(open arrows)* produce a soft tissue density pancake ("omental cake") separating bowel from the anterior abdominal wall.

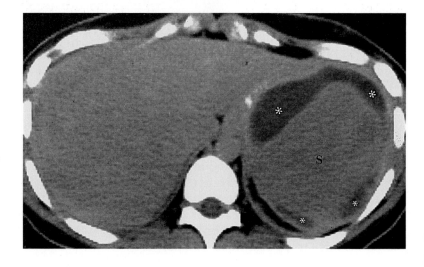

Figure 9–4. Left subphrenic abscess. An abscess in the left subphrenic recess of the peritoneal cavity is seen as loculations of the fluid density (*) surrounding the spleen (S).

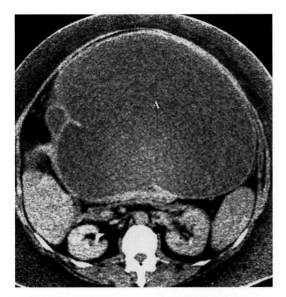

Figure 9–5. Huge abdominal abscess. Image obtained through the mid abdomen in a very obese patient demonstrates a huge cystic mass (A) with well-defined thick walls. This mass contained 14 liters of purulent green fluid that grew *Streptococcus agalactiae*.

1. Loculated fluid collection, often with internal debris, fluid–fluid levels, and septations
2. Common definable walls, often irregularly thickened
3. Presence of gas within the fluid collection
4. Thickening of fascia and obliteration of fat planes due to inflammation
5. Ascites, pleural effusions, and lower lobe pulmonary infiltrates

Any fluid collection within the abdomen is suspect in patients in whom abscess is suggested. Fine-needle aspiration is a safe and definitive way to exclude or confirm the diagnosis.

Cystic Abdominal Masses

Cystic masses in the abdomen commonly present challenges in diagnosis (Fig. 9–5). Differential considerations include

1. Abscess
2. Loculated ascites
3. Pancreatic pseudocyst
4. Ovarian cyst/cystic tumor
5. Lymphocele—a cystic mass containing

lymphatic fluid that occurs as a complication of surgery or trauma that disrupts lymphatic channels. It may be of any size and appear days to years after surgery.

6. Cystic lymphangioma—a congenital counterpart of lymphocele believed to arise due to congenital obstruction of lymphatic channels. Most are thin walled and multiloculated. Attenuation ranges from water to fat density. *Mesenteric cysts* are cystic lymphangiomas of the mesentery. *Omental cysts* are less common cystic lymphangiomas of the greater omentum.

7. Enteric duplication cysts are lined with gastrointestinal mucosa and are usually attached to normal bowel.

8. Cystic teratoma may arise in the retroperitoneum, mesentery, or omentum. CT shows a complex cystic and solid mass with areas of water and fat attenuation and calcifications.

VESSELS

Anatomy

The abdominal aorta descends anterior to the left side of the spine to its bifurcation at the level of the iliac crest. The normal aorta does not exceed 3 cm in diameter and tapers progressively as it proceeds distally. The inferior vena cava lies to the right of the aorta. Its shape varies from round to oval to slitlike depending on breath holding technique and intravenous fluid balance. The common iliac arteries and veins appear oval in cross section as they diverge from the midline. The common iliac vessels bifurcate at the pelvic brim, which is identified by noting the shape of the sacrum change from convex anteriorly (the sacral promontory) to concave. The external iliac vessels course anteriorly to the inguinal triangle, whereas the internal iliac (hypogastric) vessels have many small branches in the posterior pelvis. The iliac arteries normally do not exceed 1.5 cm in diameter.

The celiac axis originates from the anterior aspect of the aorta at the level of the aortic hiatus in the diaphragm. The superior mesenteric artery originates anteriorly from the aorta 1 cm below the celiac axis. The renal arteries arise from the lateral aspect of the aorta within 1 cm of the superior mesenteric artery. The inferior mesenteric artery is a tiny anterior branch off the aorta just above the bifurcation.

A number of vascular anomalies must be recognized to avoid misinterpretation as abnormalities. Duplication of the inferior vena cava may be identified extending between the left common iliac vein and the left renal vein on the left side of the aorta (Fig. 9–6). Left renal veins may course posterior instead of anterior to the aorta (retroaortic left renal vein), or duplicated left renal veins may course both anterior and posterior to the aorta (circumaortic left renal vein). The intrahepatic segment of the inferior vena cava may be absent, with drainage continuing to the superior vena cava by means of the azygos system.

Technical Considerations

Scanning of the aorta and venae cavae is routinely performed using contiguous 7- to 10-mm thick slices after both oral and intravenous contrast medium enhancement. Spiral CT optimizes intravascular contrast medium enhancement. In cases of suspected aneurysm rupture or inflammatory aneurysm, both preinfusion and postinfusion scans should be obtained. Acute higher density hemorrhage is more obvious on preinfusion scans. Demonstration of enhancement of the periaortic tissue confirms the diagnosis of inflammatory aneurysm.

Aortic Aneurysm

Aneurysms are defined as circumscribed dilatations of an artery. CT provides more comprehensive evaluation of abdominal aortic aneurysms than does ultrasonography. Several types of aneurysms are defined (Fig. 9–7).

True Aneurysm. A true aneurysm involves all three layers of the arterial wall (intima, media, and adventitia). Most are due to atherosclerotic disease that weakens the vessel wall and allows it to dilate. CT findings include

1. Fusiform, saccular, or spherical dilatation of the aorta (Fig. 9–8)
2. Outer-to-outer diameter of the abdominal aorta greater than 3 cm. Risk of rupture depends on the size of the aneurysm. The risk is about 5% for abdominal aortic aneurysms less than 5 cm, 16% for those greater

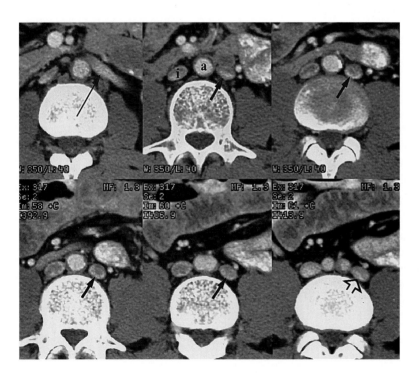

Figure 9–6. Duplication of the inferior vena cava. Selected images from an abdominal CT scan demonstrate duplication of the inferior vena cava. The persistent left inferior vena cava *(short arrows)* can be traced as the continuation of the left common iliac vein *(open arrow)* to its junction with the left renal vein *(long arrow)*. A normal right-sided inferior vena cava (i) remains present. The aorta (a) is between the two venae cavae.

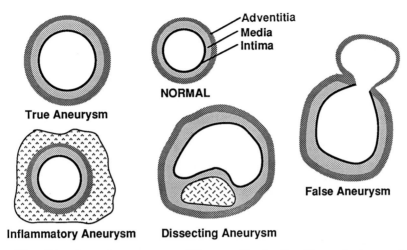

Figure 9–7. Classification of aneurysms. Diagram illustrating the major types of aneurysms.

than 6 cm, and 76% for those greater than 7 cm.

3. Diameter of an iliac artery greater than 1.5 cm (Fig. 9–9)

4. Failure of the aorta to taper distally. The normal distal aorta is 2 cm in diameter

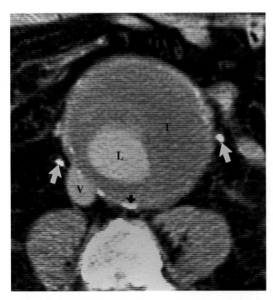

Figure 9–8. Abdominal aortic aneurysm. CT scan of a 10-cm aneurysm of the abdominal aorta lined with thrombus (T). The patent lumen (L) enhances with contrast medium. The intima can be identified by the presence of calcification *(black arrow)*. The ureters *(white arrows)* are seen in close proximity to the aneurysm. Clinically silent ureteral obstruction is one of the complications of abdominal aortic aneurysm. V = inferior vena cava.

in many patients younger than age 50 years. Distal dilatation is evidence of aneurysm even if the diameter is less than 3 cm.

5. Patent lumen enhances with intravenous contrast. Thrombus within the abdominal aortic aneurysm remains low density.

6. The proximal extent of the aneurysm must be defined. Most (90%) begin below the origin of the renal arteries (infrarenal abdominal aortic aneurysm). Origin above the renal arteries must be identified because more complicated surgical repair is required.

Pseudoaneurysm. A pseudoaneurysm, or false aneurysm, is a perforation of an artery with the hematoma confined within the adventitia or surrounding fibrous tissue. Blood continues to circulate within the confined hematoma. Pseudoaneurysms are caused by trauma, surgery, catheterization, or destruction of the arterial wall by infection (mycotic aneurysm). Mycotic aneurysms have a high risk of rupture no matter what their size. CT findings that suggest mycotic aneurysm include

1. Irregular contour
2. Little or no mural calcification
3. Surrounding soft tissue density that frequently enhances
4. Gas bubbles
5. Suprarenal location
6. Adjacent vertebral osteomyelitis

Inflammatory Aneurysm. Aneurysms with extensive perianeurysmal fibrosis are

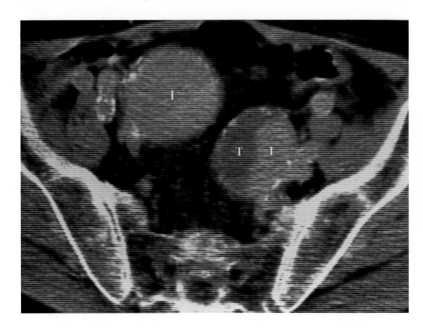

Figure 9–9. Bilateral iliac artery aneurysms. CT slice through the pelvis demonstrates bilateral aneurysms of the common iliac arteries (I). The left iliac artery aneurysm contains a larger thrombus (T).

called inflammatory aneurysms (Fig. 9–10). Surgical repair is significantly more difficult. The fibrosis is believed secondary to an autoimmune reaction to components of the atherosclerotic plaques. Some authors prefer treatment with corticosteroids before, or in place of, surgical repair. CT signs include

1. Rind of sharply defined soft tissue surrounding the aneurysm

2. Relative sparing of the posterior wall by the fibrotic process

3. Variable enhancement of the fibrosis

4. Ureters, duodenum, and small bowel may be trapped within the fibrosis

Dissecting Aneurysm. Dissection of blood into the media through a tear in the intima results in a dilated segment of artery with

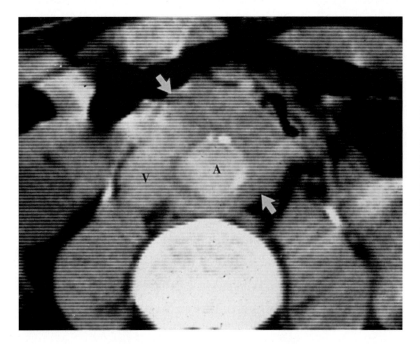

Figure 9–10. Inflammatory aneurysm. The abdominal aorta (A) is surrounded by a collar of inflammatory tissue *(arrows)*. The aorta is only minimally dilated to 3.2 cm but has a thick wall that is calcified. V = inferior vena cava.

two lumina. Branch vessels may be occluded by the process or may be fed by the new (false) lumen or the original (true) lumen. Most aortic dissections are idiopathic. Predisposing conditions include hypertension and Marfan's syndrome. Classification of aortic dissection is discussed in Chapter 3. CT findings of involvement of the abdominal aorta (Fig. 9–11) are

1. Demonstration of intimal flap separating the true and false lumina
2. Thrombosis of the false lumen—may preclude visualization of the intimal flap
3. Internal displacement of intimal plaque calcification
4. Compression of the true lumen by expanding hematoma in the false lumen
5. Ischemia or infarction of organs supplied by branch arteries.

Ruptured Aortic Aneurysm. Acute rupture of an abdominal aortic aneurysm is highly lethal (mortality = 77% to 94%). The classic presentation is abdominal pain, hypotension, and pulsatile abdominal mass.

Because ruptured abdominal aortic aneurysms are commonly confused clinically with other diseases, CT is used to confirm the diagnosis. CT findings in rupture (Fig. 9–12) are

1. Large abdominal aortic aneurysm
2. Adjacent retroperitoneal hematoma dissecting between tissue planes
3. Extension of bleeding into psoas muscles and into the peritoneal cavity

Venous Thrombosis

Venous thrombi may be bland, septic, or associated with tumor invasion. CT signs of thrombosis include increased venous diameter, low-density intraluminal filling defects, and a surrounding rim of high-density contrast medium. Flow artifacts and layering of contrast medium may mimic thrombosis. Extrinsic displacement and compression may also be difficult to differentiate from thrombosis. Tumors most likely to extend into the inferior vena cava are renal, hepatic, and adrenal carcinomas.

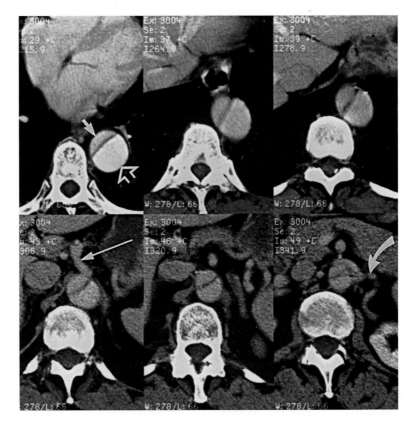

Figure 9–11. Dissecting aneurysm. Selected images from a CT examination of the chest and abdomen demonstrate a DeBakey type I (Daily type A) dissection that originated in the ascending aorta and continued into the abdominal aorta. A well-defined intimal flap separates the true lumen *(open arrow)* and the false lumen *(solid arrow)*. The celiac axis *(long arrow)* is supplied by the false lumen. The dissection extends into the origin of the left renal artery *(curved arrow)*.

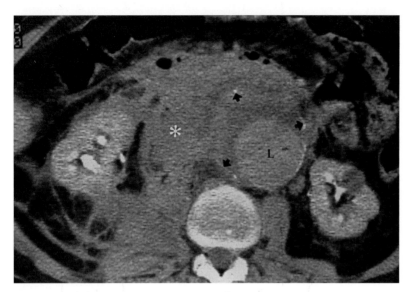

Figure 9–12. Rupture of an abdominal aortic aneurysm. Blood (*) from rupture of an aortic aneurysm dissects through the retroperitoneal space and displaces the right kidney. The wall of the aneurysm is identified by calcification in its wall *(arrows)*. The lumen (L) shows contrast medium enhancement.

NODES

Anatomy

Normal lymph nodes are oblong and homogeneous in CT attenuation. Most are oriented parallel to their accompanying vessels (see Fig. 17–3). Abdominoaortic nodal groups surround the aorta and inferior vena cava and are commonly involved in abdominal and pelvic malignancy. Visceral nodes drain adjacent organs and include mesenteric, hepatic, splenic, and pancreaticoduodenal nodal groups.

Technical Considerations

CT remains the imaging procedure of choice for detection of abdominal lymphadenopathy. Both intravenous and oral contrast agents are essential for accurate identification of nodal disease. My colleagues and I routinely scan the abdomen and pelvis with contiguous 7- to 10-mm thick slices when searching for adenopathy.

Nodal Metastases

Size is the major criterion for diagnosis of abnormal lymph nodes. Nodes are considered to be pathologically enlarged when they exceed 10 mm in short axis in the abdomen or pelvis or 6 mm in the retrocrural and porta hepatis region. Multiple 8- to 10-mm nodes in the abdomen or pelvis are considered suspicious. Interpretation must always be made in clinical context. Even minimally enlarged nodes should be viewed with suspicion when present in an area where a known malignancy is highly likely to metastasize.

Unfortunately, involvement of nodes with metastatic tumor does not usually change the CT attenuation of the node and, in some cases, will not enlarge the node sufficiently to be interpreted as pathologic by size criteria. Nodes may be enlarged due to benign disease (false-positive interpretation) or be of normal size and yet be involved (false-negative interpretation). Low attenuation within enlarged nodes is seen uncommonly and usually represents necrosis. Calcification of nodes may occur with some calcifying tumors or with tumor necrosis after treatment.

Lymphoma

Lymphomas are divided into Hodgkin's and non-Hodgkin's types. Hodgkin's lymphoma accounts for about 40% of the total and tends to spread in an orderly contiguous manner. Non-Hodgkin's lymphoma is a mixed group of diseases with a confusing array of changing names and classifications. Noncontiguous spread and involvement of the gastrointestinal tract is characteristic of non-Hodgkin's lymphoma. CT features of lymphoma in the abdomen and pelvis (Figs. 9–13 and 9–14) include

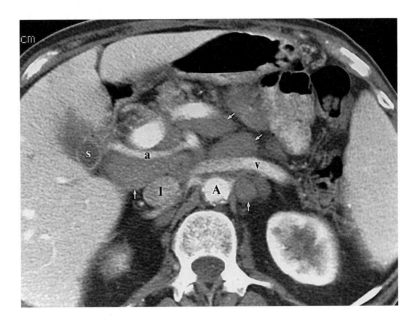

Figure 9–13. Lymphoma. CT image through the upper abdomen demonstrates enlarged nodes *(arrows)* surrounding the hepatic artery (a), left renal vein (v), aorta (A), and inferior vena cava (I). The patient also has a gallstone(s).

1. Multiple enlarged individual nodes
2. Coalescence of enlarged nodes to form rounded multilobular masses that may encase vessels, displace organs, and obstruct ureters

Conglomerate nodal masses are typical of lymphoma and are rarely seen with other conditions.

Acquired Immunodeficiency Syndrome

Acquired immunodeficiency syndrome (AIDS) is characterized on abdominal CT by signs of intraabdominal opportunistic infections, AIDS-related lymphoma, and Kaposi's sarcoma. Most CT findings are a manifestation of a complicating disease rather than human immunodeficiency virus (HIV) infection alone. The most common findings on CT are

1. Lymphadenopathy involving the retroperitoneal, pelvic, and mesenteric nodes—causes include disseminated *Mycobacterium avium-intracellulare* infection (30%), AIDS-related lymphoma (30%), Kaposi's sarcoma, or other infection. Lymph node enlargement

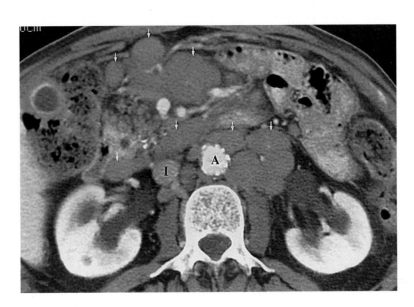

Figure 9–14. Lymphoma. Enlarged lymph nodes *(arrows)* surround the aorta (A) and inferior vena cava (I) and are seen in the small bowel mesentery.

is unlikely to be due to HIV infection alone. Unexplained adenopathy warrants biopsy.

2. Hepatosplenomegaly without focal lesions—causes include *M. avium-intracellulare* infection, histoplasmosis, and hepatocellular disease.

3. Focal small (<1 cm) low-attenuation lesions in the liver—causes include *Mycobacterium tuberculosis,* AIDS-related lymphoma, Kaposi's sarcoma, and histoplasmosis.

4. Focal small (<1 cm) low-attenuation lesions in the spleen—causes include *M. tuberculosis, M. avium-intracellulare,* coccidioidomycosis, candidiasis, bacillary peliosis, Kaposi's sarcoma, AIDS-related lymphoma, and *Pneumocystis carinii* infection.

5. Focal bowel wall thickening or focal bowel mass—cause is nearly always AIDS-related lymphoma.

6. Calcifications in spleen, lymph nodes, and liver—cause is usually *P. carinii* infection.

7. Nephromegaly with striated nephrogram after contrast agent administration—cause is HIV nephropathy.

Mycobacterial infections cause lymph node enlargement, small low-density lesions in solid organs, hepatosplenomegaly, and bowel wall thickening.

Pneumocystis carinii infections cause punctate or nodular calcifications in solid organs and lymph nodes and low-attenuation lesions in the spleen.

Kaposi's sarcoma causes adenopathy and hepatosplenomegaly. Less common findings include focal bowel wall thickening, low-density nodules in the liver, and intrahepatic low-density bands in the periportal region.

AIDS-related lymphoma must be suspected for any solid mass anywhere in the abdomen. Additional findings include multiple sites of adenopathy, bowel involvement with wall thickening and focal masses, and focal masses in the spleen, liver, and kidney.

TRAUMA CT

CT remains the imaging method of choice for diagnosis of intraabdominal injury after blunt abdominal trauma. Characterization of the precise nature of injury, or absence of injury, allows for the most appropriate treatment. CT is particularly useful in patients when physical examination of the abdomen is equivocal or unreliable, such as with head trauma or impairment of consciousness due to drugs or alcohol. CT has the advantage of evaluating the entire abdomen and pelvis in a single study. The sensitivity of CT for intraabdominal injury exceeds 90%.

Candidates for trauma CT of the abdomen are patients who have had significant blunt trauma to the abdomen and who are hemodynamically stable. Patients who are hemodynamically unstable, who have signs of peritonitis, or who have penetrating trauma to the abdomen are candidates for immediate exploratory surgery, which should not be delayed by CT. Diagnostic peritoneal lavage is a quick and simple method of detecting intraperitoneal bleeding. However, this procedure does not quantitate the amount of hemorrhage, does not identify its source, does not exclude hemorrhage into the retroperitoneal space, and is not indicated in patients with multiple abdominal surgeries and high risk of adhesions. The radiologist must know, however, if diagnostic peritoneal lavage has been performed before trauma CT because it may be the cause of free air or fluid seen in the peritoneal cavity.

Technical Considerations

An intravenous contrast medium is the most critical component of preparation for trauma CT of the abdomen. Solid organ enhancement confirms blood flow and provides the best delineation of lacerations and hematomas, which may be isodense with unenhanced organs. A contrast agent is given intravenously by power injector at 1 to 2 mL/sec for a volume of 150 mL. Rapid scans (1–2 seconds) or helical technique is used to provide contiguous 7- to 10-mm thick slices through the abdomen. The pelvis must always be included on trauma CT scans to detect and quantitate hemoperitoneum, which may settle dependently in the pelvis. Oral contrast medium is helpful in the detection of gastrointestinal injury, but most solid organ injuries may be detected without it. CT should never be delayed by extended patient preparation with oral contrast agent. Three hundred to 500 mL of contrast medium is given by mouth or through a nasogastric tube as soon as urgent trauma CT is requested. Placement of a nasogastric tube is helpful to allow post-CT aspiration of stomach contents in patients who are going to have anesthesia and surgery soon after CT.

In addition to viewing scans at standard soft tissue windows, all slices should also be viewed at lung windows to detect pneumothorax and pneumoperitoneum and at bone windows to detect skeletal injury.

Findings

CT signs of traumatic injury in the abdomen include

1. Hemoperitoneum—high-density intraperitoneal fluid (30–45 H) may be the only sign of injury and may settle in the pelvis with little blood seen in the upper abdomen (Fig. 9–15). Very high attenuation fluid (80–130 H) is a sign of active bleeding.

2. "Sentinel clot," a localized collection of clotted blood (>60 H), serves as an accurate marker of injury of the adjacent organ (Fig. 9–16).

3. Free contrast agent in the peritoneal cavity is a sign of intraperitoneal bladder rupture or bowel perforation (if oral contrast medium was administered).

4. Free air in the peritoneal cavity is a sign of bowel perforation but is present in only half the cases. The volume of free air present is frequently small and difficult to identify. Free air due to diagnostic peritoneal lavage, coexisting pneumothorax, or mechanical ventilation must also be considered.

5. Intraparenchymal hematomas are seen as rounded, low-density areas within enhanced solid organs.

6. Subcapsular hematomas are usually crescent shaped and flatten organ parenchyma.

7. Lacerations appear as jagged, linear low-density areas that extend through the organ parenchyma.

8. Individual organ injuries are discussed in the appropriate chapters.

ABDOMINAL WALL

Anatomy

CT is an excellent imaging technique for evaluation of abnormalities of the abdominal wall. The muscles of the abdominal wall are outlined by subcutaneous and extraperitoneal fat. The rectus abdominis muscles are anterior within the rectus sheath. The

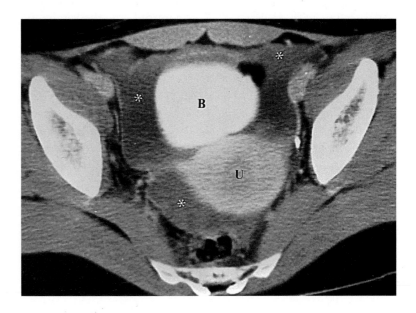

Figure 9–15. Hemoperitoneum. Free blood (*) in the peritoneal cavity pools around the uterus (U) and bladder (B) in this woman with a large liver laceration. CT of the pelvis is always needed in the setting of blunt abdominal trauma to quantitate the amount of intraperitoneal bleeding.

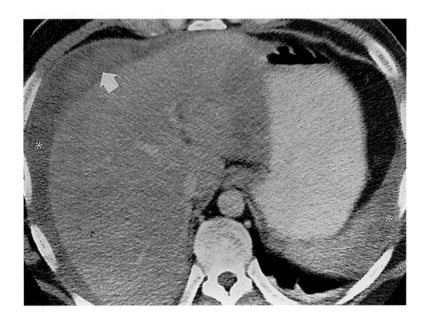

Figure 9–16. Sentinel clot. A blood clot in the intraperitoneal space adjacent to the liver *(arrow)* is an important sign of liver injury. A laceration of the left hepatic lobe, not seen on CT, was found at surgery. Free blood (*) is also evident in the peritoneal cavity.

flanks are defined by three muscle layers formed by the external and internal oblique and transversus abdominis muscles. The posterior muscles are the latissimus dorsi, the quadratus lumborum, and the paraspinal muscles.

Abdominal Wall Hernia

Obesity makes hernias of the abdominal wall difficult to detect clinically. Hernias may cause intermittent pain or bowel obstruction. Hernia sacs contain fat, which is usually omentum, bowel, and occasionally ascites. *Incisional hernias* are common ventral hernias with protrusion of abdominal contents through the abdominal wall weakened by a surgical incision. *Inguinal hernias* are classified as indirect or direct. Indirect hernias are congenital lesions seen to protrude anterior to the spermatic cord (males) or round ligament (females) and lateral to the inferior epigastric vessels. Direct inguinal hernias are always acquired and are seen to arise medial to the inferior epigastric vessels. *Paraumbilical hernias* protrude through the linea alba in the region of the umbilicus. *Spigelian hernias* are uncommon but carry a high risk of bowel incarceration and strangulation. They protrude through the linea semilunaris at the lateral edge of the rectus abdominis (Fig. 9–17).

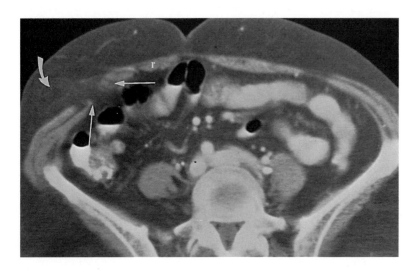

Figure 9–17. Spigelian hernia. Fat-density omentum and blood vessels *(curved arrow)* protrude through a defect *(straight arrows)* in the anterior abdominal wall at the lateral edge of the rectus abdominis (r).

Abdominal Wall Hematoma

Bleeding into the abdominal musculature may complicate bleeding disorders or anti-coagulant therapy or result from trauma. Hematomas enlarge the involved muscle, are hyperdense acutely, and progressively decrease in attenuation with time. Hematomas or seromas are commonly visualized in surgical wounds during the postoperative period. Infection results in abscess formation with increased stranding densities in subcutaneous fat, gas formation, and fluid levels. Confirmation of infection requires percutaneous aspiration.

Suggested Reading

Arrive L, Correas JM, Leseche G, et al. Inflammatory aneurysms of the abdominal aorta: CT findings. AJR 1995; 165:1481–1484.

Castelline RA. The non-Hodgkin lymphomas: practical concepts for the diagnostic radiologist. Radiology 1991; 178:315–321.

DeMeo JH, Fulcher AS, Austin RF Jr. Anatomic CT demonstration of the peritoneal spaces, ligaments, and mesenteries: normal and pathologic processes. RadioGraphics 1995; 15:755–770.

Dorfman RE, Alpern MB, Gross BH, Sandler MA. Upper abdominal lymph nodes: criteria for normal size determined by CT. Radiology 1991; 180:319–322.

Einstein DM, Singer AA, Chicote WA, Desai RK. Abdominal lymphadenopathy: spectrum of CT findings. RadioGraphics 1991; 11:457–472.

Fisher ER, Stern EJ, Godwin JD II, et al. Acute aortic dissection: typical and atypical imaging features. RadioGraphics 1994; 14:1263–1271.

Goerg C, Schwek WB. Peritoneal carcinomatosis with ascites. AJR 1991; 156:1185–1187.

Goodman P, Raval B. CT of the abdominal wall. AJR 1990; 154:1207–1211.

Hamrick-Turner JE, Chiechi MV, Abbitt PL, Ros PR. Neoplastic and inflammatory processes of the perito-

neum, omentum, and mesentery: diagnosis with CT. RadioGraphics 1992; 12:1051–1068.

Harrison LA, Keesling CA, Martin NL, et al. Abdominal wall hernias: review of herniography and correlation with cross-sectional imaging. RadioGraphics 1995;15:315–332.

Kellman GM, Alpern MB, Sandler MA, Craig BM. Computed tomography of vena caval anomalies with embryologic correlation. RadioGraphics 1988; 8:533–556.

Kuhlman JE, Fishman EK. Acute abdomen in AIDS: CT diagnosis and triage. RadioGraphics 1990; 10:621–634.

Kuhlman JE, Browne D, Shermak M, et al. Retroperitoneal and pelvic CT of patients with AIDS: primary and secondary involvement of the genitourinary tract. RadioGraphics 1991; 11:473–483.

LaRoy LL, Cormier PJ, Matalon TAS, et al. Imaging of abdominal aortic aneurysms. AJR 1989; 152:785–792.

Miller FH, Parikh S, Gore RM, et al. Renal manifestations of AIDS. RadioGraphics 1993; 13:587–596.

Radin R. HIV infection: analysis of 259 consecutive patients with abnormal abdominal CT findings. Radiology 1995; 197:721–722.

Roberts JL, Dalen K, Bosanko CM, Jafir SZH. CT in abdominal and pelvic trauma. RadioGraphics 1993; 13:735–752.

Siegel CL, Cohan RH. CT of abdominal aortic aneurysms. AJR 1994; 163:17–29.

Stoupis C, Ros PR, Abbitt PL, et al. Bubbles in the belly: imaging of cystic mesenteric or omental masses. RadioGraphics 1995; 14:729–737.

Townsend RR. CT of AIDS-related lymphoma. AJR 1991; 156:969–974.

Walkey MM, Friedman AC, Sohotra P, Radecki PD. CT manifestations of peritoneal carcinomatosis. AJR 1988; 150:1035–1041.

Wolfman NT, Bechtold RE, Scharling ES, Meredith JW. Blunt upper abdominal trauma: evaluation by CT. AJR 1992; 158:493–501.

Vogelzang RL, Gore RM, Anschuetz SL, Blei AT. Thrombosis of the splanchnic veins: CT diagnosis. AJR 1988; 150:93–96.

Zarvan NP, Lee FT Jr, Yandow DR, Unger JS. Abdominal hernias: CT findings. AJR 1995; 164:1391–1395.

Chapter

10

Liver

William E. Brant, M.D.

ANATOMY

The vascular anatomy of the liver defines the surgical approach to hepatic resection. Resectability of hepatic lesions can be determined by CT interpretation only if hepatic vascular anatomy is clearly understood. A knowledge of three-dimensional hepatic anatomy is essential to correlate lesion location with the various hepatic imaging methods. Older concepts of hepatic lobar anatomy can be ignored in favor of current anatomic considerations that relate directly to surgical resection of hepatic lesions. A key concept to remember is that the hepatic veins run in the *inter*lobar and *inter*segmental fissures, whereas the portal veins, hepatic arteries, and bile ducts course together within the *intra*segmental parenchyma. Portal veins and hepatic arteries supply the parenchyma of the segments through which they course. Portal vein flow from the gut and spleen provides about 80% of hepatic blood flow. The remainder is nutrient systemic circulation from the hepatic artery. The proportion of blood flow from the portal vein and hepatic artery to any given segment of the liver is not uniform but is determined by anatomic, hormonal, nutritional, and neural factors. The pattern of portal vein and hepatic artery blood flow determines the anatomic distribution of several disease states, such as fatty infiltration. Hepatic veins drain the segments bordering the fissures that the veins help define.

Hepatic vascular territories divide the liver into three lobes and four segments (Fig. 10–1). The right and left lobes are separated by the major lobar fissure. This fissure is defined on CT by the plane of the middle hepatic vein in the cranial third of the liver and by a line drawn from the center of the inferior vena cava through the gallbladder fossa to the liver edge in the lower portion of the liver. The right hepatic lobe is divided into anterior and posterior segments by the right intersegmental fissure. This fissure is defined by the course of the right hepatic vein in the cranial aspect of the liver and by a line drawn midway between the anterior and posterior branches of the right portal vein more caudad. The left hepatic lobe is divided into medial and lateral segments by the left intersegmental fissure marked by the left hepatic vein in the cranial aspect of the liver and by the prominent fissure of the ligamentum venosum and falciform ligament more inferiorly. The medial segment was formerly called the quadrate lobe. An international numbering system developed by Couinaud (pronounced "kwee-NO") is commonly used outside the United States and provides further subdivision of hepatic segments (Table 10–1).

Lesions confined to the right or left lobe can be surgically removed by right or left hepatic lobectomy carried up to but not including the middle hepatic vein. Lateral segmentectomy of the left lobe and technically more difficult posterior segmentectomy of the right lobe can be performed for lesions

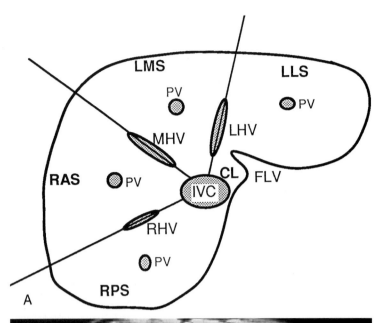

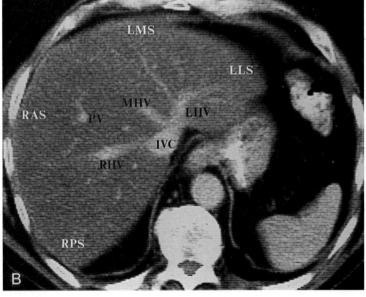

Figure 10–1. Hepatic segmental anatomy. Diagram *(A)* and CT scan *(B)* demonstrate the anatomy of the hepatic veins that serve as landmarks for the fissures that divide the liver into lobes and segments. The hepatic and portal veins are prominent on the CT scan because the liver has diffuse fatty infiltration that lowers the CT attenuation of the liver parenchyma. RPS = right lobe, posterior segment; RAS = right lobe, anterior segment; LMS = left lobe, medial segment; LLS = left lobe, lateral segment; CL = caudate lobe; RHV = right hepatic vein; MHV = middle hepatic vein; LHV = left hepatic vein; PV = portal veins; IVC = inferior vena cava; FLV = fissure of the ligamentum venosum.

confined to the corresponding segments. Extended right lobectomy, which includes removal of the medial segment of the left lobe, can be performed if the volume of hepatic parenchyma in the remaining lateral segment of the left lobe is sufficient to sustain life. Accurate localization of lesions on CT and other imaging methods is critical to surgical planning.

The caudate lobe is separated from the rest of the liver by the fissure of the ligamentum venosum anteriorly and the inferior vena cava posterolaterally. It is supplied by branches of both right and left hepatic arteries and portal veins and drains venous blood directly into the inferior vena cava by multiple small hepatic veins. The papillary process of the caudate lobe extends toward the lesser sac and may appear separate from the rest of the caudate lobe simulating a mass or enlarged lymph node.

Several fissures and ligaments deserve special mention either because they are particularly prominent or because they define important perihepatic spaces. The falciform ligament consists of two closely applied layers of peritoneum extending from the umbilicus to the diaphragm in a parasagittal plane. The caudal free end of the falciform ligament contains the ligamentum teres, which is the obliterated umbilical vein remnant. The reflections of the falciform ligament separate over the posterior dome of the liver to form the coronary ligaments that define the "bare area" of the liver not covered by peritoneum. The coronary ligaments reflect between liver and diaphragm and prevent access of ascites or other intraperitoneal fluid from covering the "bare area" of the liver. The absence of fluid over the "bare area" is an important sign in the differentiation of ascites from pleural effusion on CT. The remainder of the falciform ligament and ligamentum teres continues into the liver to form a prominent fat-filled fissure often mistaken for the main interlobar fissure. Actually, the fissure of the ligamentum teres and falciform ligament defines the left intersegmental fissure dividing the medial and lateral segments of the left lobe.

The fissure of the ligamentum venosum contains the remnant of the ductus venosus, which in fetal life carried oxygenated blood from the umbilical vein to the inferior vena cava. This fissure is commonly fat filled and prominent on CT, separating the caudate lobe and the left lobe.

The lesser omentum suspends the lesser curve of the stomach and the duodenal bulb from the inferior surface of the liver, attaching within the fissure of the ligamentum venosum. The lesser omentum is subdivided into the gastrohepatic ligament and the hepatoduodenal ligament. The gastrohepatic ligament contains coronary veins that serve as an important sign of portal hypertension when they become dilated. The right free edge of the hepatoduodenal ligament carries the portal vein, hepatic artery, and common bile duct between the porta hepatis and the duodenum. The hepatoduodenal ligament provides the anterior border of the foramen of Winslow, which opens into the lesser sac.

The normal liver is homogeneous in attenuation, measuring 40 to 70 H on unenhanced CT. The unenhanced liver parenchymal density is normally greater than that of blood vessels and 7 to 8 H greater than splenic parenchyma. Anemia lowers the CT density of blood vessels and may make the liver parenchyma appear falsely increased in density. The contour of the liver is smooth and convex adjacent to the diaphragm with a sharp inferior border and a concave undersurface. Fissures may be fat filled and prominent. The right lobe is usually larger than the left lobe and may extend far caudad as a Riedel's lobe. The left lobe is more variable in size, and its lateral segment may extend far to the left and wrap partially around the spleen. Congenital absence of the left lobe is a rare anomaly.

Liver enhancement with intravenous contrast medium enhancement is uniform. Early scans during contrast medium bolus, especially with spiral CT, show bright inho-

TABLE 10–1. **American and International Nomenclature for Anatomic Segments of the Liver**

American	International	Number
Caudate lobe	Caudate lobe	I
Left lobe		
Lateral segment	Left lateral superior subsegment	II
	Left lateral inferior subsegment	III
Medial segment	Left medial subsegment	IV
Right lobe		
Anterior segment	Right anterior inferior subsegment	V
	Right anterior superior subsegment	VIII
Posterior segment	Right posterior inferior subsegment	VI
	Right posterior anterior subsegment	VII

Adapted from Dodd GD. An American's guide to Couinaud's numbering system. AJR 1993; 161:574–575.

mogeneous enhancement of the spleen and less-dense homogeneous enhancement of the liver. Early liver enhancement is primarily due to delivery of contrast medium by means of the hepatic artery. Maximal liver parenchymal enhancement is delayed about 1 minute, relative to splenic enhancement, because of passage of the contrast medium bolus through the gut before delivery to the liver by means of the portal vein. Assessment of liver parenchymal CT density is best made on unenhanced or on portal venous phase enhanced scans.

TECHNICAL CONSIDERATIONS

Unenhanced liver CT is greatly inferior to contrast medium bolus CT for detection of most liver masses. However, on some occasions, especially with suboptimal contrast medium administration, a liver mass will be isodense with enhanced liver parenchyma and will escape detection if scans are performed only after contrast medium administration. For mass detection, a standard technique is to obtain base liver scans before contrast medium administration and then repeat the entire scan of the liver after the contrast agent is instilled. Spiral CT technique is greatly preferred because it offers superior lesion detection and characterization compared with conventional CT. Our routine technique for liver CT is a three-phase study: base liver, early arterial phase liver, and portal venous phase liver. When cavernous hemangioma is suspected, additional delayed scans are obtained at 5 and 10 minutes after contrast medium administration. Sixty percent iodine contrast agents are used in a 150-mL dose administered intravenously by power injector at 2 to 3 mL/sec. I routinely use 7-mm collimation and pitch of 1 for spiral CT. Contiguous 7-mm thick slices are reconstructed. Greater detail can be obtained by reconstructing at smaller intervals (i.e., 7-mm thick slices at 3-mm intervals) without the need for rescanning. A single spiral CT run with a single 20- to 30-second breath hold allows the entire liver volume to be scanned continuously and eliminates the risk of missing lesions owing to the misregistration that occurs with multiple breath hold scans.

Conventional CT technique uses 10-mm collimation with contiguous 10-mm reconstruction. Cluster scans, using 1- to 2-second scan times per slice and obtaining several slices per breath hold, are preferred over single-slice scans. Scanning the entire liver within the first 2 to 3 minutes after contrast bolus administration is essential to avoid masking lesions due to the equivalent contrast medium enhancement of the lesion and liver parenchyma that occurs when scans are obtained during equilibrium phase.

To further characterize the enhancement pattern of a liver mass, single-level, bolus-contrast, dynamic scanning may be performed. A single slice level through the midportion of the mass is selected. Contrast agent is given by power injector with a 100-mL dose at 2.5 mL/sec. A minimum of six scans per minute are obtained for the first 2 minutes, then three scans per minute for the next 5 minutes, and final scans at 15, 20, and 25 minutes after injection.

DIFFUSE LIVER DISEASE

Fatty Liver

Fatty infiltration of the liver is one of the most common abnormalities diagnosed by liver CT. Fatty infiltration is a nonspecific response of hepatocytes to a variety of insults, including alcoholism, obesity, diabetes, chemotherapy, corticosteroid therapy, hyperalimentation, and malnutrition. Fatty infiltration lowers the CT attenuation of the liver parenchyma, causing hepatic vessels to stand out in relief (Fig. 10–2; see also Fig. 10–1*B*). The normal CT attenuation of the liver is equal to or greater than that of the normal spleen, both before and after intravenous contrast medium administration. Fatty infiltration makes involved portions of the liver appear more lucent than the splenic parenchyma. Four major patterns of fatty infiltration are seen on CT.

Diffuse Fatty Infiltration. The entire liver is uniformly reduced in density. Vessels stand out in prominent relief especially

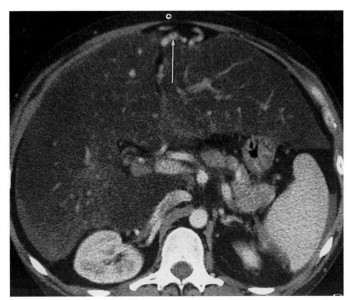

Figure 10–2. Diffuse fatty infiltration. The liver parenchyma is diffusely and markedly lower in density than the spleen parenchyma, indicating diffuse hepatocellular fatty infiltration. Enlarged paraumbilical veins *(arrow)* are evidence of portal hypertension.

after contrast medium administration but run their normal course through the liver without displacement by mass effect (see Figs. 10–1*B* and 10–2). The liver is usually enlarged, and the parenchyma enhances minimally. This pattern is the most common and is easiest to recognize.

Focal Fatty Infiltration. A geographic or fan-shaped portion of the liver shows fat infiltration whereas the remainder of the liver is of normal density (Fig. 10–3). The low density may extend to the liver surface, but no bulge in contour is seen. Vessels run

their normal course through the area of involvement.

Multifocal Fatty Infiltration. Patchy areas of decreased attenuation are scattered through the liver. Tumors may be simulated by the islands of fatty infiltration surrounded by normal parenchyma or by islands of normal parenchyma surrounded by fatty infiltration. The pattern tends to be geographic with straight margins rather than rounded masses (Fig. 10–4).

Focal Sparing. Islands of normal parenchyma are surrounded by large areas of dif-

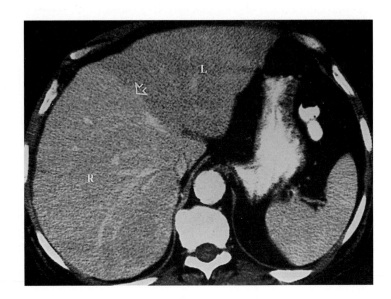

Figure 10–3. Focal fatty infiltration. The left lobe of the liver (L) is lower in density than the right lobe of the liver (R) and the spleen. A strikingly sharp boundary *(arrow)* separates the left and right lobes. This appearance is characteristic of focal fatty infiltration.

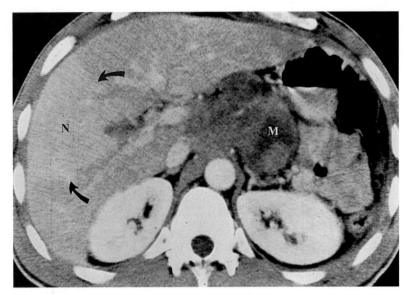

Figure 10–4. Multifocal fatty infiltration. This geographic pattern of fatty infiltration developed within 2 weeks of commencing chemotherapy in this patient with lymphoma. The higher-density wedge-shaped area (N) is normal liver parenchyma that has been spared from the process of fatty infiltration affecting the left lobe, the posterior segment of the right lobe, and the caudate lobe. Note the sharp margins of demarcation between the normal high-density and fatty low-density areas of the liver *(arrows).* A mass of adenopathy (M) is due to lymphoma.

fuse fatty infiltration and may simulate neoplasms (Fig. 10–5). The pattern of focal infiltration and focal sparing is related to variations in hepatic artery and portal venous supply to areas of the liver. Alcohol may be delivered from the stomach by the portal vein in higher concentration to some areas of the liver than others, causing

greater hepatocyte injury and resulting in greater fat deposition. A higher percentage of blood flow from the arterial circulation may promote focal sparing, especially near the gallbladder fossa and in the medial segment of the left lobe.

Focal fatty infiltration and focal sparing can be differentiated from hepatoma, metas-

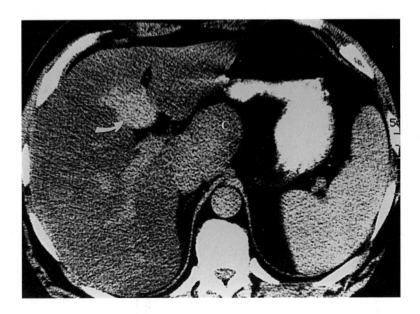

Figure 10–5. Focal sparing. An island of normal parenchyma *(arrow),* in the medial segment of the left lobe, simulates a mass lesion in a liver with extensive fatty infiltration. The caudate lobe (C) is hypertrophied. The image is photographed with narrow "liver" windows to accentuate the findings.

tases, and other tumors by the following signs:

1. Angulated geometric margins (nonspherical shape)
2. Interdigitating margins with slender fingers of normal or fatty tissue
3. Absence of mass effect and vessel displacement
4. Rapid change over time. Fatty changes can be seen within 3 weeks after the insult and can resolve within 6 days after removing the insult.

Further confirmation of fatty replacement can be provided by other imaging tests. Ultrasonography will show the areas of fatty infiltration as corresponding areas of increased parenchymal echogenicity. Technetium sulfur-colloid liver scans will show normal activity in the area of involvement because the reticuloendothelial cells are not displaced. Xenon scintigraphy will show increased uptake in the area of involvement because xenon is fat avid. Percutaneous biopsy is an option in difficult cases.

Chronic Hepatitis

Chronic hepatitis is characterized pathologically by portal and perilobular inflammation and fibrosis. CT is usually normal. The primary role of CT is to detect hepatocellular carcinoma. Hepatitis B infection carries a risk of hepatoma. Hepatitis C infection progresses to cirrhosis in 10% to 20% of patients.

Cirrhosis

Cirrhosis is a chronic diffuse liver disease characterized by progressive destruction of hepatocytes with distortion of hepatic architecture by extensive collagen deposition. The common forms of cirrhosis are Laënnec's due to alcoholism, postnecrotic due to various types of hepatitis and toxic injury to the liver, and biliary due to chronic intrahepatic cholestasis. In Western countries, alcohol abuse causes 60% to 70% of cases of cirrhosis. Patients with cirrhosis show the following CT findings:

1. Fatty infiltration with hepatomegaly (early cirrhosis) (see Fig. 10–2)
2. Nonuniform attenuation due to chronic fatty infiltration and irregular fibrosis (Fig. 10–6)
3. Irregular lobulated hepatic contour due to areas of atrophy and nodular regeneration (Fig. 10–6)
4. Intrahepatic regenerating nodules (Table 10–2; Fig. 10–7)
5. Atrophy of the right lobe with hypertrophy of the left and caudate lobes (common in alcoholic cirrhosis)
6. Decreased liver volume (chronic cirrhosis)

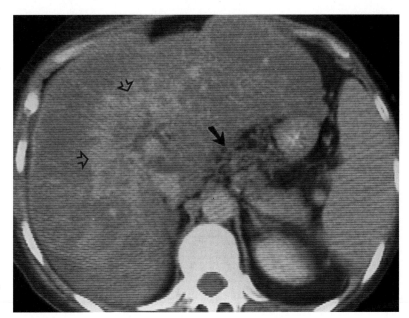

Figure 10–6. Cirrhosis. CT scan of the liver demonstrates signs of advanced cirrhosis. The periphery of the liver is lower in density than the spleen, indicating fatty replacement of the liver. The higher-density areas centrally *(open arrows)* are due to extensive scarring and collagen deposition. The contour of the liver is lobulated, and the left lobe is enlarged. A tangle of collateral vessels *(solid arrow)* in the gastrohepatic ligament indicates the presence of portal hypertension.

TABLE 10–2. **Causes of Nodules in Cirrhosis**

Regenerative nodules (nodules <10 mm)
   Collections of regenerating hepatocytes
     surrounded by fibrous septa
Adenomatous hyperplastic nodules (nodules
   >10 mm)
   Proliferative precancerous lesion
Hepatocellular carcinoma
Confluent fibrosis
   Masslike fibrosis in advanced cirrhosis
Focal fat infiltration

---

7. Increased size and prominence of the intrahepatic fissures due to shrunken liver parenchyma

8. Signs of portal hypertension

9. Ascites

Patients with cirrhosis are at high risk of developing portal hypertension and hepatocellular carcinoma. Each CT scan in patients with cirrhosis must be carefully analyzed for signs of these conditions.

Portal Hypertension

Portal hypertension results from progressive fibrosis of the hepatic vascular bed with development of portosystemic collateral vessels and eventually hepatofugal flow (i.e., flow away from, instead of into, the liver). Portal hypertension causes major morbidity in the cirrhotic patient because of the risk of hepatic encephalopathy and variceal hemorrhage. Portal hypertension can be diagnosed on CT by the presence of the following anatomic signs:

1. Portosystemic collateral vessels (Figs. 10–8 and 10–9)

2. Increased size of the portal vein (>13 mm)

3. Increased size of the splenic and mesenteric veins (>10 mm)

4. Portal vein thrombosis seen as an enlarged low density portal vein that fails to enhance (Fig. 10–10)

5. Splenomegaly due to splenic congestion

6. Ascites

The enlarged collateral vessels characteristic of portal hypertension may be subtle and easily missed or may be mistaken for other structures. You see what you look for!

Portal Vein Thrombosis

Thrombosis of the portal vein is usually found in association with cirrhosis, hepatoma, or mesenteric inflammation. Portal

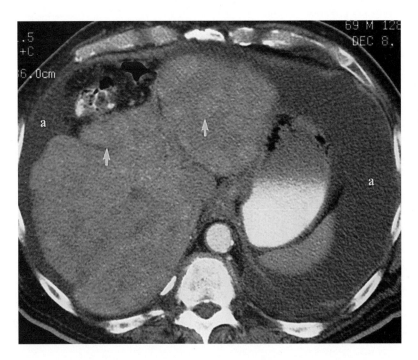

Figure 10–7. Cirrhosis with nodules. The right lobe of the liver is atrophied, and the left lobe is hypertrophied. Multiple nodules *(arrows),* larger than 10 mm, are seen in both lobes. These large nodules indicate adenomatous hyperplasia, a premalignant condition. Copious ascites (a) is present.

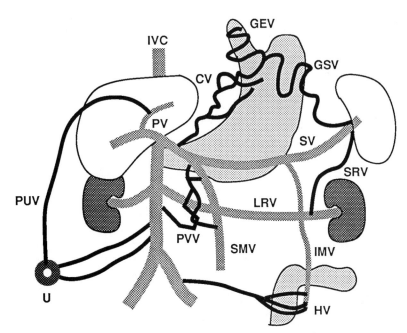

Figure 10–8. Portosystemic collateral vessels. Schematic representation of portosystemic collateral veins that may be seen in portal hypertension. IVC = inferior vena cava; PV = portal veins; SV = splenic vein; SMV = superior mesenteric vein; IMV = inferior mesenteric vein; LRV = left renal vein; HV = hemorrhoidal veins; PVV = paravertebral veins; SRV = splenorenal veins; GSV = gastrosplenic veins; GEV = gastroesophageal varices; CV = cardinal veins (in gastrohepatic ligament); PUV = paraumbilical vein; U = umbilicus.

vein thrombosis can cause or exacerbate portal hypertension. Signs of acute thrombosis (see Fig. 10–10) include

1. Increased size of the portal vein
2. Low-density, nonenhancing, intraluminal thrombus
3. Lack of contrast medium enhancement of the portal vein
4. Failure to visualize the portal vein suggests the diagnosis
5. Cavernous transformation—refers to the development of numerous periportal collateral veins in response to portal vein thrombosis, usually in patients with cirrhosis. CT demonstrates a nest of collateral vessels in the porta hepatis.
6. Calcification may be seen within the portal vein thrombus.

Passive Congestion

Passive congestion of the liver is caused by right-sided congestive heart failure and con-

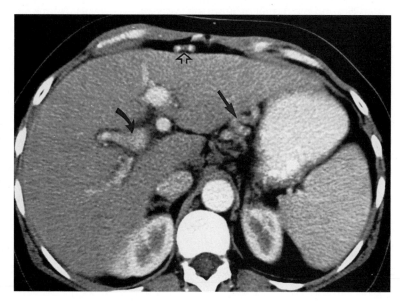

Figure 10–9. Portal hypertension. CT signs of portal hypertension are demonstrated in this slice through the porta hepatis. The portal vein *(curved arrow)* is enlarged, measuring 15 mm. Dilated and tortuous cardinal veins *(straight arrow)* are seen in the gastrohepatic ligament. The paraumbilical vein *(open arrow)* is enlarged. Visualization of a patent paraumbilical vein is the most specific CT sign of portal hypertension.

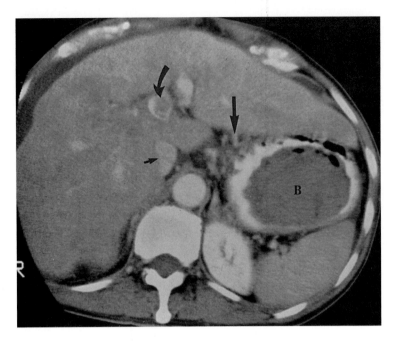

Figure 10–10. Portal vein thrombosis. Tumor thrombus causes central low density *(curved arrow)* in the portal vein. A diffusely infiltrating hepatoma causes subtle low density in the right lobe with mass effect on vascular structures. Note the subtle indentation of the inferior vena cava *(small arrow).* The tumor occupies the entire right lobe of the liver. Enlarged collateral vessels between liver and stomach *(large arrow)* indicate accompanying portal hypertension. The patient also has ascites and a bezoar (B) in his stomach.

strictive pericarditis. Chronic passive congestion may progress to cirrhosis. CT findings include dilatation of the inferior vena cava and hepatic veins, mottled liver parenchymal enhancement, and periportal edema. Pleural and pericardial effusions, ascites, cardiomegaly, and hepatomegaly are also frequently present.

Iron Deposition

Primary hemochromatosis is an autosomal recessive disorder of intestinal metabolism resulting in iron deposition within hepatocytes. Secondary hemochromatosis refers to iron deposition with reticuloendothelial cells of the liver and spleen, usually due to multiple blood transfusions. Hepatic iron deposition is usually diffuse but may be focal. On CT, iron deposition increases parenchymal attenuation to 75 to 130 H. Iron deposition may be confirmed on magnetic resonance imaging, which shows a strikingly decreased signal on T2-weighted images.

Budd-Chiari Syndrome

Budd-Chiari syndrome refers to the manifestations of hepatic venous outflow obstruction, which include severe centrilobular congestion, hepatocellular necrosis, and atrophy. Acute thrombosis of the main hepatic

veins or inferior vena cava is associated with pregnancy, oral contraceptive use, and polycythemia vera. Neoplastic obstruction of the hepatic veins or inferior vena cava occurs with hepatoma and renal cell and adrenal carcinoma. Chronic fibrosis is idiopathic and affects small sublobular and central hepatic veins. CT findings include

1. Caudate lobe enlargement (the caudate lobe is spared because of its separate hepatic vein drainage)
2. Hepatic veins and inferior vena cava that are narrowed or not visualized
3. Inhomogeneous parenchymal enhancement
4. Early enhancement of the central liver
5. Late enhancement of the peripheral liver
6. Intrahepatic collateral vessels seen as comma-shaped enhancing vessels

FOCAL LIVER MASSES

Solid Liver Masses

A primary goal of liver imaging is to differentiate significant liver masses from insignificant ones. Clinically significant liver masses include metastases, hepatoma, and hepatic adenoma. Cavernous hemangioma, hepatic cyst, and focal nodular hyperplasia are nonsurgical liver masses that must be discriminated.

Metastases. Metastases are the most common malignant tumors in the liver, outnumbering primary malignancy by a ratio of 18 to 1. Liver metastases can originate from almost any primary malignancy, but most arise from the gastrointestinal tract, especially the colon. Usually, metastases are multiple, but the greatest problems in differentiation occur when they are solitary. A wide spectrum of CT appearance is possible, including

1. Well-defined low-density solid mass with vague peripheral enhancement (most common) (Fig. 10–11)
2. High-density solid mass, especially when the liver is fatty replaced
3. Cystic/necrotic mass, especially when the primary tumor is mucinous colon carcinoma, lung, melanoma, or carcinoid tumor
4. Partially calcified mass, especially when the metastatic deposit is necrotic (Fig. 10–12)
5. Diffusely infiltrating metastases that mimic diffuse hepatic disease and not appear as distinct masses

In summary, metastases can look like almost every other lesion in the liver and must always be considered a possibility.

Hepatoma. Hepatocellular carcinoma is the most common primary hepatic malignancy. In Western countries, 80% of hepatomas arise in cirrhotic livers. Most patients are older than age 50. Elevated serum α-fetoprotein is a common clinical clue to the diagnosis. Three patterns of tumor growth are seen: solitary tumor (50%) (Fig. 10–13), diffuse infiltrative tumor (30%) (see Fig. 10–10), and multinodular tumor (20%). On CT, most are low density on unenhanced scans and enhance prominently during the arterial phase on dynamic contrast injection. Areas of tumor necrosis are common, and calcification is present in 25%. Tumor invasion of hepatic and portal veins is frequent. Fatty metamorphosis within hepatomas is common histologically and has been reported on CT.

Fibrolamellar Carcinoma. This is a slow-growing tumor that usually arises in normal liver. Patients are younger (usually <40 years) than most hepatoma patients, and α-fetoprotein is not present in serum. Prognosis is good if the tumor is completely resected. Characteristic CT findings are a well-defined hypodense mass, a central low-density scar that may calcify, and marked tumor enhancement due to hypervascularity. Fibrolamellar carcinoma may be difficult to differentiate from focal nodular hyperplasia.

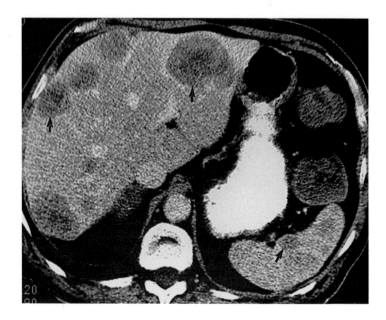

Figure 10–11. Metastases. Photography of this CT scan with narrow windows makes multiple metastases *(arrows)* in the liver and spleen more apparent. Faint peripheral enhancement of the metastatic lesions is evident. Low-density centers indicate necrosis. The primary tumor was lung carcinoma.

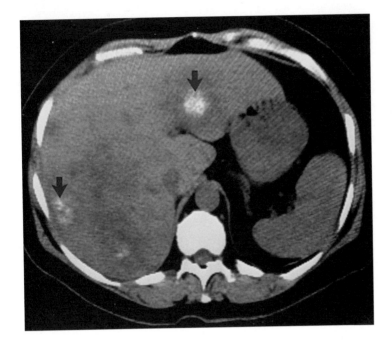

Figure 10–12. Calcified liver metastases. Metastatic deposits from mucinous adenocarcinoma of the colon cause multiple focal masses in the liver, some of which are calcified *(arrows)*. Calcified metastases are characteristic of mucinous carcinomas and necrotic tumors.

Lymphoma. The liver is involved in more than half of all patients with both Hodgkin's and non-Hodgkin's lymphoma. Diffuse infiltration is common and may cause only hepatomegaly without altering parenchymal density. Multiple well-defined, large, homogeneous low-density nodules are the most characteristic finding. The spleen is usually also involved, and abdominal adenopathy is usually present.

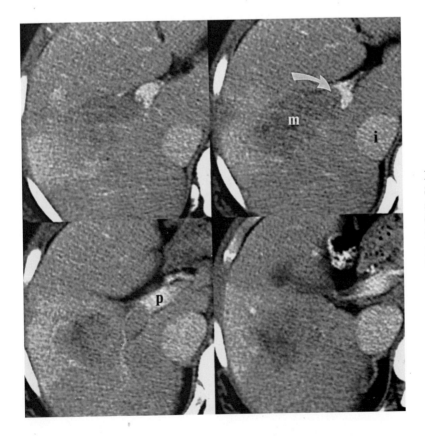

Figure 10–13. Hepatoma. Serial CT scans demonstrate an ill-defined mass (m) in the right hepatic lobe invading *(arrow)* the main portal vein (p). i = inferior vena cava.

Hepatic Adenoma. Hepatocellular adenoma is a rare, but much talked about benign tumor. It is a significant lesion because of the risk of major hemorrhage associated with its presence. Hepatic adenomas are composed of neoplastic hepatocytes. Kupffer cells are occasionally present. Most tumors are solitary. Areas of hemorrhage and necrosis are nearly always present within the tumor. Most present as an abdominal mass, gastrointestinal complaints, or hemoperitoneum due to tumor rupture. Oral contraceptive and anabolic steroid use are risk factors, both for tumor growth and for rupture. Surgical removal is recommended. The imaging findings are

1. Hypodense heterogeneous mass on unenhanced CT
2. Hemorrhage within the tumor
3. Markedly heterogeneous appearance on enhanced CT with areas of increased, normal, and decreased density within the tumor
4. Nearly always absent radionuclide uptake within the tumor on technetium-99m sulfur colloid–labeled liver scan
5. Multiple tumors in 30%

Focal Nodular Hyperplasia. In contrast to hepatic adenoma, focal nodular hyperplasia contains all the histologic elements of normal liver, including Kupffer cells. Fibrous bands and stellate fibrous scars are common, but hemorrhage and necrosis are rare. Most patients are asymptomatic, and the tumor is discovered incidentally. The tumor is benign, and no treatment is indicated. The imaging findings are

1. Hypodense homogeneous solid mass (usually <5 cm diameter) on unenhanced CT
2. Dramatic homogeneous enhancement during arterial phase of enhanced CT (Fig. 10–14)
3. Central low-density scar (one third of cases) (see Fig. 10–14)
4. Normal (40%) or increased (10%) radionuclide uptake within the tumor on technetium-99m sulfur colloid–labeled liver scan—the most specific finding
5. Cold defect on technetium-99m sulfur colloid–labeled liver scan (50%)
6. Multiple tumors in 7%

Cavernous Hemangioma. Cavernous hemangiomas are the second most common focal mass lesion in the liver, exceeded in frequency only by metastases. They are the most common benign liver neoplasm, found in up to 7% of patients in autopsy series. They are often discovered incidentally during hepatic imaging by ultrasonography or computed tomography. They may be found at any age and are more common in women. Although most are solitary, 10% of the affected patients have multiple lesions easily

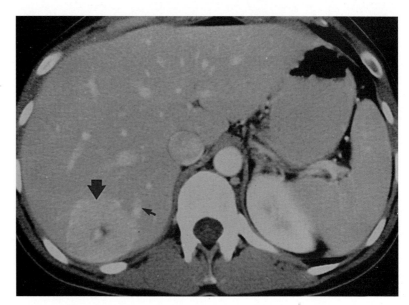

Figure 10–14. Focal nodular hyperplasia. A brightly enhancing mass *(large arrow)* in the posterior segment of the right hepatic lobe has a characteristic central low-density scar. A large draining vein *(small arrow)* indicates the hypervascular nature of the mass.

mistaken for metastases. The tumors consist of large, thin-walled, blood-filled vascular spaces lined by epithelium and separated by fibrous septa. Blood flow through the complex of vascular spaces is very slow, resulting in characteristic prolonged retention of contrast agents on CT. The majority of lesions are less than 5 cm, are asymptomatic, and pose no threat to the patient. Larger *giant cavernous hemangiomas* may cause symptoms by pressure effect, hemorrhage, or arteriovenous shunting. The imaging findings (Fig. 10–15) are

1. Well-defined hypodense mass of the same density as other blood-filled spaces, such as the portal vein, on unenhanced CT scans
2. Development of nodule-like areas of enhancement in the periphery when contrast medium is given as a rapid bolus
3. Areas of enhancement that become confluent with the entire lesion gradually becoming isodense or hyperdense relative to the liver parenchyma
4. Contrast medium enhancement usu-

ally persisting within the lesion for 20 to 30 minutes after contrast agent injection
5. Large lesions with discrete areas of fibrosis and, occasionally, calcification that remain hypodense throughout the period of enhancement

When these classic findings are observed, the CT examination can be considered diagnostic of cavernous hemangioma with a high degree of confidence. In questionable cases, tagged red blood cell scintigraphy is usually diagnostic.

CYSTIC LIVER MASSES

Simple Hepatic Cyst. Simple hepatic cysts are believed to be congenital and due to maldevelopment of bile ducts. Benign hepatic cysts are found in 5% to 10% of the population. They are usually solitary but may be multiple, especially in patients with adult polycystic disease. Simple hepatic cysts appear on CT as round, fluid-density masses with sharply defined, smooth, thin

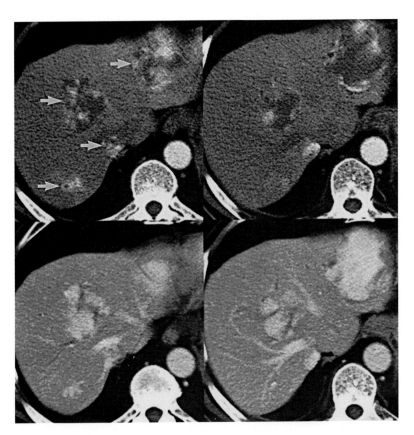

Figure 10–15. Cavernous hemangioma. Early *(top row)* and late *(bottom row)* nonequilibrium phase images from contrast-bolus–enhanced CT demonstrate the characteristic enhancement pattern of multiple cavernous hemangiomas *(arrows)*. Early contrast medium enhancement appears nodular and at the periphery. Enhancement proceeds centrally to complete opacification, except for areas of fibrous scarring in large lesions.

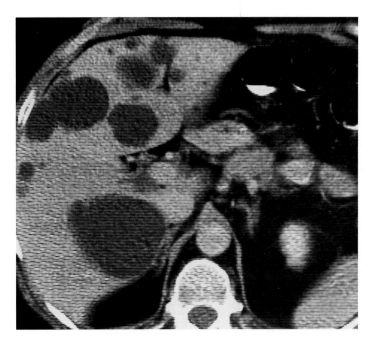

Figure 10–16. Multiple simple hepatic cysts. Simple hepatic cysts have uniform low internal density and sharp margins with the surrounding hepatic parenchyma. No cysts walls are evident. The lesions do not enhance with intravenous contrast medium.

walls (Fig. 10–16). They have no internal structure and show no enhancement with contrast medium administration. Lesions with this appearance in asymptomatic patients may be confidently diagnosed as simple hepatic cysts.

The following diseases must be considered in symptomatic patients and when the cystic hepatic lesion is not characteristic of simple hepatic cyst:

Pyogenic Abscess. Bacterial abscess is usually solitary but often multiloculated with thickened enhancing walls (Fig. 10–17). When multiple, lesions are often grouped and consist of many microabscesses. Masses are hypodense with a peripheral rim that usually enhances with contrast medium. Gas is present within the lesion in 20%. Patients are usually clinically septic and are often jaundiced. Fine-needle

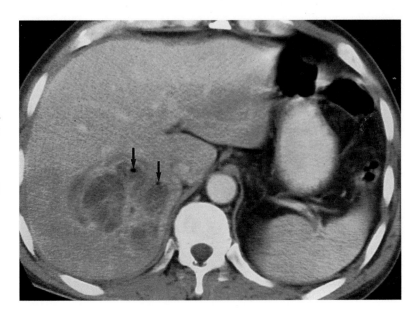

Figure 10–17. Pyogenic liver abscess. A liver abscess containing *Escherichia coli* has irregular septations and contains a few bubbles of air *(arrows)*. Because of the multiple loculations, this abscess did not respond to percutaneously placed catheter drainage but required surgical débridement.

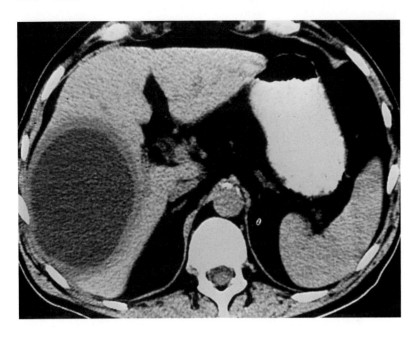

Figure 10–18. Amebic abscess. A 50-year-old American living in Thailand returned to the United States with this mass in his liver. Although the internal density is homogeneously low, a distinct thick wall is present and was observed to enhance with intravenous contrast medium administration. Serologic titers were positive for amebiasis.

aspiration is indicated for bacterial culture. Catheter or surgical drainage is needed.

Amebic Abscess. Liver abscess occurs in 3% to 7% of patients with amebiasis. The abscess is usually solitary (85%) and in the right lobe (72%) and has a well-defined, nodular, enhancing wall (Fig. 10–18). Its appearance overlaps that of pyogenic abscess, but patients are generally not septic and live in, or have a history of travel to, an endemic area. Right pleural effusion and right lower lobe infiltration are often present. Diagnosis is made by clinical and radiographic findings and is confirmed by serology. Treatment with metronidazole is usually effective (90%). Drainage is used for large and poorly responding lesions.

***Echinococcus* Cyst.** Infestation with the *Echinococcus* tapeworm results in the formation of single or multiple (60%) cystic

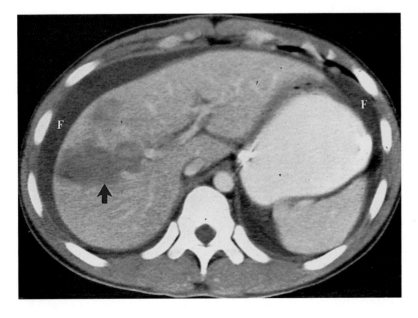

Figure 10–19. Liver laceration. A CT scan of the liver in a 16-year-old boy injured in a motor vehicle accident demonstrates a low-density band *(arrow)* through the liver. The low-density band is due to hematoma within a laceration of the liver. Fluid (F) around the liver, spleen, and stomach is free blood within the peritoneal cavity. CT is excellent in quantitating the amount of hemoperitoneum, but the entire abdomen and pelvis must be surveyed.

masses. The cysts are usually well defined, and 50% have calcification in their walls. Daughter cysts can be visualized with the parent cyst in 70%. The remainder may be difficult to differentiate from simple cysts. Drainage is the treatment of choice.

Cystic/Necrotic Liver Tumor. Necrotic, hemorrhagic, or primarily cystic tumors may mimic hepatic cysts. Most have thickened walls, nodularity, or internal debris or show evidence of contrast medium enhancement. Metastases are most common and usually multiple. Biliary cystadenomas and cystadenocarcinomas are uncommon cystic tumors. Hepatocellular carcinoma may rarely be cystic.

LIVER TRAUMA

CT accurately depicts the extent of liver injury and quantitates the amount of hemoperitoneum present after blunt abdominal trauma. Liver injuries may be classified as contusions or lacerations, with variably sized intrahepatic and subcapsular hematomas. Hemoperitoneum associated with liver injury generally implies a laceration extending through the liver capsule with bleeding and/or bile leakage into the peritoneal cavity. Lacerations may be linear or stellate and are defined on CT by blood within the area of injury (Fig. 10–19). The hematoma may be isodense with unenhanced liver parenchyma. Visualization of the hematoma and the laceration is improved by intravenous contrast agent administration, which enhances liver parenchyma.

Suggested Reading

Auh YH, Lim JH, Kim KW, et al. Loculated fluid collections in hepatic fissures and recesses: CT appearance and potential pitfalls. RadioGraphics 1994; 14:529–540.

Baker ME, Pelley R. Hepatic metastases: basic principles and implications for radiologists. Radiology 1995; 197:329–337.

Bluemke DA, Fishman EK. Spiral CT of the liver. AJR 1993; 160:787–792.

Brady AP, Malone DE, McGrath FP, Friedman L. Focal nodular hyperplasia of the liver—an imaging conundrum. Can Assoc Radiol J 1994; 45:108–116.

Brant WE, Floyd JL, Jackson DE, Gilliland JD. The radiological evaluation of hepatic cavernous hemangioma. JAMA 1987; 257:2471–2474.

Buetow PC, Pantongrag-Brown L, Buck JL, et al. Focal nodular hyperplasia of the liver: radiologic-pathologic correlation. RadioGraphics 1996;16:369–388.

Cho KC, Patel YD, Wachsberg RH, Seeff J. Varices in portal hypertension: evaluation with CT. RadioGraphics 1995; 15:609–622.

Choi BI, Takayasu K, Han MC. Small hepatocellular carcinomas and associated nodular lesions of the liver: pathology, pathogenesis, and imaging findings. AJR 1993; 160:1177–1187.

Cohen J, Edelman RR, Chopra S. Portal vein thrombosis: a review. Am J Med 1992; 92:173–182.

Dodd GD. An American's guide to Couinaud's numbering system. AJR 1993; 161:574–575.

Gore RM, Mathieu DG, White EM, et al. Passive hepatic congestion: cross-sectional imaging features. AJR 1994; 162:71–75.

Jones EC, Chezmar JL, Nelson RC, Bernardino ME. The frequency and significance of small (≤15 mm) hepatic lesions detected by CT. AJR 1992; 158:535–539.

Ito K, Honjo K, Fujita T, et al. Liver neoplasms: diagnostic pitfalls in cross-sectional imaging. RadioGraphics 1996; 16:273–293.

Marn CS, Francis IR. CT of portal venous occlusion. AJR 1992; 159:717–726.

Matsui O, Kadoya M, Takahashi S, et al. Focal sparing of segment IV in fatty livers shown by sonography and CT: correlations with aberrant gastric venous drainage. AJR 1995; 164:1137–1140.

Mergo PJ, Ros PR, Buetow PC, Buck JL. Diffuse disease of the liver: radiologic-pathologic correlation. RadioGraphics 1994; 14:1291–1307.

Morgan-Parkes JH. Metastases: mechanisms, pathways, and cascades. AJR 1995; 164:1075–1082.

Murphy BJ, Casillas J, Ros PR, et al. The CT appearance of cystic masses of the liver. RadioGraphics 1989; 9:307–322.

Parvey HR, Raval B, Sandler CM. Portal vein thrombosis: imaging findings. AJR 1994; 162:77–81.

Soyer P. Segmental anatomy of the liver: utility of a nomenclature accepted worldwide. AJR 1993; 161:572–573.

Soyer P, Bluemke DA, Bliss DF, et al. Surgical segmental anatomy of the liver: demonstration with spiral CT during arterial portography and mulitplanar reconstruction. AJR 1994; 163:99–103.

Taylor AJ, Carmody TJ, Quiroz FA, et al. Focal masses in cirrhotic liver: CT and MR imaging features. AJR 1994; 163:857–862.

Winter TC, Nghiem HV, Freeny PC, et al. Hepatic arterial anatomy: demonstration of normal supply and vascular variants with three-dimensional CT angiography. RadioGraphics 1995; 15:771–780.

11

Biliary Tree and Gallbladder

William E. Brant, M.D.

BILIARY TREE

Anatomy

The bile ducts arise as biliary capillaries between hepatocytes. Bile capillaries coalesce to form intrahepatic bile ducts. Intrahepatic ducts branch in a predictable manner corresponding to the segments of the liver. Interlobular bile ducts combine to form two main trunks from the right and left lobes of the liver. The 3- to 4-cm long common hepatic duct is formed in the porta hepatis by the junction of the main right and left bile ducts. The cystic duct runs posteriorly and inferiorly from the gallbladder neck to join the common hepatic duct and form the common bile duct. The 6- to 7-cm long common bile duct courses ventral to the portal vein and to the right of the hepatic artery, descending from the porta hepatis along the free right border of the hepatoduodenal ligament to behind the duodenal bulb. Its distal third turns directly caudad, descending in the groove between the descending duodenum and the head of the pancreas just ventral to the inferior vena cava. The common duct tapers distally as it ends in the sphincter of Oddi, which protrudes into the duodenum as the ampulla of Vater. The common bile duct and the pancreatic duct share a common orifice in 60% of cases and have separate orifices in the remainder. In any case, they are in such close proximity that tumors of the am-pullary region will generally obstruct both ducts.

Normal-sized intrahepatic bile ducts are not usually visible on routine abdominal CT. However, with thin collimation (3 to 5 mm) and dynamic bolus intravenous contrast medium enhancement, normal intrahepatic ducts may be visualized in up to 40% of patients. Normal intrahepatic ducts are 2 mm diameter in the central liver and taper progressively toward the periphery. The common hepatic duct is usually seen in the porta hepatis, and the common bile duct is routinely visualized descending adjacent to the descending duodenum. It is fair to use the generic term *common duct* to refer to both the common hepatic and the common bile ducts because the cystic duct junction marking their anatomic partition is not routinely visualized on CT. The normal common duct does not exceed 6 mm in diameter in most adult patients. In elderly patients the normal common duct diameter increases about 1 mm per decade (i.e., 7 mm is normal for patients in their 70s, and 8 mm is normal for those in their 80s). Contrast medium enhancement improves identification of both normal and dilated bile ducts by enhancing blood vessels and the surrounding parenchyma. Bile ducts are seen as lucent branching tubular structures. The bile ducts may be difficult to differentiate from blood vessels without contrast agent administration. Gas (Fig. 11–1) or contrast media from the gastrointestinal tract that refluxes into the biliary tree may be associ-

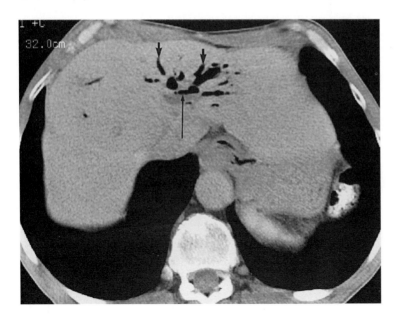

Figure 11–1. Air in the biliary tree. Air is seen in the bile ducts *(short arrows)* of the left lobe of the liver in this patient with a choledochojejunostomy performed as part of a Whipple procedure. Air fills the left hepatic bile ducts in a supine patient and the right hepatic bile ducts in a prone patient. Note the air–bile level *(long arrow).*

ated with a number of conditions (Table 11–1).

Biliary Obstruction

CT is about 96% accurate in determining the presence of biliary obstruction, 90% accurate in determining its level, and 70% accurate in determining its cause. The major causes of biliary obstruction are gallstones, tumor, stricture, and pancreatitis. A rare but interesting cause of biliary obstruction is Mirizzi syndrome. A gallbladder stone impacted in the cystic duct induces cholangitis or erodes into the common duct to cause obstructive jaundice (Table 11–2).

CT diagnosis of biliary obstruction depends on the demonstration of dilated bile ducts. The biliary tree dilates proximal to the point of obstruction, whereas bile ducts below the obstruction remain normal or are reduced in size. When cirrhosis, cholangitis, or periductal fibrosis prohibit dilatation of the bile ducts in obstructive jaundice, the CT will be falsely negative. The CT findings of biliary obstruction are

1. Multiple branching, round or oval, low-density tubular structures representing dilated intrahepatic biliary ducts coursing toward the porta hepatis (Fig. 11–2)

2. Dilatation of the common duct in the porta hepatis seen as a tubular or oval fluid density tube greater than 7 mm in diameter

TABLE 11–1. **Reflux of Gas or Bowel Contrast into Biliary Tree**

Iatrogenic
Sphincterotomy
Choledochojejunostomy
Gallstone fistula
Cholecystoduodenal fistula
Perforated ulcer
Choledochoduodenal fistula
Carcinoma
Choledochoenteric fistula

TABLE 11–2. **Causes of Obstructive Jaundice in Adults**

Gallstone impacted in bile duct
Bile duct stricture
Traumatic/surgery/instrumentation
Chronic pancreatitis
Sclerosing cholangitis
Oriental cholangiohepatitis
Acquired immunodeficiency syndrome–associated cholangitis
Malignancy
Pancreas carcinoma
Duodenal/ampullary carcinoma
Cholangiocarcinoma
Metastases
Parasites (*Ascaris, Clonorchis*)
Choledochal cyst

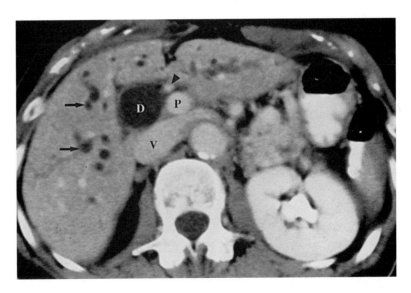

Figure 11–2. Dilated bile ducts. The greatly dilated common bile duct (D) is seen anterior to the inferior vena cava (V) and to the right of the hepatic artery *(arrowhead)* and portal vein (P). Dilated intrahepatic bile ducts *(arrows)* are seen as low-density branching tubular structures adjacent to enhancing portal veins within the liver.

3. Dilatation of the common duct in the pancreatic head seen as a round fluid density tube larger than 7 mm

4. Enlargement of the gallbladder to greater than 5 cm diameter, when the obstruction is distal to the cystic duct

Clues to the cause of biliary obstruction (Fig. 11–3) include

1. Abrupt termination of a dilated extrahepatic biliary duct, which is characteristic of a malignant process even in absence of a visible mass. Common tumors causing biliary obstruction are pancreatic carcinoma, ampullary carcinoma, and cholangiocarcinoma. A mass is often visible on CT at the point of biliary obstruction.

2. Gradual tapering of a dilated duct seen most commonly with benign disease such as inflammatory stricture or pancreatitis. Calcifications in the pancreas are a clue to the presence of chronic pancreatitis (Fig. 11–4).

3. Gallstones obstructing the bile ducts and seen as calcific, soft tissue, or fat density structures within the bile duct surrounded by a crescent of fluid density bile (Fig. 11–5). Some stones are isodense with bile and are not detectable by CT.

Cholangiocarcinoma

Cholangiocarcinoma is a slow-growing primary adenocarcinoma of the bile ducts. Although it may arise anywhere in the biliary tree, it occurs most commonly in the common bile duct between the cystic duct and the ampulla of Vater. This tumor is frequently small at the time of discovery because it causes jaundice early in its course. Focal or generalized biliary dilatation extends to the point of tumor obstruction. The tumor itself may be isodense with surrounding parenchyma or be too small to see on CT. When visible, it is generally hypodense to liver parenchyma and infiltrates surrounding tissues. CT findings of cholangiocarcinoma vary with location:

1. Intrahepatic (20%–30%): hypodense mass with irregular enhancement, obstructed intrahepatic bile ducts, noncirrhotic liver

2. Hilar (Klatskin's tumor, 10%–20%): small, hypodense mass at the confluence of dilated right and left hepatic ducts

3. Distal (50%–70%): short stricture or small polypoid mass in the common duct with proximal biliary dilatation.

Sclerosing Cholangitis

Sclerosing cholangitis is a fibrosing inflammation of the biliary tree resulting in biliary dilatation due to destruction and fibrous obliteration of large intrahepatic bile ducts. CT demonstrates beaded dilatation of intrahepatic and extrahepatic bile ducts alternating with multiple segmental strictures and thickening (2–5 mm) of the bile duct walls (Fig. 11–6). Most cases are con-

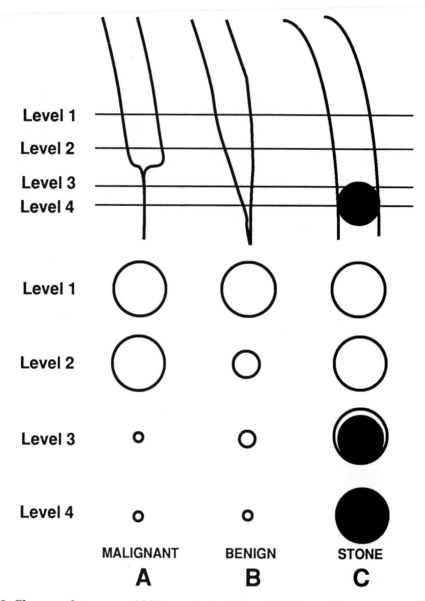

Figure 11–3. Clues to the cause of biliary obstruction. *A,* Malignant tumors cause abrupt termination of the distal common bile duct. *B,* Inflammatory strictures and pancreatitis cause progressive tapering of the distal common bile duct. *C,* Impacted gallstones may be seen as rounded structures in the distal common bile duct. The CT density of gallstones varies from calcific density to fat density.

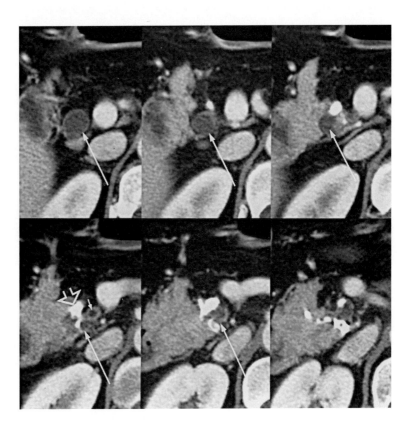

Figure 11–4. Benign stricture of common bile duct due to chronic pancreatitis. Serial CT images demonstrate progressive tapering of the distal common bile duct *(long arrows)* as it passes through the head of the pancreas. The pancreatic head is deformed, and multiple calcifications *(open arrow)* and cystic changes *(short arrow)* indicate chronic pancreatitis.

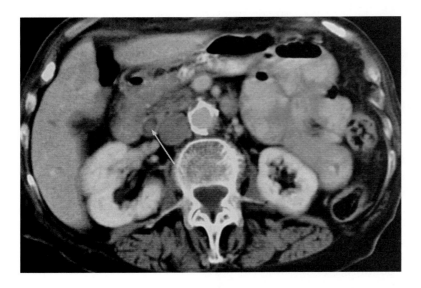

Figure 11–5. Obstructing gallstone in common bile duct. A gallstone *(arrow)* is seen in the distal common bile duct in this patient with biliary obstruction. The stone is partially surrounded by a crescent of lower-density bile.

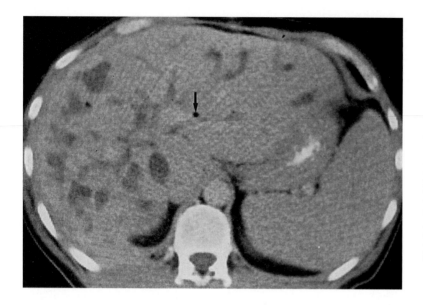

Figure 11–6. Recurrent cholangitis. Dilated bile ducts are seen as low-density oval and tubular structures within the liver. Note the marked variation in diameter of the ducts in the periphery of the liver that is found in both recurrent cholangitis and Caroli's disease. This patient has had a choledochojejunostomy and has a bubble of air *(arrow)* in the biliary tree.

sidered to be "primary" and of unknown etiology, although some cases are associated with ulcerative colitis. Acquired immunodeficiency syndrome–associated cholangitis demonstrates a similar CT appearance but is due to opportunistic infection with *Cryptosporidium* or cytomegalovirus.

Oriental Cholangiohepatitis

Recurrent pyogenic cholangitis with propensity to form pigmented stones in the intrahepatic and extrahepatic biliary tree is endemic in Southeast Asian and Chinese populations and is seen predominantly in immigrants in Western countries. Infestations with *Clonorchis sinensis* and *Ascaris lumbricoides*, malnutrition, and portal vein bacteremia all seem to play a role in its etiology. CT signs include

1. Dilated bile ducts filled with stones and pus
2. Abrupt tapering of dilated ducts indicating strictures
3. Contrast medium enhancement of bile duct walls
4. Fatty infiltration and atrophy of hepatic parenchyma in the segments affected

Caroli's Disease

Caroli's disease is a rare congenital anomaly of the biliary tract characterized by saccular dilatation of the intrahepatic biliary tree,

cholangitis, and gallstone formation in the absence of cirrhosis or portal hypertension. CT demonstrates cystic dilatation of the intrahepatic biliary tree with focal areas of tubular and saccular enlargement (see Fig. 11–6). Patients are at greatly increased risk of bile duct carcinoma (7% of patients).

Choledochal Cyst

Choledochal cyst is a congenital segmental dilatation of the common bile duct. Three major types have been described: (1) symmetric ectasia of the entire common duct (most common) (Fig. 11–7), (2) diverticulum of the common bile duct, and (3) localized fusiform dilatation of the distal common bile duct (choledochocele). On CT, choledochal cyst appears as a well-defined fluid-filled structure separate from the gallbladder and associated with dilatation of the intrahepatic biliary tree. Identification of bile ducts joining the cystic mass proves the diagnosis. Complications include gallstones and carcinoma of the common bile duct and gallbladder.

GALLBLADDER

Anatomy

The gallbladder lies in a fossa formed by the junction of the right and left lobes of the liver. Although the position of the fundus varies, the neck and body of the gallbladder are invariably related to the porta hepatis and major interlobar fissure. The gallbladder is in close proximity to the duodenal bulb and hepatic flexure of the colon. The normal gallbladder is 3 to 5 cm in diameter and 10 cm in length and has a capacity of roughly 50 mL. Agenesis of the gallbladder is extremely rare (<0.02%) and duplication of the gallbladder occurs in about 1 in 4000 individuals. Folds in the gallbladder, producing a phrygian cap deformity, are common (1%–6% incidence) and not clinically significant.

Ultrasonography, not CT, is the primary modality for imaging the gallbladder. However, significant gallbladder pathology may be diagnosed by CT, especially when screening the acutely ill patient. Normal bile is of fluid density (0–20 H) on CT. Higher-density bile suggests bile stasis (sludge), hemorrhage, or infection (pus). The gallbladder wall enhances avidly with bolus contrast agent administration.

Gallstones

Although gallstones may be detected by CT, the sensitivity of CT is only 80% to 85%, much less than that of ultrasonography or oral cholecystography. Gallstones vary in CT density from negative numbers, indicating fat density of cholesterol stones, to high positive numbers of calcified stones (Fig. 11–8). Fissured stones may contain linear streaks of air. Some gallstones may not be seen on CT because they are isodense with bile or because they are too small. Contrast medium enhancement in adjacent bowel loops may obscure, or mimic, gallstones.

Acute Cholecystitis

Acute cholecystitis is usually diagnosed clinically or by ultrasonography or radionuclide hepatobiliary scan. Cases are studied with CT usually because they are atypical or suspected to be complicated. Gangrenous cholecystitis may lead to perforation, abscess, fistula, or peritonitis. Acalculous cholecystitis occurs most commonly in critically ill patients, especially after surgery, trauma, or burns or in patients on hyperalimentation. Emphysematous cholecystitis is a severe form of cholecystitis that tends to occur in the elderly and in diabetics. It may produce deceptively mild symptoms but carries a high morbidity and mortality. The CT findings in acute cholecystitis (Fig. 11–9) are

1. Gallstones in 95%
2. Distended gallbladder lumen greater than 5 cm
3. Thickening of the gallbladder wall more than 3 mm

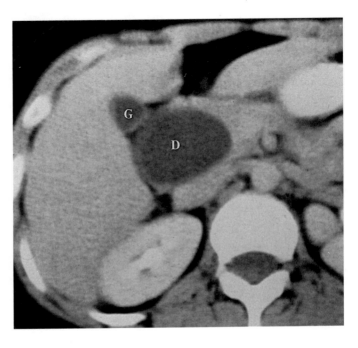

Figure 11–7. Choledochal cyst. The common bile duct (D) is massively enlarged. The neck of the gallbladder (G) is seen adjacent to the dilated common bile duct.

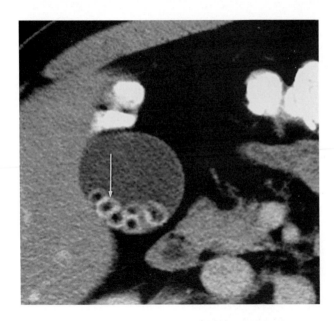

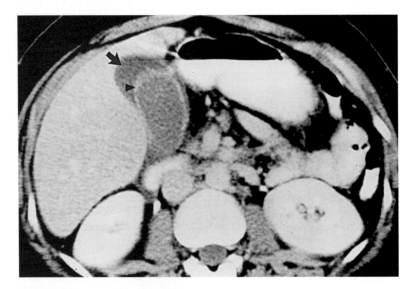

Figure 11–8. Gallstones. Gallstones *(arrow)* settle dependently in the gallbladder. These stones demonstrate low-density centers of high cholesterol content and calcified outer margins.

Figure 11–9. Acute cholecystitis. The gallbladder wall *(arrowhead)* enhances brightly after intravenous contrast medium administration in this patient with acalculous cholecystitis. Note the pericholecystic fluid *(arrow)*.

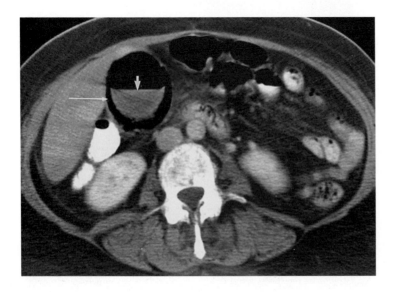

Figure 11–10. Emphysematous cholecystitis. Gas infiltrates the wall *(long arrow)* of the gallbladder and forms an air–fluid level *(short arrow)* with bile in the gallbladder lumen.

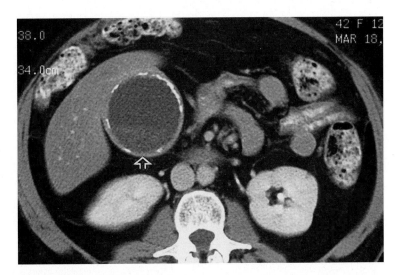

Figure 11–11. Porcelain gallbladder. The wall of the gallbladder *(arrow)* is thickened and calcified. A faint fluid level is seen in the gallbladder lumen owing to chronic bile stasis.

4. Halo of subserosal edema in the gallbladder wall

5. Pericholecystic fluid collection associated with perforation

6. Increase in bile density (above 20 H) due to biliary stasis, intraluminal pus, hemorrhage, or cellular debris

7. Air in the gallbladder wall or lumen with emphysematous cholecystitis (Fig. 11–10)

Porcelain Gallbladder

Calcification of the gallbladder wall, in association with chronic cholecystitis, is termed *porcelain gallbladder.* The calcification may be broad and continuous or multiple and punctate (Fig. 11–11). Gallstones are nearly always present. Gallbladder carcinoma may develop in 25% of patients with porcelain gallbladder. Cholecystectomy is advocated even when the patient is asymptomatic.

Gallbladder Carcinoma

Primary carcinoma of the gallbladder is commonly misdiagnosed preoperatively. CT provides an excellent method of evaluation. Chronic cholelithiasis is the major risk factor for this tumor. CT findings in gallbladder carcinoma are

1. Intraluminal soft tissue mass (Fig. 11–12)

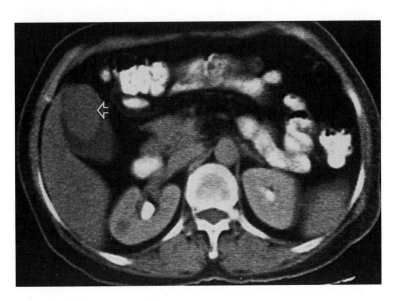

Figure 11–12. Gallbladder carcinoma. Adenocarcinoma of the gallbladder is seen as a polypoid intraluminal soft tissue mass *(arrow).*

2. Focal or diffuse thickening of the gall-bladder wall

3. Subhepatic mass replacing the gall-bladder

4. Gallstones (80%)

5. Calcification of the gallbladder wall

6. Extension of tumor into liver, subhepatic space, extrahepatic bile ducts, or adjacent bowel

Suggested Reading

Burrell MI, Zeman RK, Simeone JF, et al. The biliary tract: imaging for the 1990s. AJR 1991; 157:223–233.

Kim OH, Chung HJ, Choi BG. Imaging of choledochal cyst. RadioGraphics 1995; 15:69–88.

Lim JH. Oriental cholangiohepatitis: pathologic, clinical, and radiologic features. AJR 1991; 17:1–8.

Miller WJ, Sechtin AG, Campbell WL, Pieters PC. Imaging findings in Caroli's disease. AJR 1995; 165:333–337.

Rege RV. Adverse effects of biliary obstruction: implications for treatment of patients with obstructive jaundice. AJR 1995; 164:287–293.

Rizzo RJ, Szucs RA, Turner MA. Congenital abnormalities of the pancreas and biliary tree in adults. RadioGraphics 1995; 15:49–68.

Rooholamini SA, Tehrani NS, Razavi MK, et al. Imaging of gallbladder carcinoma. RadioGraphics 1994; 14:291–306.

Soyer P, Bluemke DA, Reichle R, et al. Imaging of intrahepatic cholangiocarcinoma: 1. peripheral cholangiocarcinoma. AJR 1995; 165:1427–1431.

Soyer P, Bluemke DA, Reichle R, et al. Imaging of intrahepatic cholangiocarcinoma: 2. Hilar cholangiocarcinoma. AJR 1995; 165:1433–1436.

Chapter

12

Pancreas

William E. Brant, M.D.

ANATOMY

The pancreas is positioned within the anterior pararenal compartment of the retroperitoneal space, behind the left lobe of the liver and the stomach, and in front of the spine and great vessels (Fig. 12–1). The peritoneum-lined lesser sac forms a potential space between the stomach and pancreas. The pancreas somewhat resembles a question mark turned on its left side with the hook portion formed by the pancreatic head and uncinate process as they lie cra-

dled in the duodenal loop. The portal vein fills the center of the hook. The uncinate process cradles the superior mesenteric vein and tapers to a sharpened point beneath it. The body and tail taper as they extend toward the splenic hilum. The pancreas is usually directed upward and to the left, although it may form an inverted U shape with the tail directed caudad. Sequential CT slices must be mentally summated to assess the shape and size of the pancreas. The entire gland is 12 to 15 cm long. Maximum dimensions for width are 3.0 cm for the

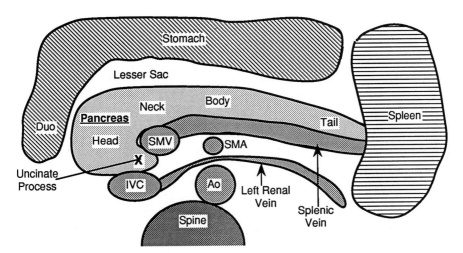

Figure 12–1. Pancreas anatomy. This diagram illustrates the CT landmarks for identification of the pancreas. The portal vein is formed behind the neck of the pancreas by the confluence of the splenic and superior mesenteric veins. The uncinate process of the pancreas extends between the superior mesenteric vein and the inferior vena cava. The lesser sac is a peritoneal-lined space between the stomach and the pancreas. SMV = superior mesenteric vein; SMA = superior mesenteric artery; IVC = inferior vena cava; Ao = aorta; Duo = descending duodenum.

head, 2.5 cm for the body, and 2.0 cm for the tail. The gland is larger in young patients and progressively decreases in size with age. The CT attenuation is uniform and approximately equal to muscle. Progressive infiltration of fat between the lobules of the pancreas gives it a feathery appearance with advancing age. The pancreatic duct is best visualized with thin slices (5 mm). It measures a maximum of 3 to 4 mm in diameter in the head and tapers smoothly to the tail.

The complex vascular anatomy about the pancreas must be understood to correctly interpret pancreatic CT. The splenic vein runs a relatively straight course in the dorsum of the pancreas from the splenic hilum to its junction with the superior mesenteric vein just posterior to the neck of the pancreas. The plane of fat between the splenic vein and pancreas is commonly mistaken for the pancreatic duct. The splenic artery runs an undulating course through the pancreas from the celiac axis to the spleen. Atherosclerotic calcifications are common in the splenic artery and are easily mistaken for pancreatic calcifications. The superior mesenteric artery arises from the aorta dorsal to the pancreas and courses caudad surrounded by a collar of fat. The superior mesenteric vein courses craniad, just to the right of the superior mesenteric artery, until it joins the splenic vein to form the portal vein. The pancreatic head entirely surrounds this junction with the uncinate process extending beneath the superior mesenteric vein. The portal vein courses upward and rightward with the hepatic artery and common bile duct to the porta hepatis.

TECHNICAL CONSIDERATIONS

Complete filling of the stomach and duodenal loop with contrast medium, air, or water is essential for high-quality pancreatic CT. Eight to 16 ounces of oral contrast agent is given immediately before scanning. Glucagon, 0.1 mg by intravenous injection, may be given to stop peristalsis in the duodenum and aid with bowel opacification. Intravenous contrast agent (150 mL) given rapidly

by mechanical injector is needed to (1) enhance the normal pancreatic parenchyma, (2) enhance peripancreatic vessels for identification and assessment of patency, and (3) enhance the liver parenchyma to detect involvement by pancreatic disease. Scanning is best performed with helical technique using 5-mm collimation and a pitch of 1. Reconstruction is performed at 3- to 5-mm intervals. Conventional CT is performed using contiguous 5- to 10-mm thick slices. Detection of functioning islet cell tumors requires dynamic helical scanning with rapid contrast agent infusion.

ACUTE PANCREATITIS

Inflammation of the pancreas damages acinar tissue and leads to focal disruption of

TABLE 12–1. **Causes of Pancreatitis**

Alcohol abuse—most common cause of chronic pancreatitis
Gallstone passage/impaction—most common cause of acute pancreatitis
Metabolic disorders
Hereditary pancreatitis—autosomal dominant
Hypercalcemia
Hyperlipidemia—types I and V
Malnutrition
Trauma
Blunt abdominal trauma
Surgery
Endoscopic retrograde cholangiopancreatography
Penetrating ulcer
Malignancy
Pancreatic adenocarcinoma
Lymphoma
Drugs—corticosteroids, tetracycline, furosemide, many others
Infection
Viral—mumps, hepatitis, infectious mononucleosis, acquired immunodeficiency syndrome
Parasitic—ascariasis, clonorchiasis
Structural
Choledochocele
Pancreas divisum
Idiopathic—20% of cases of acute pancreatitis

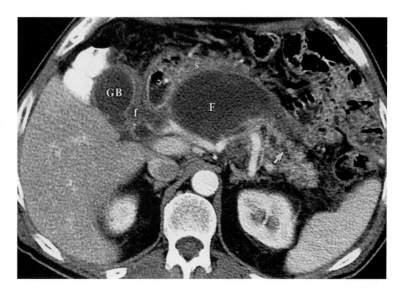

Figure 12–2. Acute pancreatitis. Fluid collections (f) resulting from acute pancreatitis extend from the necrotic pancreas into the lesser sac (F) compressing the stomach (s) and evident around the gallbladder (GB). The distal pancreatic duct *(arrow)* is dilated.

small ducts, resulting in leakage of pancreatic juice. The absence of a capsule around the pancreas allows easy access of pancreatic secretions to surrounding tissues. Pancreatic enzymes digest through fascial layers to spread to multiple anatomic compartments. The causes of pancreatitis are listed in Table 12–1.

The diagnosis of pancreatitis is made clinically. CT may be normal in mild cases. The role of CT is to document the presence and severity of complications. CT findings are

1. Pancreatic changes
   a. Focal or diffuse enlargement of the pancreas
   b. Decrease in density due to edema
   c. Blurring of the margins of the gland due to inflammation

2. Peripancreatic changes
   a. Stranding densities in fat and blurring of fat planes
   b. Thickening of retroperitoneal fascial planes
3. Complications
   a. Phlegmon: masslike edema and inflammation, seen as ill-defined heterogeneous soft tissue and fluid densities (20–40 H) in and around the pancreas
   b. Fluid collections: nonencapsulated homogeneous collections of fluid with water density (10–20 H) in the pancreatic bed, the retroperitoneum, and often widespread throughout the abdomen (Figs. 12–2 and 12–3; see also Fig. 13–5)

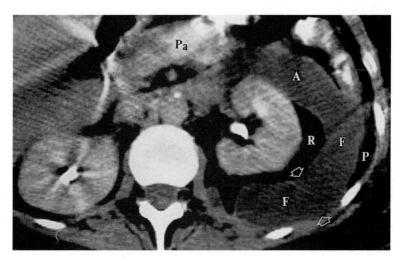

Figure 12–3. Acute pancreatitis. Pancreatic fluid (F) and inflammation extend from the pancreas (Pa) in the anterior pararenal space (A) to a retrorenal position between the leaves of the posterior renal fascia *(open arrows)*. Note that the perirenal space (R) and the posterior pararenal space (P) are spared. Compare with Figure 14–1.

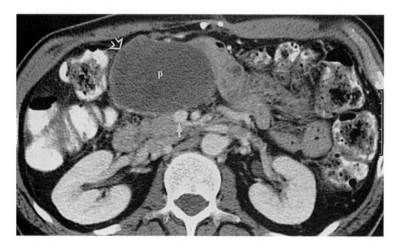

Figure 12–4. Pseudocyst. A pseudocyst (p) with a thin capsule *(open arrow)* persists 8 weeks after an episode of acute pancreatitis. The pseudocyst compressed the superior mesenteric vein *(small arrow)* and portal vein, resulting in dilatation of portosystemic collateral vessels.

c. Pseudocyst: well-defined round or oval fluid collection with clearly identifiable fibrous capsule (Fig. 12–4)

d. Necrosis: liquefaction of portions of the gland identified by lack of contrast medium enhancement (Fig. 12–5)

e. Abscess: bacterial growth within necrotic tissues seen as a loculated fluid collection; it may contain gas, and percutaneous aspiration is usually needed to confirm the diagnosis (Fig. 12–6)

f. Hemorrhage: due to erosion of blood vessels or bowel and seen as high-attenuating fluid in retroperitoneum or peritoneal cavity

g. Pseudoaneurysm: due to encapsulation of arterial hemorrhage with continued communication with eroded artery (Fig. 12–7)

h. Thrombosis of splenic vein or other peripancreatic vessel

i. Pancreatic ascites: leakage of pancreatic juice into the peritoneal cavity with high amylase level in fluid.

CHRONIC PANCREATITIS

Recurrent and prolonged bouts of inflammation cause progressive parenchymal atrophy and proliferation of fibrous tissue. Both exocrine and endocrine function are progressively impaired. CT evidence of chronic pancreatitis (Fig. 12–8) includes

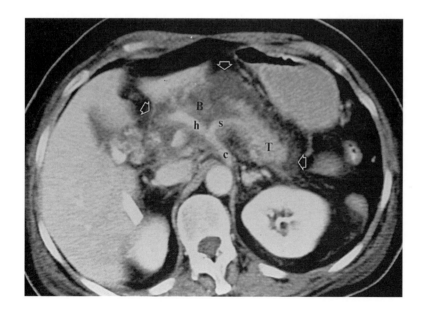

Figure 12–5. Pancreatic necrosis. The tail (T) of the pancreas enhances normally, but the head and body (B) of the pancreas have undergone liquefactive necrosis and are replaced by fluid density. Edema and inflammation *(open arrows)* cause fluid density in the pancreatic bed and in the fat surrounding the peripancreatic blood vessels. c = celiac axis; s = splenic artery; h = common hepatic artery.

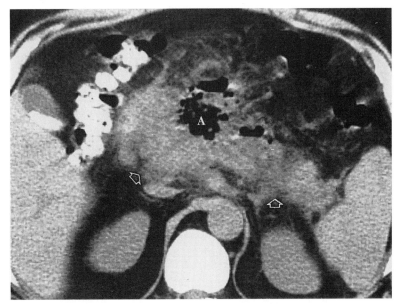

Figure 12–6. Pancreatic abscess. A penetrating duodenal ulcer resulted in pancreatitis, pancreatic abscess, and pancreaticoduodenal fistula. An extensive gas collection (A) occupies the pancreatic bed. The margins of the pancreas are blurred by the inflammatory process *(open arrows).*

1. Dilatation of the pancreatic duct, often in a beaded pattern
2. Decrease in visible pancreatic tissue due to parenchymal atrophy
3. Calcifications, varying from tiny stippled to coarse
4. Fluid collections, both intrapancreatic and extrapancreatic
5. Focal enlargement of the pancreas due to benign inflammation and fibrosis (Fig. 12–9)
6. Dilatation of the biliary duct due to fibrosis or mass in the pancreatic head
7. Fascial thickening and stranding in the peripancreatic fat

Differentiating an inflammatory mass from pancreatic carcinoma is frequently difficult and often requires biopsy (see Fig. 12–9). Pancreatic calcifications occur most frequently in hereditary pancreatitis and in chronic pancreatitis due to alcoholism.

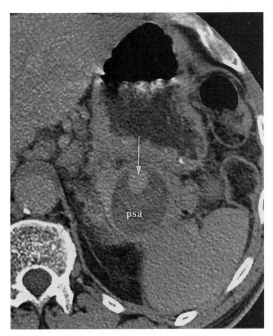

Figure 12–7. Pseudoaneurysm. A pseudoaneurysm (psa) of the splenic artery, developing as a complication of recurrent pancreatitis, is identified by a nodule of enhancement *(arrow).* The remainder of the pseudoaneurysm was low-density, indicating thrombus.

PANCREATIC CARCINOMA

Pancreatic adenocarcinoma is a highly lethal tumor with surgical resection offering only the slightest hope of long-term cure. Only 3% of afflicted patients survive 5 years. CT plays a pivotal role in preoperative staging, separating those patients whose disease is obviously not resectable from the 10% to 15% whose disease is potentially resectable. Unfortunately, most of those who undergo aggressive resection still

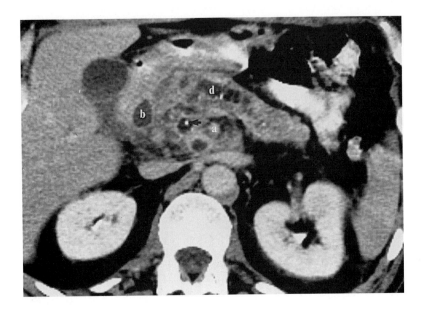

Figure 12–8. Chronic pancreatitis. The pancreatic duct (d) is enlarged, tortuous, and beaded in contour. The common bile duct (b) is also dilated. Speckled calcifications *(arrow)* are seen within the pancreas. Inflammatory changes cause increased density in the fat surrounding the superior mesenteric artery (a).

eventually die of their disease. CT signs of pancreatic carcinoma include

1. Hypodense mass that enhances minimally compared with normal pancreatic parenchyma
2. Focal enlargement of the pancreas with loss of surface lobulation
3. Blunting of the normally tapered uncinate process
4. Dilated pancreatic duct and/or common bile duct

5. Atrophy of the pancreas proximal to the tumor
6. Signs of pancreatitis proximal to the tumor
7. Signs of potential resectability (Fig. 12–10):
   a. Isolated pancreatic mass with or without dilatation of the bile and pancreatic ducts
   b. Combined bile–pancreatic duct dilatation without an identifiable pancreatic mass (pancreatic duct >5 mm in

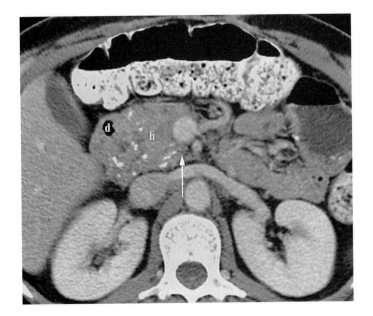

Figure 12–9. Mass due to chronic pancreatitis. Chronic pancreatitis causes enlargement of the pancreatic head (h) and blunting of the tip of the uncinate process *(arrow)*. The mass partially encases the duodenum (d). A benign etiology is suggested by the presence of calcifications, which are common with chronic pancreatitis and rare with pancreatic carcinoma. Compare with Figures 12–10 and 12–11.

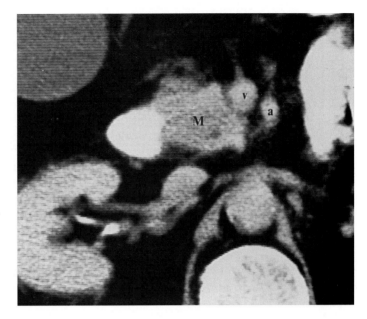

Figure 12–10. Potentially resectable pancreatic carcinoma. This small tumor (M) caused obstruction of both the pancreatic and common bile ducts in a 72-year-old man presenting with painless jaundice. The collar of fat surrounding the superior mesenteric artery (a) is uninvolved. The superior mesenteric vein (v) enhances normally, indicating patency.

head or >3 mm in tail; common bile duct >9 mm)
8. Signs of unresectability (Fig. 12–11):
   a. Extension of tumor beyond the margins of the pancreas

b. Tumor tissue invasion of adjacent organs (spleen, stomach, duodenum)
c. Enlarged regional lymph nodes (>1.5 cm)
d. Involvement of celiac axis, superior

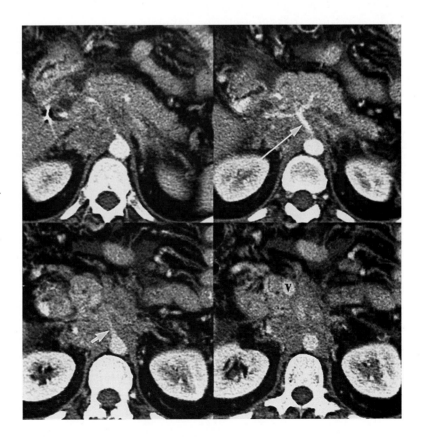

Figure 12–11. Unresectable pancreatic carcinoma. Four images from a helical CT examination demonstrate tumor encasement of the celiac axis *(long arrow)* and its branches and the superior mesenteric artery *(short arrow)* and vein (v). Tumor extensively infiltrates the retroperitoneal fat.

mesenteric artery, or portal, splenic, or superior mesenteric veins. Signs include

(1) Thickening of the vessel walls
(2) Soft tissue obscuring the normally sharp definition of the vessel by perivascular fat
(3) Deformity of the vessel by adjacent tumor
(4) Enlargement of collateral vessels
(5) Absence of vessel enhancement

e. Metastases to the liver (usually hypodense and poorly enhancing)

f. Ascites, which is presumptive evidence of peritoneal carcinomatosis

Because focal chronic pancreatitis may closely simulate malignancy in the pancreas, biopsy is frequently needed to confirm the diagnosis.

ISLET CELL TUMORS

Most islet cell tumors produce identifiable hormones and present as specific endocrine syndromes. Hormones secreted by islet cells include insulin (70% of secreting tumors), gastrin, glucagon, somatostatin, and vasoactive intestinal polypeptide. The tumors are generally small (0.4–4.0 cm) and require meticulous attention to CT technique to be detected. Most small islet cell tumors cannot be identified on precontrast scans. The characteristic feature of small tumors is transient circumscribed contrast medium enhancement that follows bolus contrast agent administration (Fig. 12–12). Rapid scan acquisition is needed to maximize contrast effect. This technique takes advantage of the hypervascularity demonstrated by most tumors. Cystic changes and necrosis are uncommon in small tumors. Functioning islet cell tumors may be either benign or malignant (90% of insulinomas and 50% of gastrinomas are benign).

Nonfunctioning islet cell tumors are larger (6–20 cm) and present clinically with mass effect. About 25% are malignant. Cystic degeneration and necrosis are frequent. Features that differentiate islet cell malignancy from pancreatic adenocarcinoma are unusually large tumor size, the presence of calcifications (in 20%), and contrast medium enhancement of the tumor.

CYSTIC LESIONS

Pseudocyst. By far the most common cystic lesions in and around the pancreas, pseudocysts are collections of pancreatic fluid that have become encapsulated within

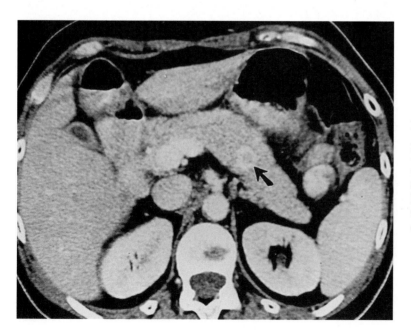

Figure 12–12. Insulinoma. A 1.8-cm insulin-producing islet cell tumor *(arrow)* is seen as a circular area of intense enhancement in the distal body of the pancreas. The patient presented with episodes of hypoglycemia.

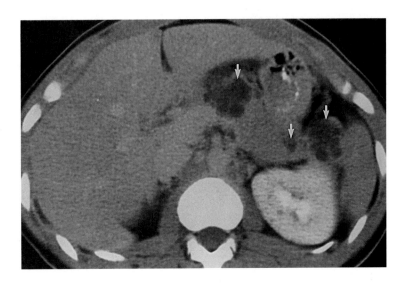

Figure 12–13. von Hippel-Lindau syndrome. Multilocular and unilocular cysts *(arrows)* are seen in the pancreas in this patient with von Hippel-Lindau syndrome.

fibrous walls. On CT they appear as low-density collections of fluid, cellular debris, and blood with well-defined walls of variable thickness and occasional calcifications (see Fig. 12–4).

Abscess. Any fluid collection in or around the pancreas is a potential abscess in a patient with fever. The CT appearance may be indistinguishable from sterile pseudocyst, although abscesses tend to have less distinct walls. Air within the fluid collection is strong evidence of the presence of infection. Diagnosis is confirmed by aspiration.

True Pancreatic Cyst. True cysts are rare, are congenital, and have an inner lining of epithelium. They are unilocular or multilocular, well-defined, fluid-filled (0–20 H), non-enhancing masses with walls of variable thickness. Multiple true cysts are seen in the pancreas in patients with autosomal dominant polycystic disease and von Hippel-Lindau syndrome (Fig. 12–13).

Cystic Tumors. Cystic tumors of the pancreas are uncommon (5%–15% of pancreatic cysts). Islet cell tumors may appear cystic owing to extensive necrosis. Cystic teratomas rarely arise in the pancreas and usually have characteristic hair, fat, calcifications, and cystic and solid components.

Microcystic adenoma is a benign hypervascular tumor usually seen in elderly women or in patients with von Hippel-Lin-

dau syndrome. It accounts for about half of the cystic neoplasms of the pancreas and has no malignant potential. The tumor consists of a honeycomb network of innumerable cysts ranging from millimeters up to 2 cm. Lining epithelial cells are rich in glycogen. CT shows a well-demarcated, usually large (10 cm average), low-density mass with enhancing septations (Fig. 12–14). Central scars, which may calcify, are evident in 20% of cases. The tumor may occur anywhere in the pancreas.

Mucinous cystic neoplasm may be a benign mucinous cystadenoma or a malignant cystadenocarcinoma. Differentiating benign from malignant tumors is difficult with imaging studies. Most (70%–95%) occur in the tail or body of the pancreas and are multilocular and hypovascular. They contain mucin and have thick walls and septations with papillary projections of solid tissue. CT demonstrates a mass composed of six, or fewer, cysts of 2 cm or greater (Fig. 12–15). Unilocular mucinous cystic neoplasms may closely resemble pancreatic pseudocysts.

TRAUMA

Traumatic injury to the pancreas is uncommon but has a high morbidity and is commonly clinically occult. Most (75%) pancreatic injuries are due to knife and gunshot wounds. Blunt abdominal trauma, often due

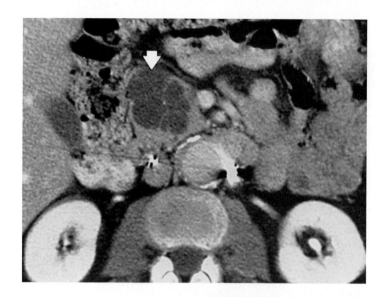

Figure 12–14. Microcystic adenoma. Multiple small cysts are evident in this microcystic adenoma *(arrow)* arising in the head of the pancreas. Thin, contrast medium–enhancing septations are evident.

Figure 12–15. Mucinous cystic adenocarcinoma. A cystic mass *(arrow)* with irregular thick walls is seen in the tail of the pancreas. Although no septations are identifiable by CT, several were evident on the pathologic specimen.

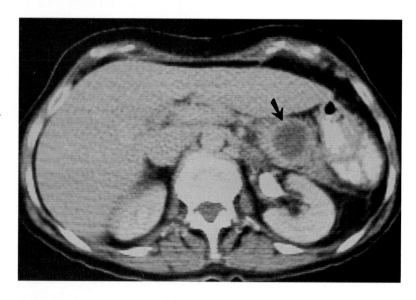

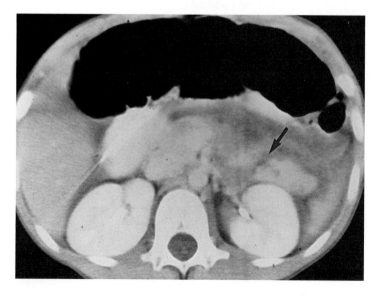

Figure 12–16. Pancreas laceration. A lucent defect *(arrow)* separates the body and tail of the pancreas in this 7-year-old boy struck by a car. Bleeding causes infiltration of the pancreas and the peripancreatic tissues.

to child abuse, is the most common cause of pancreatitis in children. The body of the pancreas may be compressed against the spine and is prone to contusion, laceration, transection, pancreatitis, and focal hemorrhagic necrosis. CT signs of pancreatic injury include pancreatic enlargement, fluid collections, and lucent defects representing lacerations (Fig. 12–16). Because tissue displacement may be minimal, lacerations are difficult to identify. Unexplained thickening of the anterior renal fascia and fluid in the lesser sac or anterior pararenal space are CT clues to possible pancreatic injury.

Suggested Reading

Balthazar EJ, Freeny PC, vanSonnenberg E. Imaging and intervention in acute pancreatitis. Radiology 1994; 193:297–306.

Balthazar EJ, Robinson DL, Megibow AJ, Ranson JH. Acute pancreatitis: value of CT in establishing prognosis. Radiology 1990; 174:331–336.

Bluemke DA, Cameron JL, Hruban RH, et al. Potentially resectable pancreatic adenocarcinoma: spiral CT assessment with surgical and pathologic correlation. Radiology 1995; 197:381–385.

Buck JL, Hayes WS. Microcystic adenoma of the pancreas. RadioGraphics 1990; 10:313–322.

Buetow PC, Parrino TV, Buck JL, et al. Islet cell tumors of the pancreas: pathologic-imaging correlation among size, necrosis and cysts, calcification, malignant behavior, and functional status. AJR 1995; 165:1175–1179.

Freeny PC, Marks WM, Ryan JA, Traverso LW. Pancreatic ductal adenocarcinoma: diagnosis and staging with dynamic CT. Radiology 1988; 166:125–133.

Hough DM, Stephens DH, Johnson CD, Binkovitz LA. Pancreatic lesions in von Hippel-Lindau disease: prevalence, clinical significance, and CT findings. AJR 1994; 162:1091–1094.

Johnson CD, Stephens DH, Charboneau JW, et al. Cystic pancreatic tumors: CT and sonographic appearance. AJR 1988; 151:1133–1138.

Luetmer PH, Stephens DH, Ward EM. Chronic pancreatitis: reassessment with current CT. Radiology 1989; 171:353–357.

Megibow AJ. Pancreatic adenocarcinoma: designing the examination to evaluate the clinical questions. Radiology 1992; 183:297–303.

Murr MM, Sarr MG, Oishi AJ, van Heerden JA. Pancreatic cancer. CA Cancer J Clin 1994; 44:304–318.

Procacci C, Graziani R, Bicego E, et al. Intraductal mucin-producing tumors of the pancreas: imaging findings. Radiology 1996; 198:249–257.

Ros PR, Hamrick-Turner JE, Chiechi MV, et al. Cystic masses of the pancreas. RadioGraphics 1992; 12:673–686.

Ward EM, Stephens DH, Sheedy PF II. Computed tomographic characteristics of pancreatic carcinoma: an analysis of 100 cases. RadioGraphics 1983; 3:547–565.

13

Spleen

William E. Brant, M.D.

ANATOMY

The spleen occupies a relatively constant position in the left upper quadrant of the abdomen. It is a soft and pliable organ that conforms to the shape of adjacent structures. The diaphragmatic surface is smooth and convex, conforming to the dome of the diaphragm, whereas the visceral surface has concavities for the stomach, kidney, and colon. The splenic artery and vein course in close relationship with the pancreas to the splenic hilum where each vessel divides into multiple branches. The normal spleen has lobulations, notches, and clefts that may be mistaken for abnormalities (Fig. 13–1). Lobulations in the splenic contour can generally be identified on serial slices as part of the spleen.

The CT density of the normal spleen is always less than, or equal to, the CT density of the normal liver. Normal spleen attenuation unenhanced is 40 to 60 H, which is 5 to 10 H less than the normal unenhanced liver. Most splenic lesions are seen best on contrast medium–enhanced CT scans. The spleen enhances irregularly in the early phase after bolus injection of contrast

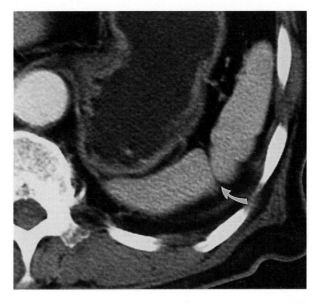

Figure 13–1. Normal cleft. A prominent, but normal, cleft is evident *(arrow)* in the spleen of a 72-year-old man.

agents, creating transient pseudomasses due to variable rates of blood flow through its pulp (Fig. 13–2).

TECHNICAL CONSIDERATIONS

The spleen is best examined using contiguous 7- to 10-mm thick slices obtained after intravenous injection of contrast agents. Unenhanced scans add little diagnostic information. When splenic pseudomasses due to early nonuniform contrast medium distribution (see Fig. 13–2) are suspected, rescanning the spleen a few minutes later will usually demonstrate uniform enhancement.

ANOMALIES

Accessory Spleen

Accessory spleens are nodules of normal splenic tissue that are formed separately from the main spleen. They are present in 10% to 30% of individuals and may be solitary or multiple. They appear (Fig. 13–3) as round or oval masses up to 2 to 3 cm in diameter, most commonly located in the hilum of the spleen and beside the tail of the

pancreas. They have the same CT density and tissue texture as the main spleen. Accessory spleens may hypertrophy after splenic resection. A radionuclide liver-spleen scan using technetium-99m sulfur colloid can confirm a hypertrophied accessory spleen as functioning splenic tissue.

Wandering Spleen

Wandering spleen refers to a normal spleen that is found outside the left upper quadrant of the abdomen. Congenital laxity of the ligaments, often associated with anomalies of intestinal fixation, cause the spleen to be freely mobile and be located anywhere in the abdomen. Wandering spleens are usually asymptomatic but may be a cause of a palpable abdominal mass and are more susceptible to traumatic injury. Diagnosis is made by noting the absence of a normal spleen in its typical location and that the ectopic mass is supplied by splenic vessels.

Splenic Regeneration

Accessory spleens or remnants of splenic tissue after splenic injury may hypertrophy after splenectomy, resulting in single or multiple left upper abdominal masses. The diagnosis is suggested clinically when a patient, with a history of splenectomy, has no Howell-Jolly bodies on peripheral blood

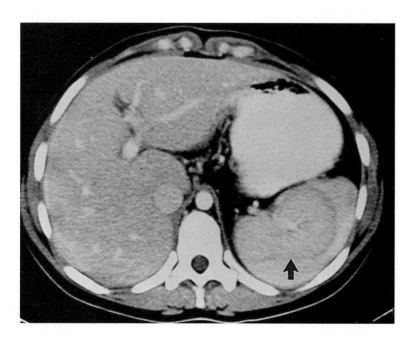

Figure 13–2. Transient pseudomass. Inhomogeneous enhancement of the spleen produces a pseudomass *(arrow)* during the early stage of intravenous contrast medium administration using a power injector. Images obtained a few minutes later *(not shown)* demonstrated uniform density of the spleen.

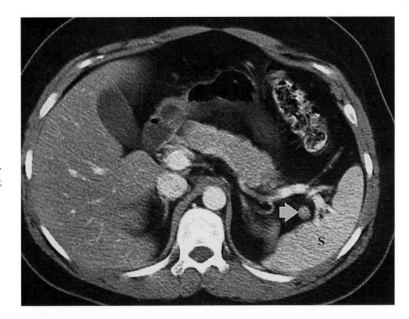

Figure 13–3. Accessory spleen. An accessory spleen *(arrow)* is evident near the hilum of the spleen (S) adjacent to the splenic vein.

smear. Howell-Jolly bodies are remnants of nuclear material in red blood cells that are usually removed from the circulating blood by the spleen. Regenerative splenic remnants have the CT appearance of normal splenic tissue. The presence of splenic tissue is confirmed by technetium-99m sulfur colloid radionuclide imaging.

SPLENOMEGALY

Spleen size varies with age, body habitus, state of hydration, and nutrition. Average maximal spleen dimensions in adults are 12 cm in length, 7 cm in breadth, and 3 to 4 cm in thickness. The spleen normally decreases in size with age. Judging spleen size is largely subjective. Size greater than 12 cm in any dimension and extension of the spleen below the costal margin, anterior to the midclavicular line, or substantially below the upper pole of the left kidney are CT signs of enlargement. The causes of splenomegaly are exhaustive but generally fall into myeloproliferative, infectious, congestive, and infiltrative categories. Most conditions do not affect CT density of the spleen, so differentiation is based on other CT findings or clinical evaluation.

CYSTIC LESIONS

Cysts

Posttraumatic cysts (Fig. 13–4) result from previous hemorrhage, infarction, or infection. They are false cysts without a true epithelial lining and make up the majority (80%) of splenic cysts. Internal debris and fluid levels are common. Calcification is found in the wall in 30% to 40%.

Congenital epidermoid cysts are true cysts with epithelial-lined walls. They are well-defined, spherical, and usually unilocular with thin walls. Internal debris is sometimes present. No contrast medium enhancement occurs. Calcification is found in the walls in about 5% of cases.

Echinococcal cysts may be indistinguishable from traumatic and epidermoid cysts but are rare in the United States. They appear as a larger mother cyst containing smaller daughter cysts near the periphery. Ringlike calcification of the walls of the mother cyst and the internal daughter cysts is common. Hydatid sand appears as internal debris of increased density. Less than 2% of patients with hydatid disease have splenic involvement.

Pancreatic pseudocysts result from pancreatitis with fluid gaining access to the splenic parenchyma from the pancreas by dissection through the splenic hilum (Fig.

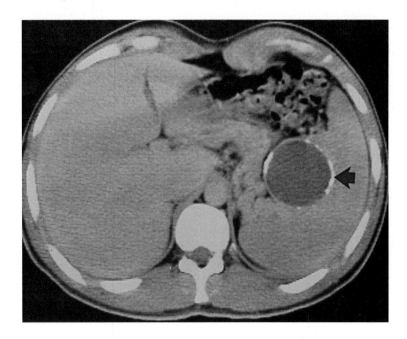

Figure 13–4. Posttraumatic cyst. Liquefaction of an old hematoma resulted in formation of this cystic mass *(arrow)* in the splenic hilum. Note the calcification in the wall.

13–5). CT demonstrates findings of pancreatitis in association with subcapsular splenic fluid.

Abscesses

Bacterial abscesses occur uncommonly but have a high mortality when untreated. Signs and symptoms may be vague. Diseased spleens are particularly susceptible to abscess formation when organisms are delivered hematogenously from distant foci of infection. Abscesses may also result from spread of infection from adjacent organs or from suppuration in a traumatic hematoma. CT demonstrates single or multiple low-density areas with ill-defined walls, which may be thickened and enhance with contrast medium. Internal attenuation is 20 to 40 H. Abscesses may contain gas or demonstrate fluid levels. Diagnosis is confirmed by aspiration. Treatment is splenectomy or catheter drainage.

Microabscesses occur in patients with the

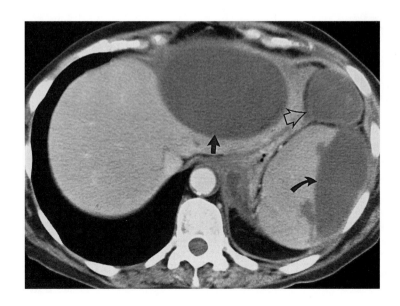

Figure 13–5. Pancreatic pseudocysts. Subcapsular fluid collections associated with acute pancreatitis are evident in the spleen *(curved arrow)* and liver *(straight arrow)*. Loculated fluid is also seen in a recess of the lesser sac *(open arrow)*. High amylase content of the fluid was confirmed by CT-guided aspiration and drainage.

acquired immunodeficiency syndrome and in those with immunocompromise due to chemotherapy, lymphoma, leukemia, or organ transplantation. CT demonstrates multiple low-density defects in the spleen that are usually 5 to 10 mm but may be up to 20 mm (Fig. 13–6). The causes of microabscesses include fungi (*Candida, Aspergillus, Cryptococcus, Histoplasma*), tuberculosis, *Pneumocystis carinii*, and cytomegalovirus. Differential diagnosis of multiple, small, low-density splenic defects (Table 13–1) includes lymphoma, Kaposi's sarcoma, sarcoidosis, and metastases.

SOLID LESIONS

Lymphoma

The spleen is the largest lymphoid organ in the body, so it is hardly surprising that involvement by lymphoma is common (Fig. 13–7). Lymphoma of the spleen may cause splenomegaly (by diffuse infiltration), a large solitary mass (lymphomatous aggregation), or multiple focal nodules (miliary pattern of lymphoma nodules). Extensive necrosis may result in a cystic appearance. Lesions do not enhance with contrast medium. However, lymphoma, especially

TABLE 13–1. **Multiple Small (<10 mm) Low-Density Defects in the Spleen**

Microabscesses (immunocompromised patient)
  Fungi
    Candida
    Aspergillus
    Cryptococcus
  Tuberculosis
    Mycobacterium tuberculosis
    M. avium-intracellulare
  Pneumocystis carinii
  Cytomegalovirus
Multiple bacterial abscesses
Histoplasmosis
Lymphoma
Kaposi's sarcoma (associated with acquired immunodeficiency syndrome)
Sarcoidosis
Metastases
  Breast carcinoma
  Lung carcinoma
  Ovarian carcinoma
  Gastric carcinoma
  Malignant melanoma
  Prostate carcinoma

Hodgkin's lymphoma, may involve the spleen and not be detectable by CT. Adenopathy in the splenic hilum and elsewhere in the abdomen is frequent.

Infarction

Infarction classically appears as a wedge-shaped hypodense area in the periphery of the spleen. However, because infarcts are often multiple, vary in size, and frequently fuse with each other, the wedge shape is often lost. The key finding is extension of the low-density area to the capsule of the spleen without causing mass effect (Fig. 13–8). The infarcted areas progressively atrophy, eventually resulting in notching of the splenic contour and, occasionally, calcification. Infarction may be due to arterial occlusion (emboli, arteritis, pancreas carcinoma) or venous sinusoid thrombosis (usually in patients with massive splenomegaly). Sickle cell and cardiac disease, lymphoma, and metastases are predisposing conditions to

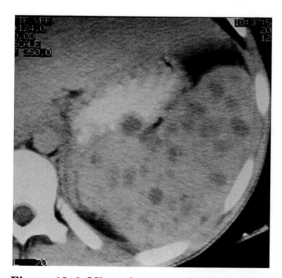

Figure 13–6. Microabscesses. Many low-density lesions are seen in the spleen in this patient with acute myelogenous leukemia. The lesions were due to *Candida albicans* sepsis.

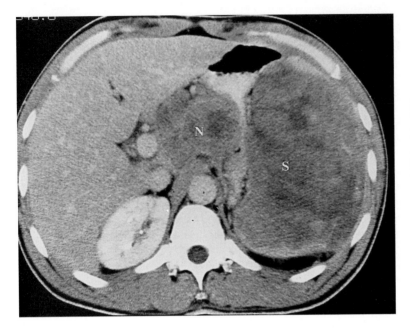

Figure 13–7. Lymphoma.
The spleen (S) is greatly enlarged and the parenchyma is mostly replaced by a diffuse, mottled low-density lesion representing non-Hodgkin's lymphoma. A mass of adenopathy (N) compresses the stomach and abuts the portal vein.

splenic infarction. Infarcts provide fertile soil for abscess formation.

Hematoma

Splenic hematomas usually occur as a result of trauma but may evolve spontaneously in a diseased spleen. CT can be effectively used to judge the severity of splenic injury in acute trauma but is not predictive of which patients need surgery or their eventual outcome.

Subcapsular hematoma appears as a crescentic area of hypodensity along the margin of the spleen flattening or indenting the splenic parenchyma. The splenic capsule may be thickened. The CT density of the hematoma gradually decreases with time.

Splenic lacerations are rents that extend through parenchyma and the splenic cap-

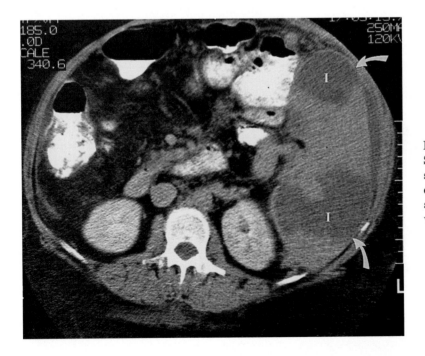

Figure 13–8. Infarction.
Splenic infarctions (I) are seen as low-density lesions extending to the splenic capsule *(arrows)* in this patient with massive splenomegaly.

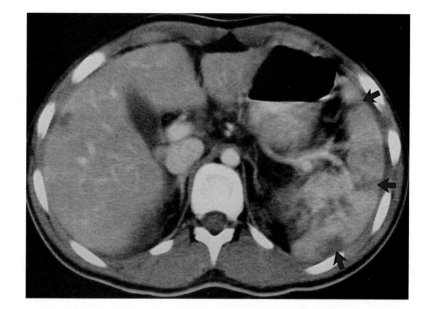

Figure 13–9. Shattered spleen. Multiple lacerations produce low-density bands *(arrows)* extending through the spleen of this patient injured in a motor vehicle accident.

sule, resulting in perisplenic hematomas and hemoperitoneum. CT findings may be subtle. Lacerations are usually seen as low-density bands or clefts traversing the splenic parenchyma (Fig. 13–9). Occasionally, the only findings are indistinct splenic margins and a perisplenic sentinel blood clot.

Intrasplenic hematoma and splenic contusions appear as low-density intrasplenic masses. Splenic hematomas resolve gradually over months, with some leaving behind

fibrous scars, calcifications, or posttraumatic cysts.

Metastases

Malignant melanoma, lung, breast, and ovarian carcinoma are the most common sources of splenic metastases. Metastases are surprisingly uncommon and are seen in only 7% of patients with widespread malignancy. Malignant melanoma is the source of 50% of the splenic metastases detected

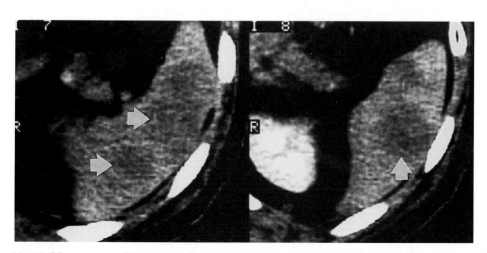

Figure 13–10. Metastases. Metastases from malignant melanoma produce poorly marginated low-density masses *(arrows)* in the spleen.

radiographically. Most appear as ill-defined low-density nodules (Fig. 13–10), but some form well-defined cystic masses. Peripheral enhancement is common.

Primary Tumors

Primary splenic tumors are rare. *Hemangiomas* are the most common. They consist of a tangle of vascular channels lined by a single layer of endothelium and filled with slow-flowing blood. They are pathologically identical to hemangiomas found in the liver. Most are asymptomatic, but very large ones may cause pain and splenomegaly. They vary from homogeneous solid to multicystic lesions. Unenhanced CT shows a low-density mass. With intravenous contrast medium enhancement the lesions show slow nodular enhancement from the periphery. Calcification may be mottled and central or peripheral and curvilinear (Table 13–2). *Angiosarcomas* are heterogeneous masses with mixed solid and cystic components.

Suggested Reading

Beahrs JR, Stehens DH. Enlarged accessory spleens: CT appearance in postsplenectomy patients. AJR 1980; 135:483–486.

Becker CD, Spring P, Glättli A, Schweizer W. Blunt splenic trauma in adults: can CT findings be used to determine the need for surgery? AJR 1994; 162:343–347.

Dachman AH, Ros PR, Murari PJ, et al. Nonparasitic splenic cysts: A report of 52 cases with radiologic-pathologic correlation. AJR 1986; 147:537–542.

Do HM, Cronan JJ. CT appearance of splenic injuries managed nonoperatively. AJR 1991; 157:757–760.

TABLE 13–2. **Multiple Splenic Calcifications**

Histoplasmosis
Tuberculosis
Healed *Pneumocystis carinii* (associated with acquired immunodeficiency syndrome)
Phleboliths
Hemangiomas

Dodds WJ, Taylor AJ, Erickson SJ, et al. Radiologic imaging of splenic anomalies. AJR 1990; 155:805–810.

Franquet T, Montes M, Lecumberri FJ, et al. Hydatid disease of the spleen: imaging findings in nine patients. AJR 1990; 154:525–528.

Freeman JL, Jafri SZH, Roberts JL, et al. CT of congenital and acquired abnormalities of the spleen. RadioGraphics 1993; 13:597–610.

Miles KA, McPherson SJ, Hayball MP. Transient splenic inhomogeneity with contrast-enhanced CT: mechanism and effect of liver disease. Radiology 1995; 194:91–95.

Mirvis SE, Whitley NO, Gens DR. Blunt splenic trauma in adults: CT-based classification and correlation with prognosis and treatment. Radiology 1989; 171:33–39.

Rabushka LS, Kawashima A, Fishman EK. Imaging of the spleen: CT with supplemental MR examination. RadioGraphics 1994; 14:307–332.

Ros PR, Moser RP Jr, Dachman AH, et al. Hemangioma of the spleen: Radiologic-pathologic correlation in ten cases. Radiology 1987; 162:73–77.

Taylor AJ, Dodds WJ, Erickson SJ, Stewart ET. CT of acquired abnormalities of the spleen. AJR 1991; 157:1213–1219.

Urrutia M, Mergo PJ, Ros LH, et al. Cystic masses of the spleen: radiologic-pathologic correlation. RadioGraphics 1996; 16:107–129.

Chapter

14

Kidneys

William E. Brant, M.D.

ANATOMY OF THE RETROPERITONEAL SPACE

Detailed understanding of the retroperitoneal fascial planes and compartments is a prerequisite for accurate interpretation of abdominal CT. The retroperitoneal space between the diaphragm and the pelvic brim is divided into anterior pararenal, perirenal, and posterior pararenal compartments by the anterior and posterior renal fascia (Fig. 14–1).

The *anterior pararenal space* extends between the posterior parietal peritoneum and the anterior renal fascia. It is bounded laterally by the lateroconal fascia, which is the continuation of the posterior lamina of the posterior renal fascia. The pancreas, duodenal loop, and ascending and descending portions of the colon are within the anterior pararenal space.

The anterior and posterior renal fascia encompass the kidney, renal pelvis, proximal ureter, adrenal gland, and perirenal fat within the *perirenal space*. The anterior renal fascia is thin and consists of one layer of connective tissue. The posterior renal fascia is thicker and consists of two layers of connective tissue. The anterior layer of the posterior renal fascia is continuous with the anterior renal fascia. The posterior layer of the posterior renal fascia is continuous with the lateroconal fascia forming the lateral boundary of the anterior pararenal space. The anterior and posterior layers of the pos-

terior renal fascia may be separated by inflammatory processes extending from the anterior pararenal space (see Fig. 12–3). The perirenal space is discontinuous across the midline owing to fusion of the renal fascial layers with connective tissues surrounding the aorta and inferior vena cava. The perirenal compartment narrows as it extends inferiorly to form an inverted cone shape. The ureter passes through the apex of the cone.

The *posterior pararenal space* is a potential space, usually filled only with fat, extending from the posterior renal fascia to the transversalis fascia. The posterior pararenal fat continues into the flank as the properitoneal fat stripe seen on plain films of the abdomen. The compartment is limited medially by the lateral edge of the psoas and quadratus lumborum muscles.

The kidneys are covered by a tight fibrous capsule that produces a sharp margin defined by perirenal fat on CT. Subcapsular collections of fluid or blood will compress and distort the renal parenchyma, often without affecting the perirenal fat. The perirenal fat extends into the renal sinus outlining blood vessels and the renal collecting system. Connective tissue septa extend between the kidney and the renal fascia. These septa may be seen as prominent stranding densities in the perirenal fat when they are thickened by inflammation, hemorrhage, or ischemia. The renal arteries and veins can generally be identified from the great vessels to the kidneys. The right

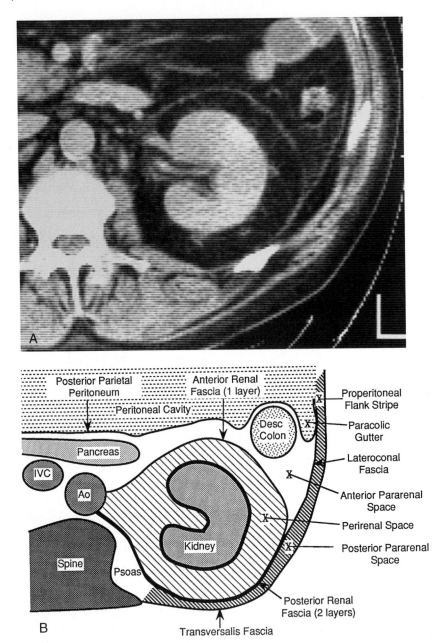

Figure 14–1. Retroperitoneal anatomy. CT image of the left kidney *(A)* and a diagram *(B)* demonstrate the fascial planes and compartments of the retroperitoneal space.

renal artery courses behind the vena cava. The left renal vein crosses between the aorta and the superior mesenteric artery.

Anatomic variants such as *horseshoe kidney* can be easily recognized on CT. With horseshoe kidney the lower poles are joined by an isthmus of fibrous tissue or functioning parenchyma. The kidneys are low in position and have an abnormal axis, with the lower poles directed medially instead of laterally.

TECHNICAL CONSIDERATIONS

Because the kidneys actively concentrate contrast medium within the parenchyma, most renal abnormalities are best seen on CT after intravenous contrast medium administration. Unenhanced CT is performed to demonstrate calcifications and calculi that may be obscured by a contrast agent. Helical CT is optimal for renal evaluation and is the current technique of choice. Our dedicated renal CT protocol includes a nonenhanced renal scan followed by two postcontrast helical series using 5-mm collimation with pitch equal to 1. A contrast agent is administered intravenously by power injector at a rate of 2.0 mL/sec for a total bolus of 150 mL of 60% contrast agent. The first contrast series is begun 40 seconds after onset of contrast medium injection. The kidneys demonstrate bright enhancement of the cortex with little or no enhancement of the medulla. The second series duplicates the first and is obtained immediately after completion of the first contrast series. This second pass through the kidneys is obtained in nephrogram phase when contrast medium enhancement of the parenchyma is uniform and contrast opacification of the collecting system has occurred (Fig. 14–2).

Protocols for nonhelical CT include a precontrast scan and a postcontrast scan with contiguous 5-mm thick slices. The longer scan acquisition time usually precludes obtaining two postcontrast series.

RENAL TUMORS

Renal Cell Carcinoma

Most solid renal masses in adults are renal cell carcinomas. Surgery (radical nephrectomy) is the only effective therapy, so preoperative CT staging of the extent of disease is important (Table 14–1). CT is inaccurate in differentiating stage I and stage II lesions; however, because both stages are treated with radical nephrectomy, the inaccuracy is of limited significance. Significant CT findings include

1. A solid renal mass is evident (see Fig. 14–2).

Figure 14–2. Renal carcinoma. Noncontrast *(A)*, cortical phase *(B)*, and nephrogram phase *(C)* images from a helical CT study demonstrate a small renal carcinoma *(arrows)* arising from the right kidney. The tumor is near isointense with the renal parenchyma on the base study. Early arterial enhancement of the tumor coincides with enhancement of the renal cortex on *B*. The tumor is hypointense compared with the renal parenchyma during nephrogram phase.

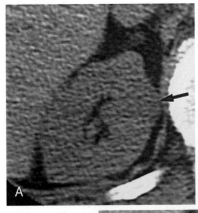
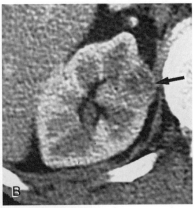
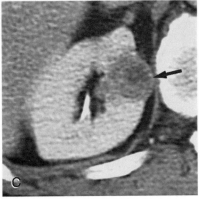

TABLE 14–1. **Staging of Renal Cell
Carcinoma**

Stage	Description
I	Tumor confined to the kidney
II	Tumor growth through the capsule into the perirenal space
IIIA	Tumor involves main renal vein
IIIB	Tumor involves regional lymph nodes
IIIC	Tumor involves main renal vein and regional lymph nodes
IVA	Tumor extends through renal fascia into adjacent organs
IVB	Hematogenous or lymphatic metastases to distant sites

2. Hemorrhage, necrosis, and calcification within the tumor are common (Fig. 14–3).

3. Most lesions are hypervascular and enhance inhomogeneously.

4. Cystic and complex multicystic variants are identified by thickened enhancing walls and septations or by a solid tumor nodule.

5. Tumor growth may be into the main renal vein (30%) and inferior vena cava (10%). Involved veins are enlarged, enhance poorly, and are filled with visible tumor thrombus seen as nodular low density within the vein (Fig. 14–4). Tumor thrombus may extend into the right atrium.

6. Local extension is seen as strands or nodules of low density extending into the perirenal fat and to adjacent organs.

7. Lymphatic spread is evidenced by enlargement of renal hilar, pericaval, and periaortic nodes to 15 mm or more.

8. Hematogenous spread favors lung, bone, liver, adrenal, and the opposite kidney. CT of the chest and radionuclide bone scans are routine components of preoperative evaluation.

Interestingly, distant metastases will occasionally melt away with removal of the primary tumor. Late appearance of metastases, as long as 20 years after "cure," is also seen. Preoperative biopsy of potentially resectable renal carcinomas may adversely affect patient survival. Percutaneous biopsy is indicated only for tumors that are obviously metastatic. Tissue diagnosis is best obtained by needle biopsy of a metastatic lesion, rather than the often necrotic renal mass.

Oncocytoma

Oncocytoma is a benign solid tumor that arises from the proximal renal tubule. Most are seen in men in their 60s. Unfortunately, no imaging test can reliably differentiate these benign tumors from renal cell carcinoma. Treatment is surgical. Exploration with limited tumor excision may be sug-

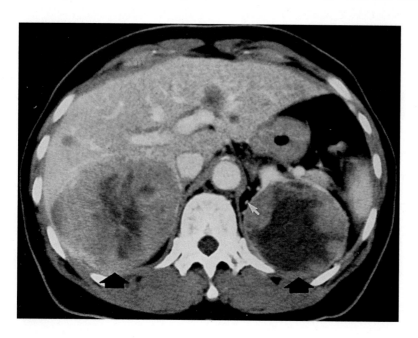

Figure 14–3. Bilateral renal carcinoma. Renal cell carcinomas *(black arrows)* arise from the upper poles of both kidneys. The low-density regions within the tumors are areas of necrosis and hemorrhage. Enhancing tumor vessels *(white arrow)* are seen in the perirenal fat.

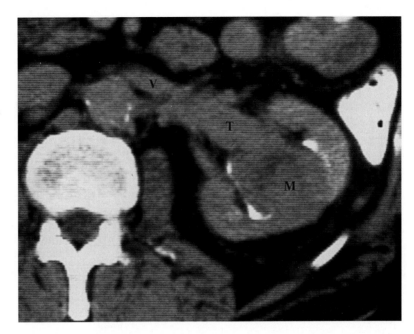

Figure 14–4. Renal carcinoma invading renal vein. A renal cell carcinoma (M) arising within the renal sinus of the left kidney extends into the left renal vein (T). The renal vein is of normal size (V) anterior to the aorta but is enlarged and nodular in the portion of the vein containing tumor (T). This tumor did not extend into the perirenal fat.

gested if CT findings suggest the possibility of oncocytoma:

1. Sharply defined solid renal mass
2. Central stellate scar

Transitional Cell Carcinoma

Tumors arising from the epithelium of the renal collecting system account for 5% to 10% of renal tumors. Most (85%) are transitional cell carcinoma. The remainder are squamous cell carcinoma or adenocarcinoma (<1%). Because hematuria is common, these tumors usually present earlier than renal cell carcinoma and thus are frequently smaller at the time of diagnosis. CT findings include

1. Soft tissue density filling defect is within the renal pelvis, or within the renal sinus, distorting and compressing collecting structures (Fig. 14–5). Unenhanced CT attenuation (8–30 H) is greater than unopacified urine but much less than even radiolucent calculi (100–300 H).
2. Enhancement is poor (18–55 H) and calcifications are rare.
3. Local spread is seen as low-density tumor extension into or through the renal parenchyma and from the sinus into the perirenal fat.
4. Lymphatic spread is seen as enlargement of regional nodes.

5. Synchronous tumors in the ipsilateral ureter and bladder should be searched for carefully.

Angiomyolipoma

CT reflects the composition of this benign tumor made up of varying quantities of thick-walled blood vessels (*angio*), smooth muscle (*myo*), and fat (*lipo*). In 20% of cases, the angiomyolipomas are multiple, are bilateral, and occur in patients with tuberous sclerosis. In 80%, the tumor is solitary and unilateral and the patient is usually a middle-aged woman. Hemorrhage is the most frequent complication of the tumor. CT diagnosis is based on demonstration of fat; however, the absence of fat does not exclude the diagnosis. Rare cases of fat density in renal cell carcinoma and Wilms' tumor have been reported, but most of these cases show other CT evidence of malignant disease. CT features of angiomyolipoma (Fig. 14–6) are

1. Fatty areas of tumor have attenuation values of −80 to −120 H.
2. Smooth muscle and vascular components of the tumor appear as nodules, whorls, and strands of soft tissue density within the fatty mass.
3. Hypervascular areas of the tumor may show striking contrast medium enhancement.

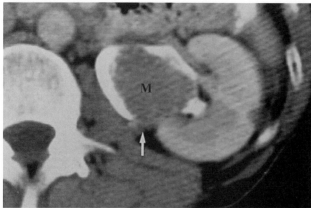

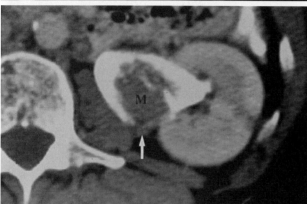

Figure 14–5. Transitional cell carcinoma. Two sequential images of the left kidney demonstrate a transitional cell carcinoma (M) occupying the renal pelvis. The tumor extends through the renal pelvis into the perirenal fat *(arrows).*

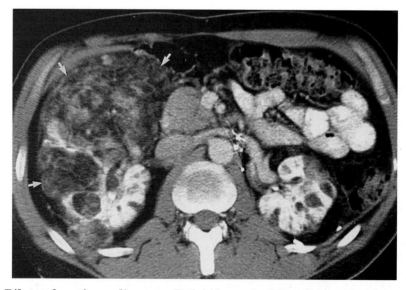

Figure 14–6. Bilateral angiomyolipomas. Both kidneys, in this patient with tuberous sclerosis, are extensively replaced by angiomyolipomas. The tumor *(arrows)* arising from the right kidney extends all the way to the anterior abdominal wall. Low-density areas within the tumor are identical in density to subcutaneous and intraabdominal fat, confirming the diagnosis of angiomyolipoma. Soft tissue density nodules and strands correspond to smooth muscle components of the tumor. Functioning renal parenchyma enhances brightly with contrast medium enhancement.

4. Tumors are commonly as small as 1 cm but may reach 20 cm and extend into perirenal tissues and lymph nodes.

Tiny angiomyolipomas (<1 cm) are a frequent incidental finding with high-resolution imaging.

Renal Lymphoma

Lymphoma may present in the kidney as multiple parenchymal nodules (50% of cases), invasion from perirenal disease, a solitary solid mass, or diffuse infiltration causing renal enlargement. Signs that suggest lymphoma include bilaterality, extensive adenopathy, and splenomegaly. Lymphoma is usually homogeneous and enhances moderately. Burkitt's and acquired immunodeficiency syndrome–related lymphomas are the most common types of lymphoma to involve the kidneys.

Metastases

Metastases to the kidney, especially from lung carcinoma, are common on autopsy series but uncommonly seen clinically. Most patients with renal metastases will soon die of their primary disease. Metastases appear as multiple, bilateral renal masses, usually seen in association with metastases in other organs.

RENAL CYSTIC DISEASE

Cystic Renal Masses

Cystic renal masses are an extremely common finding on abdominal CT. The challenge is to separate the ubiquitous simple cyst from a host of other cystic lesions.

Simple Cyst. Simple renal cysts are benign nonneoplastic, fluid-filled masses that affect half the population older than age 55. Small cysts are asymptomatic incidental findings. Large cysts (>4 cm) occasionally cause hypertension, hematuria, pain, or ureteral obstruction. Multiple and bilateral cysts are common. Strict criteria that allow confident CT diagnosis of a renal mass as a simple cyst (Fig. 14–7) are

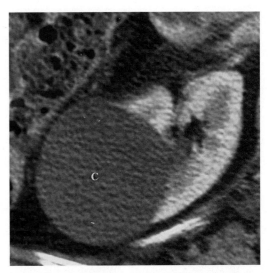

Figure 14–7. Simple renal cyst. A large cyst (C) arising from the left kidney demonstrates the classic CT features of a simple renal cyst. No further evaluation is necessary.

1. Sharp margination with the renal parenchyma
2. No perceptible wall
3. Homogeneous attenuation near water density (−10 to +15 H)
4. No evidence of enhancement after intravenous contrast medium administration

Cysts smaller than 1 cm cause a problem in diagnosis because of volume averaging. Most of these can be confirmed as simple cysts by rescanning using thinner slices, by ultrasonography, or by follow-up CT demonstrating no change. Thick walls may be simulated by imaging a beak of normal renal parenchyma abutting the cyst or by the increased enhancement observed in compressed renal parenchyma adjacent to a cyst.

When a renal mass appears cystic but does not meet the criteria for simple cyst the following lesions should be considered:

Complicated Simple Cyst. Simple cysts may be complicated by hemorrhage, infection (Fig. 14–8), or calcification within the wall. Some may have internal septations. Multiple simple cysts adjacent to each other may appear as a complex mass. If septa are thin, smooth, and regular, a diagnosis of benign cyst can be made. Thin calcification

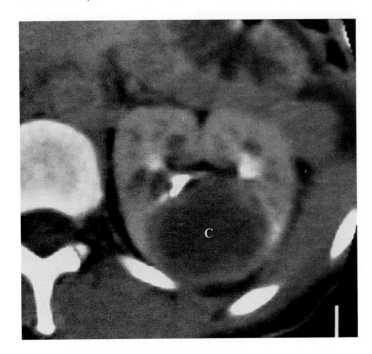

Figure 14–8. Infected renal cyst.
This cystic renal mass (C) has poorly defined margination with the renal parenchyma and thickened, poorly defined walls. Percutaneous aspiration confirmed bacterial infection of a simple renal cyst.

of the wall of a cyst, or of a septation, is still compatible with benign cyst. Small cysts (<3 cm), which are uniformly hyperdense (25–90 H) on noncontrast CT, may also be considered benign when they have other CT characteristics of simple cyst.

Indeterminate Cystic Mass. The following findings indicate an indeterminate cystic mass, which may be a cystic renal carcinoma, other cystic tumor, or a cyst complicated by infection or hemorrhage:

1. Regular or irregular thickening of the wall
2. Solid components within a cystic mass
3. Enhancement of the wall or septations
4. Irregular margins
5. Inhomogeneous cyst fluid

Surgical exploration or percutaneous aspiration biopsy may be required.

Renal Abscess. Pyelonephritis complicated by suppuration and liquefaction may result in formation of an abscess requiring drainage. On CT, abscesses appear as thick-walled, low-density fluid collections within the renal parenchyma. Gas is sometimes seen within the pus collection. The wall commonly enhances with contrast medium administration. Extension of infection into the perirenal space is common.

Renal Cell Carcinoma. Some renal carcinomas are composed of multiple fluid-filled noncommunicating cystic spaces. Malignant tumor cells line the loculations. Rarely, renal carcinoma may arise within or adjacent to a simple renal cyst.

Multilocular Cystic Nephroma. This is an uncommon benign renal neoplasm composed of cysts of varying size separated by connective tissue septa. The septations usually enhance after contrast medium administration. They are seen most commonly in infants, young children, and middle-aged women. Surgical removal is usually necessary to differentiate from renal carcinoma.

Multiple Renal Cysts

When multiple renal cysts are encountered, the following conditions should be considered:

Multiple Simple Cysts. Simple cysts increase in frequency with age and are commonly multiple and bilateral. Patients older than age 50 with no cysts in other organs and who have no family history of renal cystic disease are most likely to have multiple simple cysts.

Autosomal Dominant Polycystic Disease.

The cortex and medulla of both kidneys are progressively replaced by multiple noncommunicating cysts of varying size in this common hereditary disorder. Although this disease may be detected in childhood, most cases present clinically with hypertension and renal failure at ages 30 to 50. CT findings become more pronounced as the disease progresses. Diagnostic findings (Fig. 14–9) include

1. Progressive replacement of renal parenchyma with cysts of varying size
2. Progressive bilateral increase in renal volume
3. Multiple cysts in the liver in 30% to 50%
4. Multiple cysts in the pancreas in 10%

The renal cysts are commonly complicated by bleeding or infection, which causes thickening of the cyst walls and an increase in density of cyst fluid. Berry aneurysms are present in the circle of Willis in 10% to 15%. Autosomal dominant ("adult") polycystic disease is differentiated from other conditions by the presence of cysts in other organs, positive family history, presence of renal failure, and hypertension.

Multicystic Dysplastic Kidney.

This is a nonhereditary renal dysplasia in which the kidney consists of multiple, thin-walled cysts held together by connective tissue. The involved kidney is functionless. At birth the involved kidney is greatly enlarged. With age the kidney progressively shrinks and often becomes calcified. Rarely, only a portion of one kidney may be involved. Bilateral multicystic dysplastic kidneys occur but are fatal at birth. The opposite kidney is affected by ureteropelvic junction obstruction or another anomaly in 30% of cases.

von Hippel-Lindau Disease.

This is an autosomal dominant disorder characterized by retinal angiomas and cerebellar hemangioblastomas associated with abdominal cysts and tumors. Central nervous system abnormalities usually predominate. Abdominal findings (Fig. 14–10; see also Fig. 12–13) include multiple renal and pancreatic cysts, small renal adenomas, multiple and bilateral renal adenocarcinomas (24%–45% of patients), and pheochromocytoma (7%–18% of patients).

Tuberous Sclerosis.

This autosomal dominant syndrome combines multiple renal cysts and multiple and bilateral renal angiomyolipomas (see Fig. 14–6) with cutaneous, retinal, and cerebral hamartomas. The

Figure 14–9. Autosomal dominant polycystic disease. An unenhanced CT image of the upper abdomen demonstrates innumerable cysts (C) in the liver and replacing and enlarging both kidneys *(black arrowheads).* Residual renal parenchyma is seen as islands of higher density *(white arrow)* surrounded by cysts. Because renal failure is progressive, these patients are usually studied without intravenous contrast medium enhancement to avoid its nephrotoxic effects.

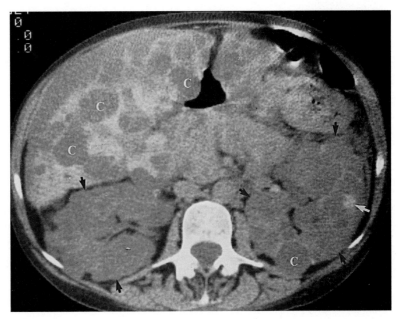

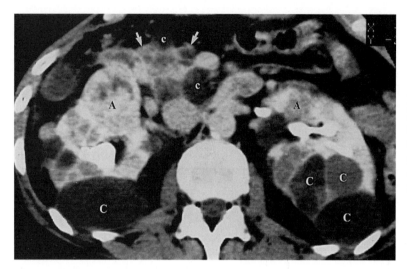

Figure 14–10. von Hippel-Lindau disease. Both kidneys demonstrate multiple cysts (C) and multiple renal adenomas (A). Cysts (c) are also evident within the head of the pancreas *(arrows).*

renal lesions are commonly detected in infancy and childhood.

Acquired Renal Cystic Disease. Patients on long-term hemodialysis commonly develop multiple cysts in their native kidneys. Multicentric renal adenomas and carcinomas develop in as many as 9% of patients.

STONES AND OBSTRUCTION

Stones

The major use of CT in renal stone disease is to differentiate radiolucent calculi from other causes of filling defects in the renal collecting system, such as tumor or hematoma. Even uric acid, xanthine, or cystine stones that are radiolucent on plain film appear as high density on CT images photographed for soft tissues. Calculi have attenuation values in the range of 100 to 600 H (Fig. 14–11). Uroepithelial tumors have attenuation values of 8 to 30 H unenhanced and 18 to 55 H enhanced. Blood clots have attenuation values of 50 to 65 H, do not enhance with contrast medium administration, may be observed to move with changes in patient position, and disappear with time.

CT is a poorer detector of small calcified renal stones than is plain film because of lesser spatial resolution and volume averaging. When contrast medium is administered, stones in the renal collecting system are often obscured by contrast concentration in the urine. CT for renal calculi should be performed without contrast medium enhancement and with thin slices (5 mm or less).

Obstruction

The dilated collecting structures occurring with obstruction are readily demonstrated by CT, either without or with contrast medium enhancement. Dependent layering of unopacified urine over heavier contrast material is commonly observed within dilated collecting structures. The affected kidney may show delayed excretion of contrast agent. CT is effective in determining both the level and the cause of obstruction by demonstrating calculi, tumor, or extrinsic mass. CT shows the parenchymal thinning that occurs with chronic obstruction.

INFECTION

CT is indicated when complications of renal infection are suspected. Predisposing conditions, including urinary calculi, neurogenic bladder, immune system compromise, diabetes, intravenous drug abuse, or chronic debilitating disease, increase the risk of complications that require intervention. Most urinary tract infections are caused by gram-negative bacilli, but the incidence of fungal and tuberculous infections is increasing.

Acute Bacterial Infection

Acute Pyelonephritis. Acute pyelonephritis is a multifocal infection of one or both kidneys. Patients with uncomplicated pyelonephritis usually resolve all symptoms within 72 hours of institution of appropriate antibiotic therapy. Patients who fail to improve should be imaged to detect complications. CT signs of acute bacterial infection include

1. A wedge-shaped area of mottled decreased parenchymal enhancement is seen. The CT appearance is very similar to renal infarction (see Fig. 14–16).
2. A striated pattern of linear alternating increased and decreased densities on enhanced scans is particularly characteristic.
3. High-density area of parenchyma on nonenhanced scans indicates hemorrhagic pyelonephritis.
4. Stranding densities in the perirenal fat and thickening of the renal fascia occur.

These findings overlap those of renal infarction. Diagnosis is made by the presence or absence of pyuria and bacteriuria.

Acute Focal Bacterial Nephritis. Acute focal bacterial nephritis (lobar nephronia) describes a severe localized infection that produces a phlegmon. CT reveals a low-density mottled mass without encapsulation or liquefaction. These phlegmons may resolve completely, result in a scar, or evolve into an abscess.

Abscess. Abscess refers to a collection of pus and liquefied tissue within the kidney or with spread into the perirenal space (Fig. 14–12). CT demonstrates a fluid collection (10–30 H) with an enhancing rim. Gas may be present within the collection, especially in patients who are diabetic. Abscesses generally require catheter or surgical drainage.

Emphysematous Pyelonephritis. Emphysematous pyelonephritis is a severe type of diffuse pyelonephritis that occurs in diabetics and patients with urinary obstruction. Gas is produced by metabolism of glucose by gram-negative bacteria. CT shows gas in the renal parenchyma (Fig. 14–13) and the additional signs of renal inflammation. Emergency nephrectomy is usually the treatment of choice.

Pyonephrosis. Pyonephrosis is acute infection with pus within an obstructed collecting system. Renal destruction is rapid, and urgent drainage is required. CT demonstrates a calculus or other cause of obstruction and high-density layering fluid within a dilated collecting system.

Figure 14–11. Uric acid stone. A CT scan of the right kidney obtained without contrast medium enhancement demonstrates a pure uric acid stone *(arrow)* as a high-density oval object in the renal sinus. CT attenuation measured 240 H. The stone appeared as an entirely radiolucent filling defect on an excretory urogram.

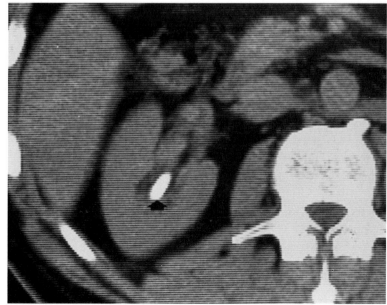

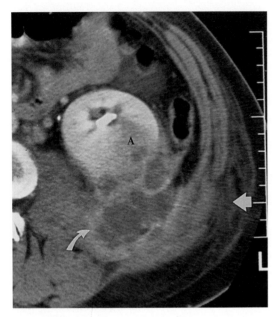

Figure 14–12. Renal and perirenal abscess.
A bacterial abscess (A) complicating acute pyelonephritis has spread through the renal capsule
into the perirenal space *(curved arrow)*. Edema
and inflammation also involve the muscles and
subcutaneous tissues *(large arrow)* of the flank.

Chronic Infection

Tuberculosis. Renal tuberculosis has once
again become common. The hallmarks are
progressive parenchymal destruction, cavity
formation, fibrosis and stricture, granuloma
formation, and calcification. End-stage tuberculous kidneys may be hydronephrotic
sacs or calcified nubbins.

Xanthogranulomatous Pyelonephritis.
Xanthogranulomatous pyelonephritis results from a combination of chronic renal
obstruction and chronic infection. The renal
parenchyma is progressively destroyed and
replaced by lipid-filled macrophages. A
staghorn calculi results in involvement of
the entire kidney. Solitary calculi or infun-
dibular stricture often results in focal
involvement. CT reveals low-density enlargement of the entire kidney or the affected area and the obstructing calculus.
Extension of the infective process into the
perirenal tissues is common (Fig. 14–14).

TRAUMA

CT effectively demonstrates the exact nature and extent of renal injury and associated hematoma in trauma. Dynamic
contrast medium–enhanced studies demonstrate the abnormalities best.

Renovascular Injury. Failure of all, or a
portion of, the kidney to enhance after intravenous contrast administration is evidence of vascular injury. If the entire kidney
fails to enhance, occlusion of the renal artery due to intimal flap is suspected. Collateral arterial supply from capsular arteries
results in a "cortical rim" sign (Fig. 14–15).
Immediate surgical repair is needed. Angiography may be indicated because CT can-

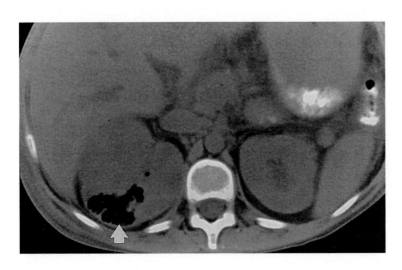

**Figure 14–13. Emphysema-
tous pyelonephritis.** Noncontrast CT demonstrates gas
pockets *(arrow)* in the right renal parenchyma. The right kidney is enlarged owing to diffuse edema.

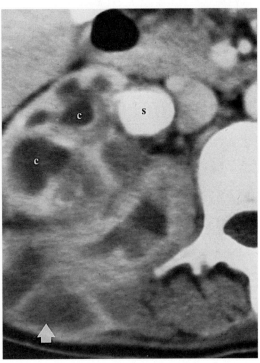

Figure 14–14. Xanthogranulomatous pyelone-phritis. A large stone (s) fills the renal pelvis and causes obstruction, resulting in dilatation of the collecting system (c). The chronic infective process extends from the kidney through the perirenal space and into the subcutaneous soft tissues *(arrow)*. A nephrectomy was performed and yielded *Proteus* organisms on bacterial culture.

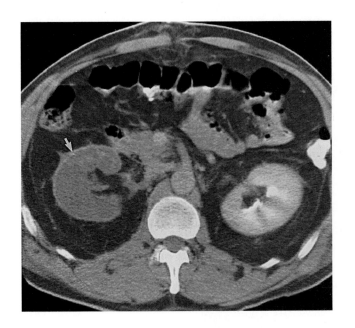

Figure 14–15. Renal pedicle injury. Occlusion of the right renal artery is evidenced by lack of enhancement of the renal parenchyma, associated with a thin rim of enhancement of the peripheral cortex, the cortical rim sign *(arrow)*. An intimal tear was confirmed at surgery. The left kidney enhanced normally. The cause of injury was a high-speed automobile accident.

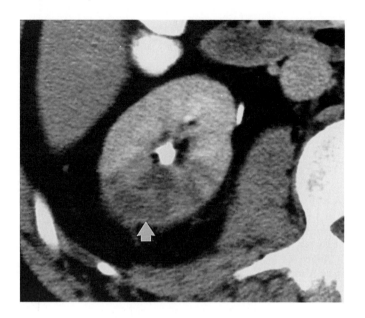

Figure 14–16. Infarction. An angiographic misadventure caused an embolus to the right kidney occluding an intrarenal artery. The resulting infarction is seen as a wedge-shaped area of diminished renal enhancement *(arrow)*. A very similar CT appearance is caused by acute renal infection (lobar nephronia).

not demonstrate the specific anatomic lesion. Traumatic segmental infarction due to occlusion of an intrarenal artery is seen as a wedge-shaped area of absence of contrast medium enhancement (Fig. 14–16). Infarctions heal as a deep parenchymal scar.

Renal Contusion. A patchy or "moth-eaten" pattern of enhancement that may be diffuse, lobar, or focal is evidence of renal contusion. The kidney is edematous. Contrast medium excretion into the collecting system is delayed. This injury can be treated conservatively.

Subcapsular Hematoma. This is the most frequent type of renal injury due to blunt trauma. Blood collects beneath the renal capsule and flattens adjacent renal parenchyma. The perirenal space remains normal. This minor injury is managed conservatively. A Page kidney is a delayed complication, present when the hematoma induces capsular fibrosis and parenchymal

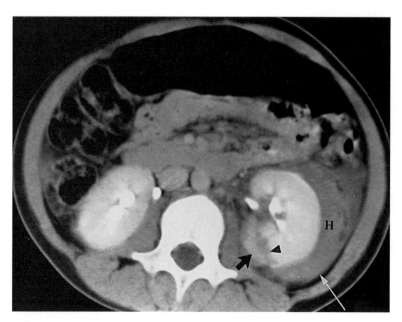

Figure 14–17. Renal laceration. A CT scan of a 10-year-old boy injured in an automobile accident demonstrates a laceration of the left kidney. Blood (H) is seen within the perirenal space confined by the renal fascia *(white arrow)*. The renal fracture *(arrowhead)* is seen as a ragged lucent cleft in the renal parenchyma. A fragment *(black arrow)* of the fractured kidney enhances poorly, indicating impairment of its blood supply.

compression results in systemic hypertension.

Renal Laceration/Fracture. Blood in the perirenal space is evidence of renal laceration or fracture disrupting the renal capsule (Fig. 14–17). A lucent defect may be seen extending through the parenchyma. The kidney may be separated into two or more portions. Multiple clefts and fragments indicate a *shattered kidney*. Lack of enhancement of the renal fragments implies loss of blood supply to those fragments. If the collecting system is disrupted, contrast medium and urine spill into the perirenal space. The resulting fluid collection is often confined between the anterior and posterior leaves of renal fascia. Treatment depends on the extent of injury and the condition of the patient.

Suggested Reading

Amendola MA, Bree RL, Pollack HM, et al. Small renal cell carcinomas: resolving a diagnostic dilemma. Radiology 1988; 166:637–641.

Bosniak MA. The current radiological approach to renal cysts. Radiology 1986; 158:1–10.

Choyke PL, Glenn GM, Walther MM, et al. von Hippel-Lindau disease: genetic, clinical, and imaging features. Radiology 1995; 194:629–642.

Curry NS. Small renal masses (lesions smaller than 3 cm): imaging evaluation and management. AJR 1995; 164:355–362.

Fanney DR, Casillas J, Murphy BJ. CT in the diagnosis of renal trauma. RadioGraphics 1990; 10:29–40.

Hartman DS, Davis CJ, Sanders RC, et al. The multiloculated renal mass: considerations and differential features. RadioGraphics 1987; 7:29–52.

Joseph RC, Amendola MA, Artze ME, et al. Genitourinary tract gas: imaging evaluation. RadioGraphics 1996; 16:295–308.

Korobkin M, Silverman PM, Quint LE, Francis IR. CT of the extraperitoneal space: normal anatomy and fluid collections. AJR 1992; 159:933–941.

Leder RA, Dunnick NR. Transitional cell carcinoma of the pelvicalyces and ureter. AJR 1990; 155:713–722.

LeRoy AJ. Diagnosis and treatment of nephrolithiasis: current perspectives. AJR 1994; 163:1309–1313.

Lowe LH, Zagoria RJ, Baumgartner BR, Dyer RB. Role of imaging and intervention in complex infections of the urinary tract. AJR 1994; 163:363–367.

Meyers MA. Dynamic Radiology of the Abdomen: Normal and Pathologic Anatomy, 4th ed. New York, Springer-Verlag, 1994.

Mindell HJ, Mastromatteo JF, Dickey KW, et al. Anatomic communications between the three retroperitoneal spaces: determination by CT-guided injections of contrast material in cadavers. AJR 1995; 164:1173–1178.

Saunders HS, Dyer RB, Shifrin RY, et al. The CT nephrogram: implications for evaluation of urinary tract disease. RadioGraphics 1995; 15:1069–1085.

Zeman RK, Cronan JJ, Rosenfield AT, et al. Computed tomography of renal masses: Pitfalls and anatomic varients. RadioGraphics 1986; 6:351–372.

Zagoria RJ, Bechtold RE, Dyer RB. Staging of renal adenocarcinoma: role of various imaging procedures. AJR 1995; 164:363–370.

Chapter

15

Adrenal Glands

William E. Brant, M.D.

ANATOMY

The adrenal glands lie within the cone of renal fascia surrounded by the fat of the perirenal space. The right adrenal gland projects posteriorly from the inferior vena cava at the level where the vena cava enters the liver (Fig. 15–1). The right adrenal is medial to the right lobe of the liver and lateral to the right crus of the diaphragm, just above the upper pole of the right kidney. The left adrenal (Fig. 15–2) lies medial and anterior to the upper pole of the left kidney, just lateral to the left crus of the diaphragm and posterior to the pancreas and splenic vessels.

On CT the adrenal glands have the shape of an inverted V or Y. Each limb is smooth in outline and uniform in thickness with straight or concave margins. Each limb is 5 to 7 mm in thickness and up to 3 cm in length. The entire gland is of uniform soft tissue density.

A major problem of adrenal CT is identifying normal and abnormal structures that simulate adrenal masses (Fig. 15–3). Masses arising from the upper pole of the kidney, tortuous splenic vessels, periadrenal portosystemic collateral blood vessels, pancreatic masses, and prominent splenic lobulations must all be differentiated from adrenal tumors. Strict attention to CT technique is the key to avoiding errors. Thin slices (3–5 mm), helical CT volume acquisition, and optimal administration of oral and in-travenous contrast agents usually permit distinction of these various conditions.

TECHNICAL CONSIDERATIONS

CT detects lesions as small as 5 mm and remains the imaging method of choice for most adrenal evaluations. The adrenal glands are usually well demonstrated on routine CT of the abdomen using 7- to 10-mm collimation. However, for fine detail and detection of small tumors, collimation should be reduced to at least 5 mm with slice reconstruction at contiguous 3- or 5-mm intervals. Oral and intravenous contrast agents are helpful in excluding pseudolesions. We give 150 mL of 60% contrast medium by mechanical injector set at 2 mL/sec for helical CT. Scanning of the adrenals is begun 50 seconds after initiation of injection. Helical scan technique is preferred to provide volume data acquisition and to avoid anatomic misregistration.

ADRENAL HYPERPLASIA

Hyperplasia typically enlarges both adrenal glands symmetrically without altering their shape. The limbs of both glands are thickened and elongated without focal masses

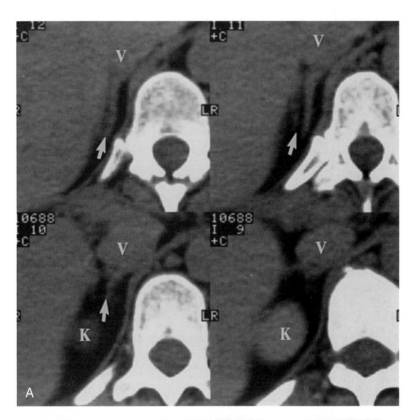

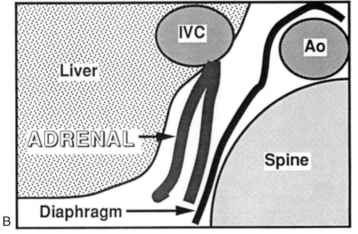

Figure 15–1. Normal right adrenal gland. The right adrenal gland *(arrows)* extends posteriorly from the inferior vena cava (V, IVC) between the right lobe of the liver and the right crus of the diaphragm, above the level of the upper pole of the right kidney (K). *A,* Sequential 5-mm thick CT scan of a normal right adrenal gland. *B,* Diagram of the CT landmarks for the right adrenal gland. Ao = aorta.

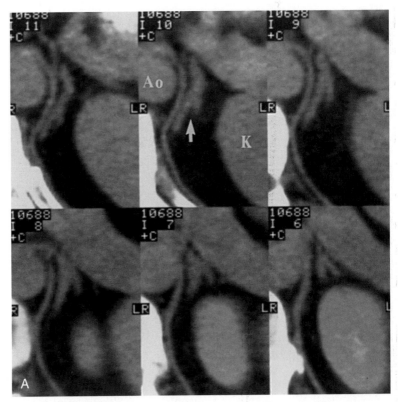

Figure 15–2. Normal left adrenal gland. The left adrenal *(arrow)* is imaged between the upper pole of the left kidney (K) and the aorta (Ao). *A,* Sequential 5-mm thick CT images of a normal left adrenal gland. *B,* Diagram of the CT landmarks for the left adrenal gland.

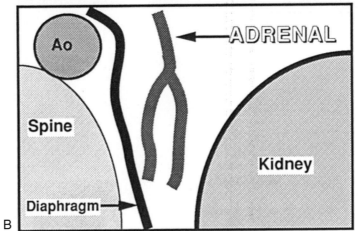

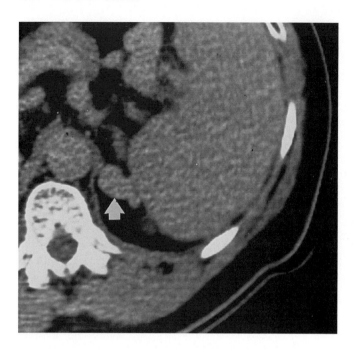

Figure 15–3. Perisplenic vessels. Enlarged portosystemic collateral blood vessels *(arrow),* in this patient with cirrhosis and portal hypertension, simulate a left adrenal mass. Differentiation is made by optimizing intravenous contrast medium administration and carefully examining sequential images.

(Fig. 15–4). However, it is important to realize that the adrenal glands may be hyperfunctional in hormone secretion and may even be hyperplastic histologically, without appearing enlarged or abnormal on CT. In long-standing Cushing's disease, a macronodular form of adrenal hyperplasia may be present, with multiple nodules, up to 3 cm, superimposed on normal-sized, or enlarged, glands.

Besides adrenal hyperplasia, enlarged adrenal glands may be caused by metastatic disease, granulomatous disease (tuberculosis or histoplasmosis), or bilateral adenomas in multiple endocrine neoplasia syndromes.

ADRENAL ADENOMA

Adrenal cortical adenomas may secrete hormones and be responsible for one of the

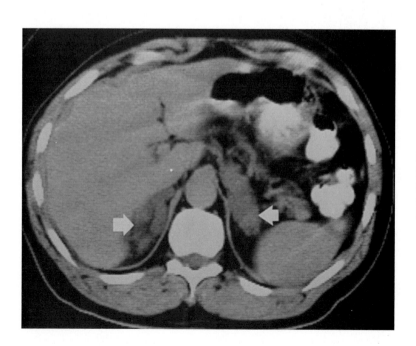

Figure 15–4. Adrenal hyperplasia. Both adrenal glands *(arrows)* demonstrate marked thickening of their limbs without focal masses.

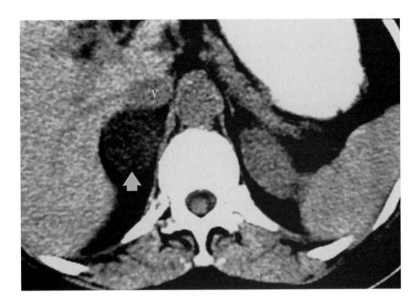

Figure 15–5. Benign adrenal adenoma—Conn's tumor. An aldosterone-producing benign adenoma *(arrow)* of the right adrenal is seen as a low-density mass extending posteriorly from the inferior vena cava (V) between the liver and the right crus of the diaphragm. High cholesterol content of this functioning tumor is believed to be responsible for its relatively low CT density.

syndromes discussed subsequently or be nonhyperfunctioning and present as an incidental adrenal mass (1% of the general population). Hormone hypersecretion cannot be determined from the CT appearance, although high cholesterol content makes some adenomas appear relatively lucent (as low as − 20 H) (Fig. 15–5). CT features of benign adrenal adenoma (Fig. 15–6) are

1. Small size, less than 3 cm diameter
2. Smooth, round, well-defined contour
3. Uniform tissue density without evidence of hemorrhage or necrosis (− 20 to + 30 H).
4. Unenhanced attenuation less than 10 H has about 95% sensitivity for benign adenoma
5. Minimal contrast enhancement
6. Calcification uncommon

Nonhyperfunctioning adrenal adenomas increase in incidence with age and are commonly detected on routine CT examinations.

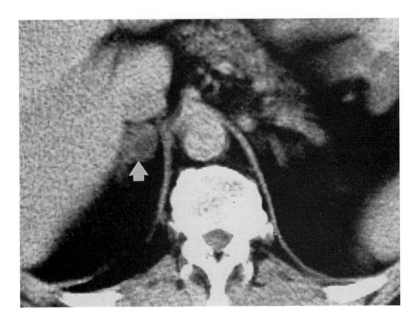

Figure 15–6. Benign adrenal adenoma. CT staging of a patient with squamous carcinoma of the lung revealed a small mass of the right adrenal gland *(arrow)*. Its benign nature was confirmed by percutaneous, CT-guided, fine-needle aspiration biopsy. Benign adrenal adenomas are common, even in patients with known malignancy.

Adrenal tumors that are less than 6 cm and have the appearance just described can be considered benign and incidental if there is no evidence of excess hormonal function and no history of malignant disease. Routine follow-up at 3- to 6-month intervals for growth or change in appearance is recommended. Metastatic disease must be ruled out by percutaneous fine-needle biopsy in patients with known malignancy. Adrenal masses larger than 6 cm should be considered for surgical removal because of risk of carcinoma.

ADRENAL CARCINOMA

Adrenal carcinomas are rare but highly malignant tumors with an extremely poor prognosis. Five-year survival is almost zero. Thirty to 50% are functional, most commonly producing Cushing's syndrome. About 10% are bilateral. The CT appearance of adrenal carcinoma (Fig. 15–7) is

1. Large size, averaging 12 cm median diameter, rarely smaller than 6 cm
2. Irregular, poorly defined contour
3. Large areas of internal hemorrhage and necrosis in most
4. Calcification present in 30%
5. Rapid growth with invasion of adjacent

organs and veins, including the inferior vena cava

ENDOCRINE SYNDROMES

Cushing's Syndrome

Cushing's syndrome results from excessive production of glucocorticoids. Approximately 70% of cases are due to adrenal hyperplasia resulting from adrenocorticotropic hormone (ACTH)–secreting pituitary adenoma or ectopic ACTH produced by small cell lung carcinoma or bronchial carcinoid. About 20% are due to adrenal adenoma, and 10% are due to adrenal carcinoma (see Fig. 15–7). Most adenomas causing Cushing's syndrome are 2 to 3 cm or larger and are easily demonstrated on CT. About 80% of all patients are women, most commonly aged 20 to 40. An additional finding common with Cushing's syndrome is increased fat deposition in the subcutaneous tissues, abdomen, and liver.

Conn's Syndrome

Primary hyperaldosteronism is diagnosed clinically by the presence of hypertension, persistent hypokalemia, increased aldosterone, and decreased renin in the plasma.

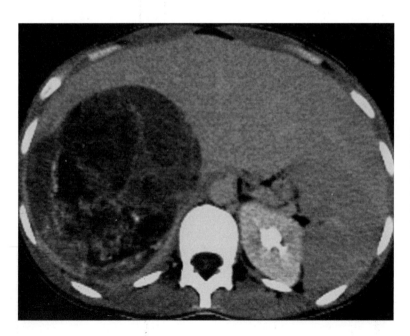

Figure 15–7. Adrenal carcinoma. This huge necrotic tumor replacing the right adrenal gland was discovered during evaluation for Cushing's syndrome in a 27-year-old woman.

Figure 15–8. Pheochromocytoma. A large, heterogeneous, necrotic tumor *(arrow)* arises from the right adrenal gland in this 19-year-old woman who presented with hypertensive crisis during childbirth.

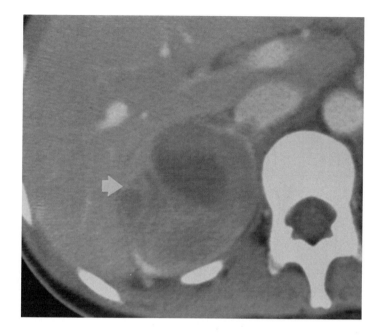

The role of CT is to identify the lesion. Solitary adrenal adenoma is the cause of 80% of cases (see Fig. 15–5), whereas 20% are due to idiopathic bilateral adrenal hyperplasia. Surgical resection of adenoma is curative, whereas patients with adrenal hyperplasia are treated medically. Adenomas causing Conn's syndrome tend to be small, with an average size of 1.8 cm. Optimal CT technique is required to demonstrate these small tumors.

Pheochromocytoma

Pheochromocytoma secretes catecholamines responsible for the clinical syndrome of hypertension, headaches, palpitations, and excessive sweating. Like primary hyperaldosteronism, the diagnosis is made by laboratory evaluation and the causative lesion is identified radiographically before surgery. Elevated total plasma catecholamines (norepinephrine, epinephrine) or elevated catecholamine metabolites (metanephrine) in the urine make the diagnosis. Ninety percent of tumors arise from the adrenal medulla. The tumor follows the "rule of 10s"; 10% are extra-adrenal, 10% are bilateral, and 10% are malignant. Most adrenal lesions can be demonstrated by CT (Fig. 15–8):

1. Well-defined tumor is usually larger than 2 cm.

2. Contrast medium enhancement may be uniform or nonuniform.

3. Cystic degeneration, hemorrhage, necrosis, and calcification are common.

Multiple and bilateral tumors are generally seen in association with multiple endocrine neoplasia or von Hippel-Lindau syndromes. Although extra-adrenal tumors (paragangliomas) have been found everywhere along the sympathetic chain from skull base to pelvis, most (98%) are in the abdomen along the course of the aorta, especially arising from the organ of Zuckerkandl near the aortic bifurcation (Fig. 15–9). CT evaluation before clinical confirmation of the diagnosis is not indicated. The most appropriate CT strategy is to scan the adrenal glands initially. If no lesion is apparent, then additional scanning of the abdomen, bladder, and chest is performed.

Addison's Disease

Adrenal insufficiency occurs after destruction of 90% of the adrenal cortex. The most common causes are idiopathic adrenal atrophy and destruction by tuberculosis or disseminated fungal disease, hemorrhage, lymphoma, or metastases. CT findings depend on the cause of adrenal dysfunction:

1. Tiny adrenal glands with primary cortical atrophy may be difficult to detect.

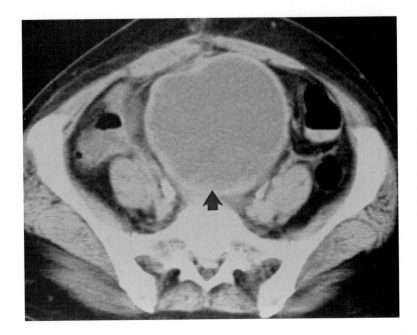

Figure 15–9. Pheochromocytoma. This pheochromocytoma *(arrow)* arose at the aortic bifurcation from the organ of Zuckerkandl. Pathologic examination revealed that the tumor was benign with a thick fibrous wall and was filled with hemorrhagic fluid.

2. Enlarged glands resemble hyperplasia in tuberculosis or histoplasmosis; calcification is common.

3. Both glands are replaced by tumor when metastases are the cause.

ADRENAL METASTASES

The adrenals are a common site of metastatic deposits from common malignancies. Bilateral adrenal masses are usually metastases (Fig. 15–10). The tumors may be any size, round or lobulated, homogeneous or inhomogeneous, calcified, or necrotic (Fig. 15–11). Despite the frequency and varied appearance of adrenal metastases, even in patients with known malignancy up to 50% of adrenal masses may be benign adenomas (see Fig. 15–6). Features that favor malignancy include

1. Size greater than 3 cm
2. Poorly defined margins

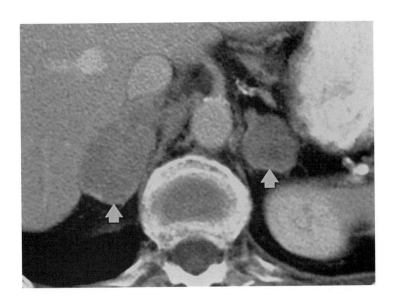

Figure 15–10. Bilateral adrenal metastases. Masses *(arrows)* arise from both adrenal glands in this patient with small cell carcinoma of the lung. The mass in the right adrenal gland exceeds 3 cm in diameter. The left adrenal mass has ill-defined margins.

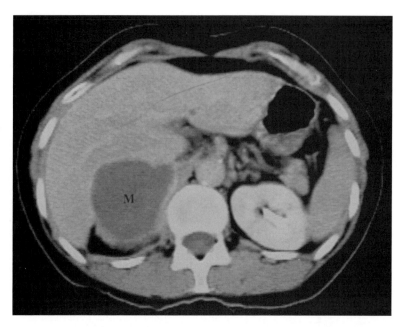

Figure 15–11. Necrotic adrenal metastasis. A large cell carcinoma of the lung metastasized to the right adrenal gland and produced this large cystic-appearing mass (M). Note the lobulated contour, ragged margins, and thick walls. Compare with the adrenal cyst in Figure 15–12.

3. Thick, enhancing rim (see Fig. 15–11)
4. Inhomogeneous attenuation
5. Invasion of adjacent structures
6. Evidence of metastases elsewhere

Percutaneous biopsy is needed for tissue diagnosis.

ADRENAL CYST

Adrenal cyst is an uncommon, benign, incidental lesion that can generally be diagnosed by CT, avoiding confusion with significant lesions. An adrenal cyst may be a true cyst with epithelial or endothelial lining or a pseudocyst that results from adrenal hemorrhage. Each is seen as an oval or round, well-defined mass of uniform water density with a thin wall (Fig. 15–12). A calcified rim may be seen with a pseudocyst. A ragged outline or thickened wall suggests necrotic tumor (see Fig. 15–10) rather than benign cyst. Because some adrenal solid tumors are low density on CT (see Fig. 15–5), ultrasonography may occasionally be needed to confirm an adrenal cyst.

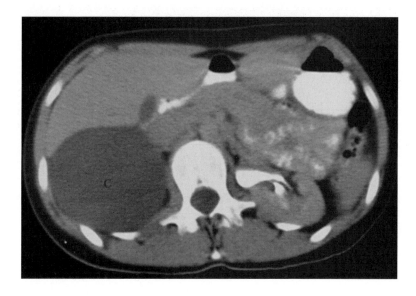

Figure 15–12. Adrenal cyst. This benign cyst (C) of the right adrenal gland has smooth well-defined margins, homogeneous low internal density, and no discernible walls. (Courtesy of Dr. James P. Dyrud, Rawlins, Wyoming.)

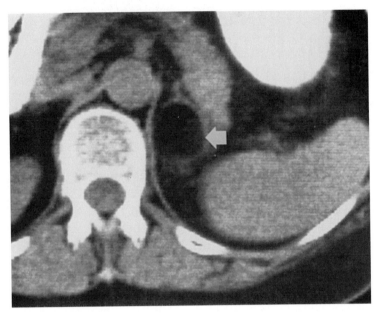

Figure 15–13. Adrenal myelolipoma. A myelolipoma *(arrow)* of the left adrenal gland has an internal low density identical to intraabdominal and subcutaneous fat.

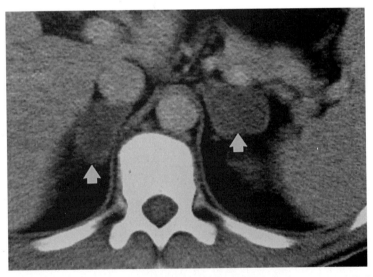

Figure 15–14. Adrenal hemorrhage. Bilateral adrenal hemorrhage is seen as ill-defined, low-density masses *(arrows)* replacing both adrenal glands. The patient had been injured in a motor vehicle accident.

ADRENAL MYELOLIPOMA

Myelolipomas are rare but radiographically interesting because usually a definitive diagnosis can be made. They are nonfunctional tumors consisting of fat and bone marrow elements with no malignant potential. Large tumors may hemorrhage, cause pain, or displace adjacent organs. Characteristic CT findings (Fig. 15–13) are

1. Well-defined adrenal mass of any size up to 30 cm
2. Diagnostic inhomogeneous central fat density (− 30 to − 100 H)
3. Calcification present in 20%
4. Relatively avascular lesion showing little or no contrast medium enhancement

Fat density, not just low density, must be demonstrated to make a firm diagnosis. Necrotic tumors and cholesterol-laden adenomas may be of low density but not of fat density.

ADRENAL HEMORRHAGE

Hemorrhage into the adrenal glands may occur as a complication of trauma or anticoagulant therapy or spontaneously in association with sepsis, hypertension, or renal vein thrombosis. In neonates, only 10% of cases are bilateral, whereas in the trauma-

TABLE 15–1. Causes of Adrenal Calcifications

Previous adrenal hemorrhage
Infection
   Tuberculosis
   Histoplasmosis
   Sepsis: Waterhouse-Friderichsen syndrome
Tumors
   Neuroblastoma
   Pheochromocytoma
   Adrenal carcinoma
   Metastasis
Metabolic disorders
   Wolman's disease: autosomal recessive
     xanthomatosis

tized adult, 25% of cases are bilateral. Bilateral hemorrhage can result in adrenal insufficiency. CT demonstrates the evolving appearance of hematoma over time:

1. Heterogeneous mass replacing the adrenal gland (Fig. 15–14)
2. Common streaky infiltrates of periadrenal fat
3. Initial hematoma of high density (50–90 H)
4. Gradual decrease in size and density (to near water)
5. Return to normal appearance or persistence as a hemorrhagic pseudocyst or residual calcification (Fig. 15–15; Table 15–1).

Hemorrhage into an adrenal tumor must also be considered.

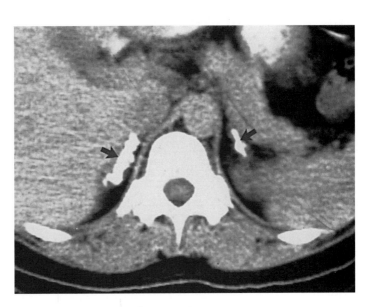

Figure 15–15. Adrenal calcification. Both adrenal glands demonstrate coarse, dense, linear calcifications *(arrows).* The patient had had bilateral adrenal hemorrhages in the newborn period.

Suggested Reading

Cyran KM, Kenney PJ, Memel DS, Yacoub I. Adrenal myelolipoma. AJR 1996; 166:395–400.

Doppman JJ, Gill JR Jr. Hyperaldosteronism: sampling the adrenal veins. Radiology 1996; 198:309–312.

Dunnick NR. Adrenal imaging: current status. AJR 1990; 154:927–936.

Francis IR, Gross MD, Shapiro B, et al. Integrated imaging of adrenal disease. Radiology 1992; 184:1–13.

Korobkin M, Dunnick NR. Characterization of adrenal masses. AJR 1995; 164:643–644.

McLoughlin RF, Blbey JH. Tumors of the adrenal gland: findings on CT and MR imaging. AJR 1994; 163:1413–1418.

Miyake H, Maeda H, Tashiro M, et al. CT of adrenal tumors: frequency and clinical signficance of low-attenuation lesions. AJR 1989; 152:1005–1007.

Musante F, Derchi LE, Zappasodi F, et al. Myelolipoma of the adrenal gland: sonographic and CT features. AJR 1988; 151:961–964.

Radin DR, Manoogian C, Nadler JL. Diagnosis of primary hyperaldosteronism: importance of correlation CT findings with endocrinologic studies. AJR 1992; 158:553–557.

Tung GA, Pfister RC, Papanicolaou N, Yoder IC. Adrenal cysts: imaging and percutaneous aspiration. Radiology 1989; 173:107–110.

Westra SJ, Zaninovic AC, Hall TR, et al. Imaging of the adrenal gland in children. Radiographics 1994; 14:1323–1340.

16

Gastrointestinal Tract

William E. Brant, M.D.

BASIC PRINCIPLES

CT complements barium examination of the gastrointestinal tract by better demonstration of intramural and extraintestinal components of gastrointestinal disease, including disease in the mesentery, peritoneal cavity, lymph nodes, and liver. CT is used to (1) diagnose the presence of gastrointestinal disease, (2) evaluate its nature and extent, and (3) demonstrate complications such as abscess, phlegmon, fistula, and perforation. CT is excellent for determining the extent of gastrointestinal disease but is seldom specific for its nature.

The gastrointestinal tract is shown on every CT of the abdomen. The intestinal lumen should be distended and opacified for routine abdominal CT by administration of 700 to 800 mL of 2% to 3% iodinated, or barium, contrast agent at least 1 hour before scanning. CT examination dedicated to evaluation of the gastrointestinal tract requires cleansing of the colon (by barium enema preparation), fasting for at least 4 hours (to keep the stomach empty), and oral contrast medium administration. Studies should be optimized by oral administration of gas-producing crystals, colon insufflation with air, and changing the patient's position to maximize gastrointestinal distention in the area of a suspected pathologic process. Intravenous contrast medium is used to assess enhancement of known lesions, demonstrate blood vessels, and evaluate the solid organs of the abdomen. Thin-section (5-mm) scans or helical scans with overlapping reconstruction (5-mm collimation at 3-mm intervals) can improve lesion definition. Short scan times (1 to 2 seconds) improve image quality by limiting motion artifact. Motion artifact from peristalsis can be inhibited by 1 mg of glucagon given intravenously just before scanning. Collapsed bowel loops without intraluminal contrast medium enhancement may mimic adenopathy and mass lesions. However, when scans are obtained during the arterial phase of bolus contrast medium enhancement, identification of enhanced bowel wall confirms the nature of nondistended bowel.

A CT hallmark of intestinal disease is thickening of the bowel wall. When fully distended, the bowel wall is 1 to 2 mm thick. When collapsed, the bowel wall should not exceed 3 to 4 mm, except in the stomach near the esophageal junction where the normal stomach wall may be 2 cm thick when collapsed. The CT appearance of wall thickening is helpful in differentiating benign from malignant wall thickening (Table 16–1). Benign, pathologic wall thickening usually does not exceed 1 cm and is homogeneous in attenuation, circumferential, symmetric, and segmental in distribution. The "double halo" and "target" appearance of the intestine in cross section is due to inflammation, edema, and hyperemia and is best demonstrated on contrast medium–enhanced scans. Neoplastic wall thickening is thicker (1 to 2 cm), asymmetric, nodular,

TABLE 16–1. **Benign vs. Malignant Bowel Wall Thickening**

Benign	Malignant
Homogeneous attenuation	Heterogeneous attenuation
Symmetric	Asymmetric
Circumferential	Eccentric
Thickening < 1 cm	Thickening > 1–2 cm
Segmental or diffuse involvement	Focal mass
	Abrupt transition
"Double-halo sign"	Lobulated contour
Dark inner ring	Spiculated contour
Bright outer ring	Narrowed bowel lumen
"Target sign"	Enlarged lymph nodes
Bright inner ring	Liver metastases
Dark middle ring	
Bright outer ring	

lobulated, or spiculated in contour and tends to narrow the intestinal lumen. Benign wall thickening is caused by inflammatory bowel disease, intestinal ischemia, and intramural hemorrhage. Neoplastic wall thickening is produced by adenocarcinoma, lymphoma, and leiomyosarcoma.

ESOPHAGUS

Anatomy

The esophagus is a muscular tube that extends from the cricopharyngeus muscle at the level of the cricoid cartilage to the stomach. The major portion of its length is within the middle mediastinum. The cervical portion extends from the level of the C6 vertebral body to the thoracic inlet. A short abdominal segment extends below the diaphragm to the gastroesophageal junction. The esophagus is lined by squamous epithelium to the gastric junction where the mucosa abruptly changes to columnar epithelium. The lack of serosal covering allows early invasion by esophageal tumors into periesophageal tissues. The musculature of the esophageal wall is striated in the upper

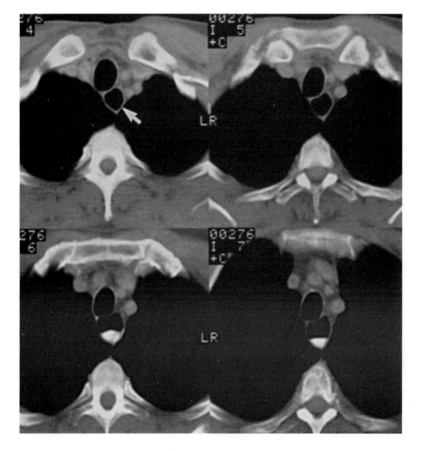

Figure 16–1. Normal esophagus. Multiple sequential slices through the normal upper esophagus in a patient with a distal obstructing tumor demonstrate the normal thin wall *(arrow)*. Oral contrast medium is seen layering in the esophagus due to distal obstruction.

one third, striated and smooth muscle in the middle third, and solely smooth muscle in the distal third.

On CT the esophagus appears as an oval of soft tissue density often containing air or contrast material within its lumen. When distended, the wall of the esophagus should not exceed 3 mm in thickness (Fig. 16–1). In the neck and upper thorax, the esophagus courses between the trachea and the spine. In the lower thorax, the esophagus courses to the right of the descending aorta between the left atrium and the spine. The esophagus enters the abdomen through the esophageal hiatus and courses to the left to join the stomach. The edges of the diaphragmatic crura forming the esophageal hiatus are seen as often prominent, teardrop-shaped structures partially surrounding the esophagus.

Technical Considerations

The esophagus is studied using contiguous 7- to 10-mm thick slices from the level of the larynx to the stomach. When esophageal tumors are evaluated, scanning is continued through the liver to look for metastases. Oral contrast agent is given to distend the stomach and the gastroesophageal junction. Intravenous contrast medium is useful to evaluate mediastinal vessels and to detect varices. Attempts to fully distend the esophagus during CT scanning are not consistently successful. Oral administration of dilute barium paste may aid in coating the esophageal mucosa.

Hiatus Hernia

Hiatus hernia is a protrusion of any portion of the stomach into the thorax. On CT, hiatus hernia appears as an air- or contrast agent–filled mass continuous with the stomach lying within and above the esophageal hiatus (Fig. 16–2). The edges of the esophageal hiatus are often widely separated, exceeding 15 mm in width. The major reason to recognize a hiatus hernia is to avoid mistaking it for a tumor.

Esophageal Carcinoma

Because of the lack of serosal covering, carcinoma spreads beyond the esophagus early

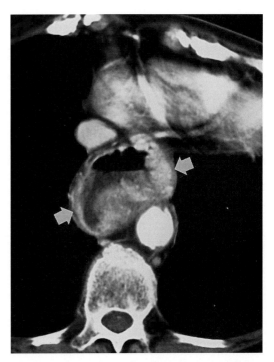

Figure 16–2. Hiatus hernia. A portion of the stomach extends through the esophageal hiatus to form a hiatal hernia *(arrows)*. Gastric folds are evident. Fluid retained within the herniated stomach forms an air–fluid level.

in its course, resulting in a poor prognosis. Ninety percent of tumors are squamous cell carcinoma, with the remaining 10% being adenocarcinoma arising in Barrett's esophagus in the distal esophagus. It must be recognized that the CT findings in esophageal carcinoma may be duplicated by benign disease. Diagnosis depends on biopsy. CT is performed to assess the extent of disease and to identify those patients whose disease cannot be resected. The CT findings in esophageal carcinoma (Fig. 16–3) include

1. Irregular thickening of the wall of the esophagus more than 3 mm
2. Intraluminal polypoid mass
3. Eccentric narrowing of the lumen
4. Dilatation of the esophagus above the area of narrowing
5. Invasion of periesophageal tissues: fat, aorta, trachea
6. Metastases to lymph nodes, liver, and other organs (Fig. 16–4)

Tumor invasion of the trachea or bronchi is suggested by tumor that displaces or in-

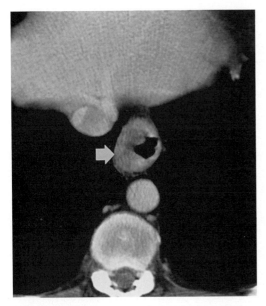

Figure 16–3. Esophageal carcinoma. Adenocarcinoma arising in the distal esophagus causes asymmetric nodular thickening *(arrow)* of the esophageal wall.

dents the posterior airway wall (90% accurate). Tumor invasion of the aorta is suggested by an arc of contact between the tumor and aorta of greater than 90°. An arc less than 45° indicates no invasion, and an arc between 45° and 90° is indeterminate. These findings are reported to be 80% accurate.

Esophageal carcinoma spreads to para-esophageal, other mediastinal, gastrohepatic ligament, and left gastric nodal chains. Microscopic disease in normal-sized nodes, and lymph node enlargement due to benign conditions, limits the CT accuracy of nodal involvement by esophageal carcinoma to 39% to 85%.

Tumor recurrence after esophagectomy is well demonstrated by CT. Tumors may recur anywhere within the mediastinum, in distant lymph nodes in the neck or abdomen, and in liver, lung, pleural space, adrenal glands, or peritoneal cavity.

Esophageal Leiomyoma

Leiomyoma is the most common benign tumor of the esophagus. Most are asymptomatic until becoming very large and causing dysphagia. Endoscopy demonstrates a submucosal mass, usually easily differentiated from carcinoma. On CT it appears as a smooth, well-defined 2- to 8-cm mass of uniform soft tissue density. The esophageal wall is eccentrically thickened, and the lumen is deformed. A large, well-defined mass is much more likely to be a leiomyoma than a carcinoma. Leiomyomas are multiple in 3% to 4% of cases.

Esophageal Varices

Varices cause scalloped thickening of the esophageal wall that may be indistinguish-

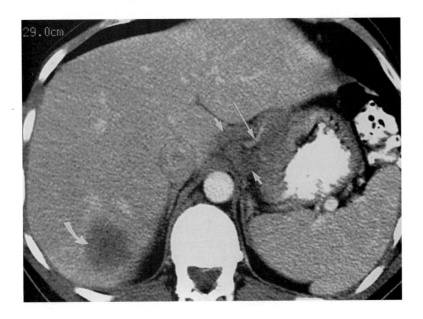

Figure 16–4. Carcinoma of the gastroesophageal junction. Carcinoma arising near the gastroesophageal junction has spread to the liver *(curved arrow)* and to lymph nodes *(short arrows)* surrounding the celiac axis *(long arrow).*

able from tumor or inflammation without the use of contrast medium enhancement. The key to CT diagnosis is vascular enhancement (Fig. 16–5), which is best demonstrated by giving bolus contrast agent injection combined with rapid CT scanning. Signs of cirrhosis, portal hypertension, and other portosystemic collateral vessels may also be present.

Esophagitis

Esophagitis results in circumferential thickening of the esophageal wall, usually without disruption of the periesophageal tissues. Strictures are seen as areas of luminal narrowing with dilatation of the esophagus above the lesion. Severe esophagitis may lead to deep ulcers, perforation, mediastinitis, and abscess. Immunosuppressed patients are prone to fungal (*Candida albicans*), viral (herpes simplex and cytomegalovirus), and tuberculous esophagitis.

Esophageal Perforation

Esophageal perforation may be traumatic, may be iatrogenic after instrumentation, or may result from neoplasm or inflammation. Because it may be lethal, prompt recognition is essential. CT signs include fluid collections, air, and contrast material within the mediastinum adjacent to the esophagus, widening of the mediastinum, and hydrothorax and pneumothorax.

STOMACH

Anatomy

The posteriorly located gastric fundus is seen on CT sections through the dome of the diaphragm. The esophagus joins the stomach a short distance below the fundus. A prominent pseudotumor, caused by thickening of the gastric wall due to incomplete distention, is often seen near the gastroesophageal junction (Fig. 16–6). Additional distention with more air or contrast agent will eliminate this pseudotumor. The body of the stomach sweeps toward the right. The antrum crosses the midline of the abdomen between the left lobe of the liver and the pancreas to join the duodenal bulb in the region of the gallbladder.

The normal gastric wall should not exceed 5 mm in thickness when the stomach is well distended. Rugal folds are commonly visualized even with good distention. Like the esophagus, both benign and malignant conditions produce similar CT findings. CT is performed to document the extent of extraluminal disease.

Technical Considerations

The stomach must be filled with positive contrast medium or distended with air or water for optimal assessment by CT. Oral contrast agent (200–300 mL) is routinely

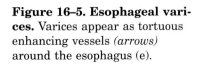
Figure 16–5. Esophageal varices. Varices appear as tortuous enhancing vessels *(arrows)* around the esophagus (e).

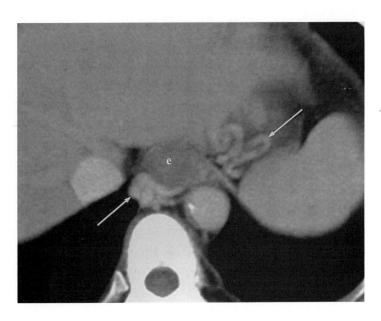

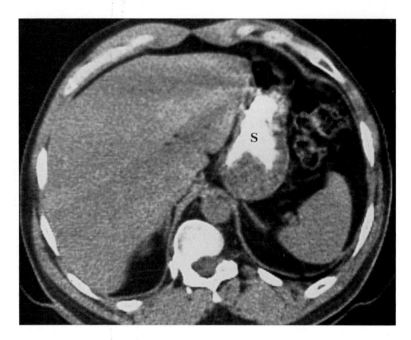

Figure 16–6. Pseudotumor at gastroesophageal junction. The wall of the stomach (S) is thickened and nodular owing to poor distention. Subsequent images, obtained after oral administration of additional contrast medium, demonstrated normal gastric wall thickness.

given to fill the stomach just before the patient lies down on the CT couch. Alternatively, distention of the stomach with air may be achieved by giving gas-producing crystals (4 to 6 g of Citrocarbonate granules with 16 to 30 mL of water) instead of the opaque contrast agent. The patient can be repositioned, in prone or decubitus positions, to optimize distention of the different portions of the stomach with air or contrast agent. Water (200–300 mL) can also be

given to distend the stomach and provide good tissue contrast between low-density lumen and the gastric wall. Scanning is performed using contiguous 7- to 10-mm thick slices.

Thickened Gastric Wall

Thickening of the gastric wall (Fig. 16–7), either focal or diffuse, is an important but nonspecific, sign of gastric disease. With

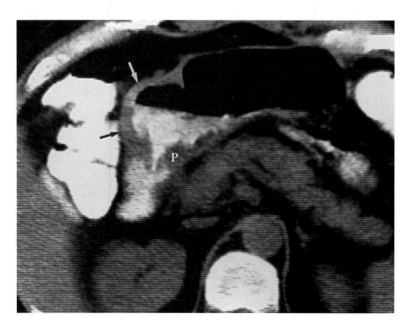

Figure 16–7. Gastric lymphoma. Lymphoma thickens the gastric wall in the region of the antrum *(arrows)*. This finding is nonspecific, and this appearance may be caused by both inflammatory and neoplastic conditions. P = pylorus.

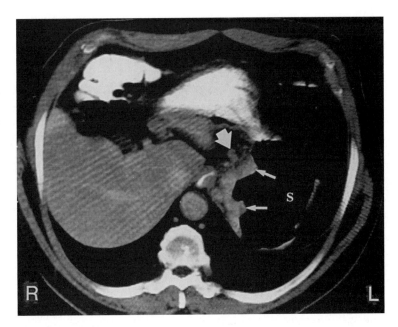

Figure 16–8. Gastric carcinoma. This patient was scanned prone to optimally distend the gastric fundus (S) after administration of gas-producing crystals. The image is inverted to maintain standard anatomic orientation. A gastric carcinoma causes nodular thickening of the gastric wall *(small arrows).* Tumor extension through the wall, suggested by the soft tissue densities *(large arrow)* in the perigastric fat, was confirmed at surgery.

good technique, which includes aggressive distention of the stomach with air or contrast agent, wall thickening greater than 5 mm can be considered abnormal. Causes include carcinoma, lymphoma, gastric inflammation (peptic or Crohn's disease), perigastric inflammation (pancreatitis), and radiation. CT may show gastric ulcers as collections of contrast agent within a thickened wall. Penetrating ulcers appear as a sinus tract, marked by contrast agent or air, extending to adjacent structures.

Gastric Carcinoma

Adenocarcinoma is the cause of 95% of gastric malignancy. CT is used to stage disease and identify patients whose disease is not surgically resectable. CT findings in gastric carcinoma (Figs. 16–8 and 16–9) include

1. Focal, nodular or irregular thickening of the gastric wall
2. Polypoid, soft tissue density, intraluminal mass
3. Diffuse wall thickening with nar-

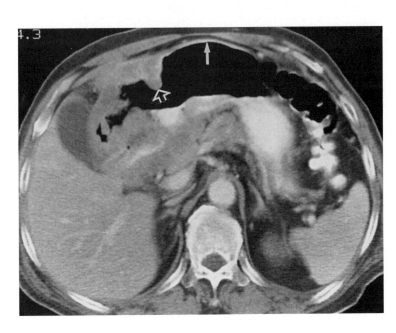

Figure 16–9. Gastric carcinoma. Nodular thickening of the wall of the gastric antrum *(open arrow)* is striking in comparison to the normal wall of the gastric body *(closed arrow).*

rowing of the lumen (scirrhous carcinoma, linitis plastica)

4. Stippled calcifications with mucinous adenocarcinoma

5. Extension of tumor into the perigastric fat—nearly always present when wall thickness exceeds 2 cm

6. Adenopathy near the celiac axis and in the gastrohepatic ligament

7. Peritoneal carcinomatosis

8. Metastases in the liver

Gastric Lymphoma

The stomach is the most common site of involvement for primary gastrointestinal lymphoma (see Fig. 16–7). Most cases (90%–95%) are non-Hodgkin's lymphoma. CT findings are similar to adenocarcinoma. Gastric lymphoma may cause a polypoid mass, diffuse wall infiltration with featureless walls, or markedly thickened walls with nodular thickened folds. CT features that favor lymphoma over carcinoma include more dramatic thickening of the stomach wall (exceeding 3 cm), involvement of more than one region of the gastrointestinal tract, transpyloric spread of tumor, and more widespread adenopathy above and below the level of the renal hilum. Luminal narrowing is typical of carcinoma but rare with lymphoma.

Gastric Leiomyoma/ Leiomyosarcoma

Leiomyoma, leiomyoblastoma, and leiomyosarcoma arise from the smooth muscle of the gastric wall and grow as submucosal, subserosal, or exophytic tumors. They grow silently and may reach a large size before presenting clinically as ulceration and gastrointestinal bleeding. Histologic criteria for differentiating benign from malignant tumors are not foolproof. The diagnosis of malignancy is based on size, gross appearance, and behavior of the tumor. Benign lesions are smaller (4 to 5 cm average size), are homogeneous in CT density, and enhance diffusely and symmetrically. Malignant lesions (Fig. 16–10) are larger (12 cm average size) and markedly heterogeneous with multiple low-density regions and irregular enhancement patterns. Deep ulcerations and cavitation with air–fluid levels may be evident. Leiomyoma is the most common benign gastric neoplasm. Mottled calcification is common. Leiomyoblastoma is usually benign (90%).

Gastric Varices

Gastric varices occur as a result of portal hypertension or splenic vein thrombosis. They appear as well-defined clusters of

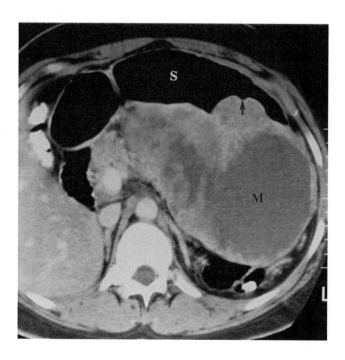

Figure 16–10. Gastric leiomyosarcoma. A huge heterogeneous mass (M) arises from the posterior wall of the stomach (S). Large low-density areas within the mass correspond to hemorrhage and necrosis. An ulcer crater *(arrow)* is identified within a nodular projection into the gastric lumen.

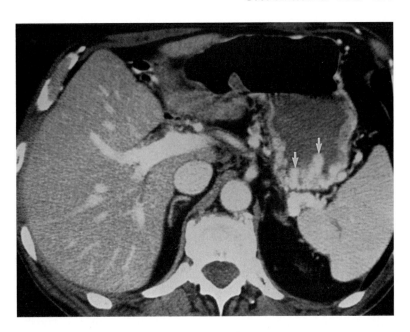

Figure 16–11. Gastric varices. Bolus intravenous contrast medium administration causes bright enhancement of varices *(arrows)* in the wall of the gastric fundus in this patient with alcoholism and portal hypertension.

rounded and tubular densities in, or adjacent to, the wall of the stomach, most commonly in the fundus (Fig. 16–11). Bright enhancement with intravenous contrast clinches the diagnosis. CT signs of liver disease and other portosystemic collateral vessels are often present.

SMALL BOWEL

Anatomy

The duodenum extends from the pylorus to the ligament of Treitz forming the familiar C-loop. The duodenum becomes retroperitoneal at the right free edge of the hepatoduodenal ligament, closely related to the neck of the gallbladder. The descending duodenum passes to the right of the pancreatic head to just below the uncinate process where the duodenum turns to the left. The horizontal portion crosses anterior to the inferior vena cava and aorta and posterior to the superior mesenteric vein and artery. The fourth portion ascends just left of the aorta to the ligament of Treitz where it becomes the intraperitoneal jejunum.

The jejunum occupies the left upper abdomen, whereas the ileum lies in the right lower abdomen and pelvis. Jejunal loops are feathery with distinct folds. Ileal loops are featureless with thin walls. Opacification of the lumen with oral contrast media is essential to adequately evaluate the bowel. Unopacified small bowel may mimic adenopathy and abdominal masses. The small bowel mesentery contains many vessels that are easily visualized when outlined by fat. The normal luminal diameter of the small bowel does not exceed 2.5 cm. The normal wall thickness is less than 3 mm.

Technical Considerations

Opacification of the small bowel with oral contrast agent is mandatory for high-quality abdominal CT. It is nearly impossible to administer too much oral contrast. A 1% to 3% concentration of oral contrast agent is optimal for CT. This concentration is obtained by adding 3 mL of 60% oral contrast solution to 100 mL of water. We give 400-mL doses of this mixture 12 hours, 2 hours, 30 minutes, and immediately before CT scanning. To study the small bowel we obtain sequential 7- to 10-mm thick slices through the abdomen and pelvis. When the duodenum is the organ of primary interest, administration of 0.1 mg of glucagon intravenously is helpful in stopping peristalsis and in distending the bowel. An intravenous contrast agent is optional for the small bowel itself but is helpful for assessment of the remainder of the abdomen.

Small Bowel Edema and Wall Thickening

Like the other portions of the gastrointestinal tract, edema and wall thickening (Fig. 16–12) are nonspecific signs seen in a wide variety of disease states. Wall thickening greater than 15 mm, or associated with mesenteric mass, suggests neoplasm. Wall thickening less than 15 mm, with normal or increased density mesenteric fat, suggests inflammatory disease or noninflammatory edema (ischemia, trauma, hypoalbuminemia, lymphatic obstruction).

Small Bowel Diverticula

Small bowel diverticula may cause unusual collections of fluid, air, contrast material, or soft tissue density in the fat and tissues adjacent to the bowel (Fig. 16–13). These must not be mistaken for abscesses, pancreatic pseudocysts, or tumors. Rescanning the patient will often demonstrate a significant change in the appearance of diverticula.

Small Bowel Tumors

Both benign and malignant small bowel neoplasms are uncommon. CT demonstrates about 73% of small bowel tumors, which appear as soft tissue mass or wall thickening. CT is useful in demonstrating extraluminal tumor growth, involvement of adjacent structures, adenopathy, and complications such as fistulas or necrosis.

Lymphomas appear as single or multiple, often large (9 cm) soft tissue masses or as nodular wall thickening (Fig. 16–14). Ulceration is common. Mesenteric or retroperitoneal adenopathy is seen in half the cases.

Carcinoids occur most commonly in the appendix (50%) and mesenteric small bowel (20%). All tumors have the potential to metastasize and are considered malignant, although some may have an indolent course. Aggressive tumors tend to be larger than 2 cm and have necrosis and ulceration. Tumor invasion of the bowel wall induces a dramatic fibrosing reaction in the mesentery that is the hallmark of CT diagnosis (Fig. 16–15). Linear strands of fibrosis radiate into the mesenteric fat from the soft tissue mass or focal wall thickening of the primary tumor. Liver metastases are always present in patients with carcinoid syndrome.

Adenocarcinoma of the small bowel occurs most commonly in the duodenum. Most tumors appear as a solitary soft tissue mass, up to 8 cm in diameter.

Leiomyosarcomas tend to be very large (11 cm) and exophytic with prominent central necrosis.

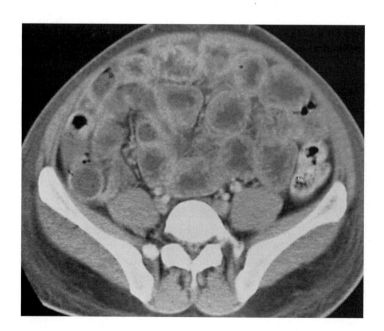

Figure 16–12. Hypoalbuminemia. Hypoalbuminemia, due to a protein-losing enteropathy, causes diffuse wall thickening and dilatation of the small bowel.

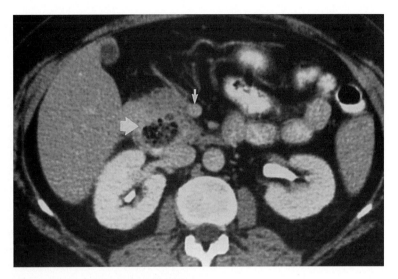

Figure 16–13. Duodenal diverticulum. A diverticulum, arising from the second portion of the duodenum, is seen as a mass *(large arrow)* containing air and fluid that displaces the superior mesenteric vein *(small arrow)*.

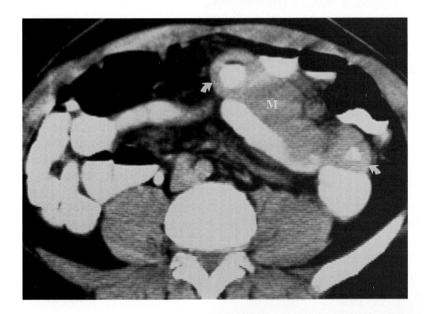

Figure 16–14. Small bowel lymphoma. CT scan through the lower abdomen demonstrates loops of ileum with markedly thickened walls *(arrows)* and adenopathy that produces a mass (M) in the small bowel mesentery.

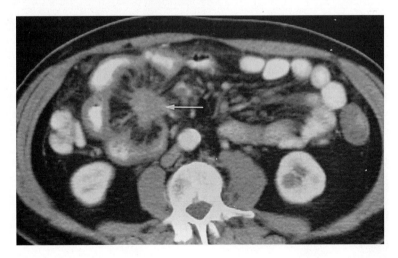

Figure 16–15. Carcinoid tumor. A carcinoid tumor arising in the ileum causes a mass *(arrow)* in the small bowel mesentery. Characteristic thick fibrotic strands radiate from the mass to the adjacent bowel. (Courtesy of Dr. James Schlund, Chico, California.)

Crohn's Disease

Crohn's disease is characterized by inflammation of the bowel mucosa, bowel wall, and mesentery with marked submucosal edema. These features are nicely reflected in the CT appearance (Fig. 16–16):

1. Circumferential thickening of the bowel wall, typically 7 to 11 mm
2. Low-density inner ring of submucosal edema ("double halo" sign)
3. Diffuse haziness and increased density of the mesenteric fat
4. "Skip areas" of normal bowel intervened between diseased segments
5. Fistulas and sinus tracts between bowel loops, or to the bladder, adjacent muscle, or the skin surface
6. Mesenteric abscesses containing fluid, air, or contrast material

CT is excellent in documenting the extraluminal manifestations of the disease.

Small Bowel Obstruction

CT is reported to be 90% to 95% sensitive for detecting small bowel obstruction and 47% to 73% sensitive in identifying its cause. The CT hallmark of small bowel obstruction is identification of a transition zone between dilated (>2.5 cm), air- or fluid-filled proximal bowel and collapsed distal bowel. Ileus may cause markedly dilated bowel (up to 5 cm diameter), but no transition zone is present. However, a totally collapsed descending colon is common in nonobstructive ileus and should not be mistaken for evidence of a transition zone.

Adhesions cause 50% of small bowel obstructions but are not directly visualized by CT. Abrupt transition from dilated to nondilated bowel without other findings suggests adhesions as the cause. Beaklike narrowing at the transition zone is characteristic of adhesions but is not common. Tumor, abscess, intussusception, inflammation, and hernia causing obstruction are identified by characteristic signs.

Closed loop obstruction has a higher morbidity and mortality than simple obstruction. Closed loop obstruction refers to a loop of bowel occluded at two adjacent points along its course, usually due to adhesions or internal hernia. The obstructed loop may twist, resulting in volvulus. *Strangulation* refers to closed loop obstruction with intestinal ischemia. Dilated bowel loops with stretched and prominent mesenteric vessels converging on a site of obstruction suggests closed loop obstruction. Strangulation is suggested by associated mild circumferential thickening of the bowel wall with the

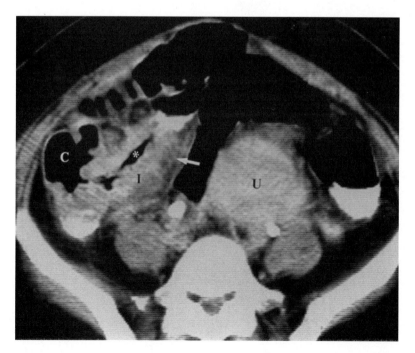

Figure 16–16. Crohn's disease. This image demonstrates the CT equivalent of the string sign that is characteristic of Crohn's disease. The wall of the terminal ileum (I) is markedly thickened, narrowing the lumen (*). The inflammatory changes extend into the surrounding fat *(arrow)*. Histologic examination, after resection, confirmed transmural inflammation with multiple granulomas. C = cecum; U = fundus of the uterus.

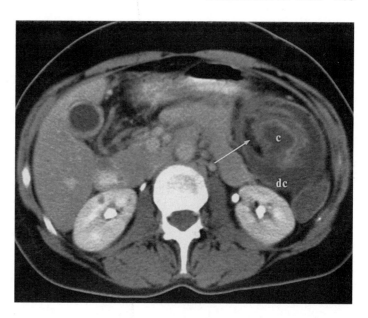

Figure 16–17. Intussusception. An adenoma arising in the cecum served as a lead mass for a cocolonic intussusception. This image demonstrates a portion of the cecum (c) inside the lumen of the descending colon (dc). Note the intraluminal crescent of fat density *(arrow),* which represents the cecal mesentery.

low-density concentric rings indicative of wall edema ("target" and "halo" signs).

Causes of *intussusception* in adults include lipoma and other benign submucosal tumors, carcinoma, metastatic disease, and lymphoma. CT demonstrates findings that are characteristic of enteroenteric, ileocolic, or colocolonic intussusception (Fig. 16–17). The distal receiving segment (intussuscipiens) is markedly dilated and has a thickened wall. Its lumen contains an eccentric, soft tissue mass (intussusceptum) with an adjacent crescent of fat density that represents the invaginated mesentery. The mass causing the intussusception can often be identified at the leading end of the intussusceptum.

Mesenteric Mass

Soft tissue masses in the small bowel mesentery are most commonly due to lymphoma (see Fig. 16–14). Lymphoma of the small bowel demonstrates focal nodular or circumferential wall thickening. Mesenteric involvement may consist of enlarged individual mesenteric nodes or large confluent masses. Lymphomatous masses characteristically "sandwich" mesenteric vessels between thin layers of spared mesenteric fat (the "sandwich" sign).

Other causes of mesenteric masses include metastases, carcinoid tumor, and mesenteric fibromatosis. Metastases tend to be multiple and small. Carcinoid tumors incite the prominent fibrotic response described previously. Mesenteric fibromatosis produces a well-defined homogeneous solid mass.

APPENDIX

Anatomy

The normal appendix can be seen on CT as a thin-walled tubular structure surrounded by mesenteric fat. It may be collapsed or filled with air, fluid, or contrast agent. The normal appendix does not exceed 6 mm in diameter and has a sharp outer contour defined by homogeneous low-density fat. The origin of the appendix is between the ileocecal valve and the cecal apex, always on the same side of the cecum as the valve. Approximately one third of appendixes course inferomedially from the cecum, whereas two thirds are retrocecal.

Appendicitis

CT has a 95% to 98% sensitivity in the diagnosis of acute appendicitis (Fig. 16–18). CT findings diagnostic of acute appendicitis are a distended appendix (>6 mm diameter), thickened walls that enhance, and periappendiceal inflammatory changes with

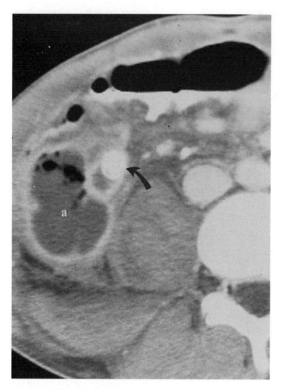

Figure 16–18. Acute appendicitis. CT demonstrates a fluid collection (a) containing air in the right lower quadrant of the abdomen. A rounded calcification nearby proved to be an appendicolith *(arrow)*. Surgery confirmed an acutely ruptured appendix with an abscess.

stranding in the fat. Complications associated with perforated appendicitis include phlegmon, seen as a periappendiceal soft tissue mass (>20 H), and abscess, seen as a fluid collection (<20 H). Phlegmons and abscesses less than 3 cm generally resolve on antibiotic treatment, whereas abscesses larger than 3 cm usually require surgical or catheter drainage. Detection of an appendicolith, appearing as a ringlike or homogeneous calcification within, or adjacent to, a phlegmon or abscess is diagnostic of appendicitis. Appendicoliths may be seen in 28% of adult patients with acute appendicitis. Additional complications that may be demonstrated by CT include small bowel obstruction, hepatic abscess, and mesenteric vein thrombosis. Differential diagnosis of right lower quadrant inflammatory change, without visualization of an abnormal appendix or appendicolith, includes Crohn's disease, cecal diverticulitis, perforated cecal

carcinoma, mesenteric adenitis, and pelvic inflammatory disease.

Mucocele of the Appendix

Mucocele refers to a distended appendix filled with mucus. Most cases are due to benign proximal obstruction, although some are due to mucus-secreting cystadenoma or cystadenocarcinoma. On CT, a mucocele appears as a well-encapsulated, cystic mass with thin walls that may be calcified (Fig. 16–19). Size is variable up to 15 cm. *Pseudomyxoma peritonei* results from implants of mucinous epithelium on peritoneal surfaces causing low-density mucinous ascites. Gelatinous implants may be seen throughout the abdomen cavity fixating bowel loops and causing mass effect.

COLON AND RECTUM

Anatomy

The colon is easily identified by its location and its haustral markings when it is distended by air or contrast agent. Mottled fecal material also serves as a marker of the colon and rectum. The scout view of the abdominal CT should be inspected to determine the general outline and course of the colon. The cecum generally occupies the iliac fossa, although, because of its variably long mesentery, it may be found almost anywhere in the abdomen. Its identity is confirmed by recognizing the ileocecal valve or appendix. The ascending colon occupies a posterior and lateral position in the right flank. The hepatic flexure makes one or more sharp bends near the undersurface of the liver and gallbladder. The transverse colon sweeps across the abdomen on a long and mobile mesentery. Because of its anterior position the transverse colon is usually filled with air when patients are supine on the CT couch. The splenic flexure makes one or more tight bends near the spleen. The descending colon extends caudad down the left flank. Remember that the ascending and descending portions of the colon are retroperitoneal. The peritoneum sweeps over their anterior surfaces and extends lat-

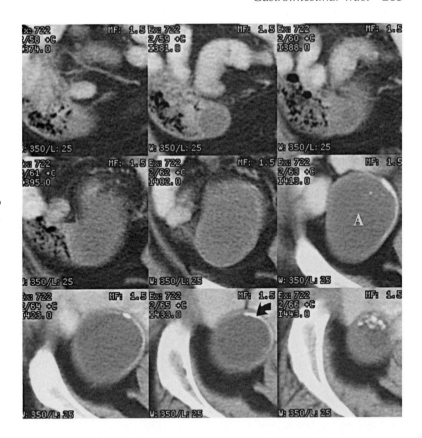

Figure 16–19. Mucocele of the appendix. Serial CT scans demonstrate a greatly dilated and fluid-filled appendix (A) with calcification *(arrow)* in its wall.

erally to form the paracolic gutters that distend with fluid when ascites is present. The sigmoid colon begins in the left iliac fossa and extends a variable distance craniad before it dives toward the rectum. The sigmoid becomes the rectum at the level of the third sacral segment. The rectum distends to form the rectal ampulla and then abruptly narrows to form the anal canal. Fat around the colon is normally uniformly of low density. Soft tissue stranding densities in the pericolic fat are indicative of inflammatory changes or neoplastic invasion.

The peritoneum covering the anterior surface of the rectum extends to the level of the vagina forming the rectovaginal pouch of Douglas. In males, the peritoneum extends to the seminal vesicles, 2.5 cm above the prostate, forming the rectovesical pouch. Three anatomic compartments are important to recognize when staging rectal carcinoma (see Fig. 17–1): (1) the peritoneal cavity above the peritoneal reflections, (2) the extraperitoneal compartment between the peritoneum and the levator ani muscle that forms the pelvic diaphragm, and (3)

the triangular ischiorectal fossa inferior and lateral to the levator ani. The lower two thirds of the rectum are extraperitoneal. On CT the thickness of the wall of the normal colon does not exceed 3 mm.

Technical Considerations

For routine scanning, the rectum and colon can usually be adequately opacified by giving contrast agents orally. However, when detailed examination of the colon is needed, air-contrast techniques are preferred. Preliminary bowel cleansing is carried out identical to preparation for a barium enema. Just before CT scanning, an enema tube is placed in the rectum after digital rectal examination. The colon is insufflated with approximately 20 puffs of air, or to the limit of patient comfort. Scanning is then carried out through the entire abdomen and pelvis. Demonstration of subtle findings is improved by narrow collimation (3–5 mm) through a defined area of abnormality. Intravenous contrast medium enhancement is optional but usually helpful. When divertic-

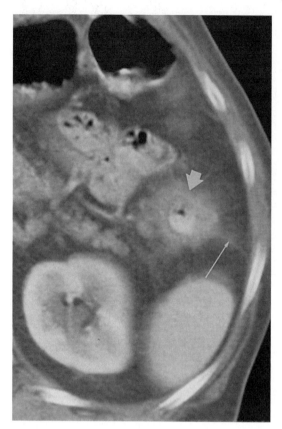

Figure 16–20. Colon carcinoma. A carcinoma of the descending colon causes thickening of the colon wall *(large arrow)* and narrowing of the lumen. Stranding densities *(long arrow)* extending into the pericolonic fat suggest tumor extension through the bowel wall.

ulitis is suspected, colon opacification is obtained entirely by oral contrast agent administration beginning 12 hours before scanning.

Colorectal Carcinoma

Seventy percent of colon cancers occur in the rectosigmoid region. The remainder are scattered fairly evenly throughout the rest of the colon. Colon cancer spreads by (1) direct extension with penetration of the colon wall, (2) lymphatic drainage to regional nodes, (3) hematogenous routes through portal veins to the liver, and (4) intraperitoneal seeding. Whereas barium enema and colonoscopy are the primary modalities for the diagnosis of colon cancer, CT has become routine for the preoperative staging. However, the accuracy of CT staging ranges from

17% from early lesions (Dukes stage B) to 81% for advanced lesions (Dukes stage D). Inaccuracies arise from nonspecific CT signs of tumor spread through the bowel wall and a high incidence of tumor-involved lymph nodes being smaller than 15 mm. CT signs of colon carcinoma (Figs. 16–20 and 16–21) include

1. Focal, lobulated, thickening of the bowel wall (>3 mm)
2. Irregular, occasionally ulcerated, luminal surface
3. Polypoid soft tissue mass in lumen
4. "Apple core" lesion with circumferential wall thickening and narrowing of the bowel lumen
5. Linear soft tissue densities extending from the colonic mass into pericolic fat suggesting, but not being diagnostic of, extension of tumor through the bowel wall
6. Regional adenopathy
7. Metastases in the liver (75%), lung (5%–50%), adrenal gland (14%), or elsewhere

The tumor is desmoplastic and commonly causes narrowing of the lumen and bowel obstruction. Additional complications in-

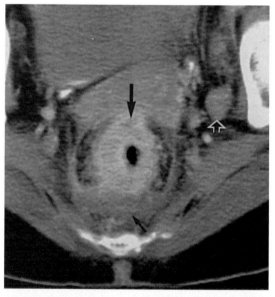

Figure 16–21. Rectal carcinoma. The rectal wall *(long arrow)* is circumferentially thickened with ill-defined outer margin. The presacral area of low density *(short arrow)* suggests focal perforation. An enlarged internal iliac lymph node *(open arrow)* is evident.

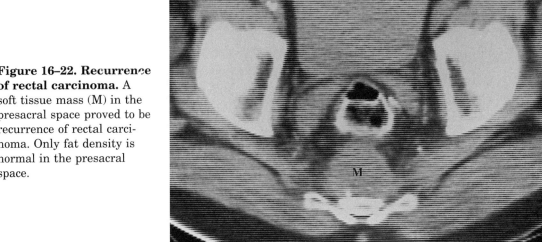

Figure 16–22. Recurrence of rectal carcinoma. A soft tissue mass (M) in the presacral space proved to be recurrence of rectal carcinoma. Only fat density is normal in the presacral space.

clude perforation and intussusception. Calcifications in the primary tumor and metastases occur with mucinous adenocarcinoma.

Recurrence. CT is more valuable in the detection of colorectal cancer recurrence than it is for initial staging. One third of patients who have undergone a colorectal cancer resection will develop recurrent disease, most (70%–80%) within 2 years. About half of the colon cancer recurrences occur at the site of the original tumor (Fig. 16–22), whereas the remainder recur at distant sites, especially in the liver. CT scans should survey the entire abdomen and pelvis to detect recurrence of colorectal cancer. The anastomotic site should be demonstrated by full air insufflation, repositioning the patient if necessary, and thin section (5-mm) scans. Because postoperative scarring and fibrosis may simulate recurrent tumor, a baseline CT scan should be obtained at 3 months after surgery with follow-up scans every 6 months for 3 years. Recurrences appear as irregular masses, often with a low-density necrotic center and an enhancing periphery. Presacral soft tissue densities, seen in patients with abdominoperineal resection (see Fig. 16–22), may be recurrent tumor or fibrosis. Percutaneous biopsy is generally required for confirmation.

Colon Lymphoma

Colon lymphoma is less common than gastric or small bowel lymphoma but has a striking and fairly characteristic CT appearance:

1. Marked thickening of the bowel wall, often exceeding 4 cm
2. Homogeneous soft tissue mass without calcification or necrosis
3. Minimal to no enhancement of the mass with intravenous contrast medium
4. Regional and diffuse adenopathy, often massive

Lymphoma characteristically causes much larger soft tissue masses than does carcinoma. The absence of desmoplastic reaction is typical; and the colon lumen is commonly dilated or normal, rather than constricted, at the site of tumor involvement. Bowel obstruction is uncommon. Patients with the acquired immunodeficiency syndrome have a much higher incidence of colon involvement with lymphoma than the general population.

Lipoma

CT can be used to make a specific and noninvasive diagnosis of gastrointestinal lipoma by demonstrating homogeneous fat density (−80 to −120 H) within a sharply defined tumor. Most lipomas are 2 to 3 cm, are round or ovoid, and are clinically silent. Some may bleed or be a cause of intussusception. Lipomas occur most commonly in the colon (65%–75%) and small bowel (20%–

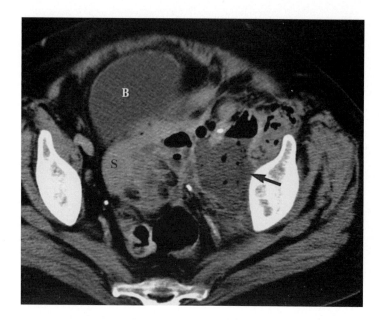

Figure 16–23. Diverticulitis and abscess. Diverticulitis of the sigmoid colon (S) has caused a large pelvic abscess *(arrow)* containing air and fluid. CT is excellent for demonstrating the nature and extent of extraluminal disease. B = bladder.

25%) and uncommonly in the stomach (5%), esophagus, and pharynx.

Diverticulitis

Because most diverticula occur along the mesenteric surface of the colon, perforation due to diverticulitis is confined initially to between the leaves of the mesocolon. The inflammatory mass that forms is both extraluminal and extraperitoneal. CT is better suited to documentation of this extraluminal disease than is barium enema. Colon opacification with a contrast agent can be achieved by oral administration without the potential trauma of an enema. Diverticula are easily visualized on CT as small, rounded collections of air, feces, or contrast material outside the lumen. Thickening of the muscular wall of the colon is common. Diverticulitis causes the following signs (Fig. 16–23):

1. Focal symmetric, usually circumferential, thickening of the bowel wall (>3 mm)
2. Pericolic inflammatory soft tissue mass, often containing fluid, air, contrast agent, or fecal material
3. Linear stranding densities in pericolic fat representing inflammatory changes

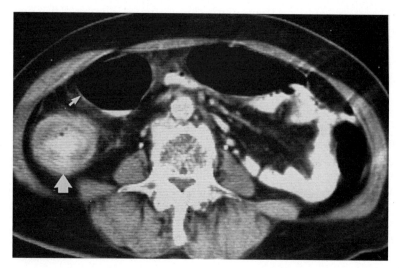

Figure 16–24. Ischemic colitis. The wall of the ascending colon *(large arrow)* is circumferentially thickened owing to bowel ischemia. Compare this area with the normal thickness of the wall of unaffected portions of the transverse colon *(small arrow)*.

4. Sinus tracts and fistulas to adjacent organs or skin, represented by linear fluid or air collections

Abscess formation may be extensive. Obstruction of the colon or urinary tract may result from the inflammatory process. A large soft tissue mass component of the inflammatory process should suggest the possibility of a colon cancer with perforation, rather than diverticulitis.

Thickening of the Colon Wall

Just as in the other portions of the gastrointestinal tract, thickening of the colon wall is nonspecific and may result from a variety of insults. The colon wall is abnormally thickened (Fig. 16–24) when it exceeds 3 mm with the lumen distended. Differential considerations include inflammatory colitis, necrotizing colitis, ischemia and bowel infarction, radiation, and tumor, including carcinoma and lymphoma. Correlation with clinical history and other findings is needed to differentiate these conditions. Gas in the bowel wall, or within the mesenteric or portal vasculature, indicates bowel necrosis.

Suggested Reading

Balthazar EJ. CT of the gastrointestinal tract: principles and interpretation. AJR 1991; 156:23–32.

Balthazar EJ. CT of small bowel obstruction. AJR 1994; 162:255–261.

Buck JL, Sobin LH. Carcinoids of the gastrointestinal tract. Radiographics 1990; 10:1081–1095.

Buetow PC, Buck JL, Carr NJ, Pantongrag-Brown L. Colorectal adenocarcinoma: radiologic-pathologic correlation. Radiographics 1995; 15:127–146.

Curtin KR, Fitzgerald SW, Nemcek AA Jr, et al. CT diagnosis of acute appendicitis: imaging findings. AJR 1995; 164:905–909.

Desai RK, Tagliabue JR, Wegryn SA, Einstein DM. CT evaluation of wall thickening in the alimentary tract. Radiographics 1991; 11:771–783.

Dudiak KM, Johnson CD, Stephens DH. Primary tumors of the small intestine: CT evaluation. AJR 1989; 152:995–998.

Gore RM, Ghahremani GG. Diagnostic imaging of diverticulitis. Radiologist 1994; 1:155–164.

Hori S, Tsuda K, Murayama S, et al. CT of gastric carcinoma: preliminary results with a new scanning technique. Radiographics 1992; 12:257–268.

Jabra AA, Fishman EK, Taylor GA. CT findings in inflammatory bowel disease in children. AJR 1994; 162:975–979.

Madwed D, Mindelzun R, Jeffrey RB Jr. Mucocele of the appendix: imaging findings. AJR 1992; 159:69–72.

McDaniel KP, Charnasangavej C, DuBrow RA, et al. Pathways of nodal metastasis in carcinomas of the cecum, ascending colon, and transverse colon: CT demonstration. AJR 1993; 161:61–64.

Noh HM, Fishman EK, Forastiere AA, et al. CT of the esophagus: spectrum of disease with emphasis on esophageal carcinoma. Radiographics 1995; 15:1113–1134.

Rubesin SE, Gilchrist AM, Bronner M, et al. Non-Hodgkin lymphoma of the small intestine. Radiographics 1990; 10:985–998.

Siewert B, Raptopoulos V. CT of the acute abdomen: findings and impact on diagnosis and treatment. AJR 1994; 163:1317–1324.

Smith C, Kubicka RA, Thomas CR Jr. Non-Hodgkin lymphoma of the gastrointestinal tract. Radiographics 1992; 12:887–899.

Taylor AJ, Stewart ET, Dodds WJ. Gastrointestinal lipomas: a radiologic and pathologic review. AJR 1990; 155:1205–1210.

Thoeni RF. Colorectal cancer: cross-sectional imaging for staging of primary tumor and detection of local recurrence. AJR 1991; 156:909–915.

Wong CH, Trinh TM, Robbins AN, et al. Diagnosis of appendicitis: imaging findings in patients with atypical clinical features. AJR 1993; 161:1199–1203.

17

Pelvis

William E. Brant, M.D.

ANATOMY

The true (lesser) pelvis is divided from the false (greater) pelvis by an oblique plane extending across the pelvic brim from the sacral promontory to the symphysis pubis. The true pelvis contains the rectum, bladder, pelvic ureters, and prostate and seminal vesicles in the male, or vagina, uterus, and ovaries in the female. The false pelvis is open anteriorly and is bounded laterally by the iliac fossae. It contains small bowel loops and portions of the ascending, descending, and sigmoid colon.

Muscle groups form prominent anatomic landmarks on CT. The psoas muscles extend from the lumbar vertebra through the greater pelvis to join with the iliacus muscles arising from the iliac fossa. The iliopsoas muscles exit the pelvis anteriorly to insert on the lesser trochanters of the femurs. The obturator internus muscles line the interior surface of the lateral walls of the true pelvis (Fig. 17–1). Involvement of these muscles by pelvic tumors precludes surgical resection of the tumor. The piriformis muscles arise from the anterior sacrum and exit the pelvis through the greater sciatic foramen to insert on the greater trochanter of the femur (see Fig. 17–6). The piriformis forms a portion of the lateral wall of the true pelvis. The pelvic diaphragm, composed of the levator ani anteriorly and the coccygeus posteriorly, stretches across the pelvis to separate the pelvic cavity from

the perineum (Fig. 17–1). The pelvic diaphragm is penetrated by the rectum, urethra, and vagina.

The pelvis is divided into three major anatomic compartments (Fig. 17–2; see also Fig. 17–1). The *peritoneal cavity* extends to the level of the vagina forming the pouch of Douglas in females or to the level of the seminal vesicles forming the rectovesical pouch in males. The *extraperitoneal space* of the pelvis is continuous with the retroperitoneal space of the abdomen. Pathologic processes from the pelvis may spread preferentially into the retroperitoneal compartments of the abdomen. The retropubic space (of Retzius) is continuous with the posterior pararenal space and the extraperitoneal fat of the abdominal wall. Fascial planes also allow communication with the scrotum and labia. The presacral space between sacrum and rectum normally contains only fat. Any soft tissue density in this space is abnormal and must be explained. The *perineum* lies below the pelvic diaphragm. On CT the most obvious portion of the perineum is the ischiorectal fossa. This fossa is seen as a triangular area of fat density extending between the obturator internus laterally, the gluteus maximus posteriorly, and the anus and urogenital region medially.

The arteries and veins define the location of the major lymphatic node chains in the pelvis. The aorta and vena cava divide to form the common iliac vessels at the level of the top of the iliac crest. The common iliac vessels divide at the pelvic brim, marked on

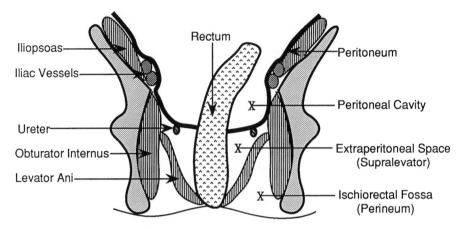

Figure 17–1. Anatomic compartments of the pelvis. Diagram of a posterior coronal section at the level of the rectum demonstrates the major anatomic compartments of the pelvis.

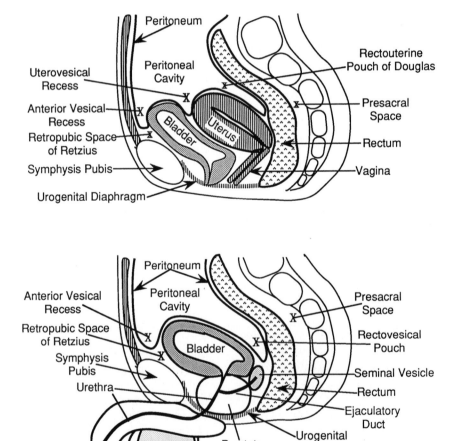

Figure 17–2. Anatomic compartments of the pelvis. Diagrams of midline sagittal planes through a female *(A)* and a male *(B)* pelvis demonstrate the pelvic compartments and peritoneal recesses and their relationships to pelvic organs.

CT by the transition between the convex sacral promontory and the concave sacral cavity. The internal iliac (hypogastric) vessels course posteriorly across the sciatic foramen dividing rapidly into smaller branches. The external iliac vessels course anteriorly adjacent to the iliopsoas to exit the pelvis at the inguinal ligament. Pelvic lymph nodes are classified with their accompanying vessels and are correspondingly named the common iliac, internal iliac, and external iliac nodal chains (Fig. 17–3). The obturator nodes are satellites of the external iliac chain and course along the midportion of the obturator internus. Inguinal nodes in the subcutaneous tissue near the common femoral vessels drain the perineum but not the true pelvis. Pelvic lymph nodes are considered pathologically enlarged when they exceed 10 mm in short axis.

The bladder is best appreciated on CT when filled with urine or contrast agent. The normal bladder wall does not exceed 5 mm in thickness when the bladder is distended. The dome of the bladder is covered by peritoneum, whereas its base and anterior surface are extraperitoneal (see Fig. 17–2). The ureters course anterior to the psoas, cross over the common iliac vessels at the pelvic brim, pass on either side of the cervix, and insert into the bladder trigone. In males, the ureters insert into the bladder just above the prostate.

The vagina is seen in cross section as a flattened ellipse of soft tissue between the bladder and rectum. An inserted tampon will outline the cavity of the vagina with air density and is useful in marking the vagina for pelvic CT. The level of the cervix is recognized by the transition from the elliptical shape of the vagina to the rounded shape of the cervix. Contrast medium–containing ureters are frequently identified in close proximity to the cervix. The uterus is seen as a homogeneous, smooth outlined, oval of soft tissue density. The myometrium is highly vascular, causing the uterus to enhance more than most pelvic organs. Assessment of the uterus is difficult on CT because of variation in position and flexion of the uterus and the amount of bladder filling. The broad ligament is a sheetlike fold of peritoneum that drapes over the uterus and extends laterally to the pelvic side walls. Between the leaves of the broad ligament is the *parametrium,* which is loose connective tissue and fat through which pass the fallopian tubes, uterine and ovarian blood vessels and lymphatics, the pelvic ureters, and the round ligament. Determination of tumor extension into the parametrium is an important part of gynecologic tumor staging. The fallopian tube forms the superior free edge of the broad ligament, best seen when outlined by ascites. The cardinal ligaments extend laterally from the cervix to the obturator internus muscles, forming the base of the broad ligament. The cardinal ligaments appear on CT as triangular densities extending laterally from the cervix. The round ligaments extend from the uterine fundus through the internal inguinal ring to terminate in the labia majora. Uterosacral ligaments extend in an arc from

Figure 17–3. Pelvic lymph node chains. Diagram of the aortic bifurcation and the iliac arteries illustrates the classification and naming of pelvic lymph nodes.

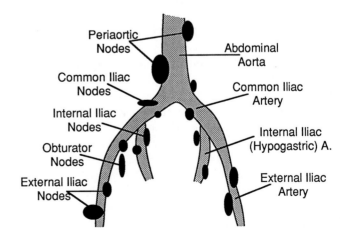

the cervix to the anterior sacrum. Uterine arteries branch from the hypogastric trunk and course in the parametrium just superior to the cardinal ligaments. Enhanced parametrial blood vessels are commonly prominent on bolus-enhanced CT scans. Normal ovaries are sometimes difficult to identify on CT. Because they are mobile, they may be anywhere in the pelvis, but they are most commonly seen adjacent to the uterine fundus. They appear as oval soft tissue densities, approximately 2 × 3 × 4 cm. The presence of cystic follicles allows positive identification of the ovaries.

The normal prostate gland is seen at the base of the bladder as a homogeneous, rounded, soft tissue organ up to 4 cm in maximal diameter. Prostate zonal anatomy is not demonstrated by CT. A well-defined plane of fat separates the prostate from the obturator internus. This fat plane may be invaded by carcinoma. Denonvilliers' fascia provides a particularly tough barrier between the prostate and rectum, usually preventing spread of disease from one organ to the other. The paired seminal vesicles produce a characteristic "bow tie"–shaped soft tissue structure in the groove between the bladder base and the prostate (see Figs. 17–2*B* and 17–5). Normal testes are easily identified in the scrotum as homogeneous oval structures 3 to 4 cm in diameter. The spermatic cord can be recognized in the inguinal canal as a thin-walled oval structure of fat density containing small dots representing the vas deferens and spermatic vessels.

TECHNICAL CONSIDERATIONS

The ideal technique for CT imaging of the pelvis requires optimal bowel opacification. We give 500 mL of dilute contrast agent orally the evening preceding the examination and repeat the dose 45 to 60 minutes before the examination. We routinely distend the colon and rectum by placing a tube in the rectum and insufflating the area with 20 puffs of air, or to the limit of patient comfort. Women are asked to place a tampon in the vagina. All patients are asked to

avoid urination for 30 to 40 minutes before the examination to allow bladder filling. Intravenous contrast medium is routinely given by mechanical injector at 2 to 3 mL/sec for a total dose of 150 mL of 60% contrast agent. Scanning through the pelvis is performed with contiguous 7- to 10-mm thick slices obtained by helical or conventional CT. We routinely scan the abdomen as well in patients with known or suspected pelvic malignancy. To optimize contrast medium enhancement of pelvic organs we often scan the pelvis first, then the abdomen.

BLADDER

Bladder Carcinoma

Bladder cancer may be superficial and confined to the mucosa. However, with invasion of the bladder wall musculature, risk of spread to regional and distant nodes increases. As the number and size of nodal metastases increases, so does the risk of hematogenous spread to bone and lung. CT is useful for the staging of advanced disease but is not accurate in defining early-stage disease (Table 17–1). Most malignant bladder tumors are transitional cell carcinomas that carry a risk of multiple synchronous tumors in the ipsilateral ureter and renal collecting system. CT findings (Figs. 17–4 and 17–5) are as follows:

1. The primary tumor appears as a focal thickening of the bladder wall or as a soft tissue mass projecting into the bladder lumen. CT is poor at differentiating superficial tumors from those that have invaded into, or minimally through, the bladder wall.

TABLE 17–1. **Staging of Bladder Carcinoma**

Stage	Description
A (T1)	Tumor involves mucosa and submucosa
B1 (T2)	Tumor invades superficial muscle layer
B2 (T3a)	Tumor invades deep muscular wall
C (T3b)	Tumor invades perivesical fat
D (T4)	Tumor involves seminal vesicles, prostate, or rectum

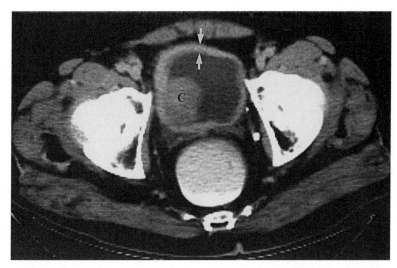

Figure 17–4. Bladder transitional cell carcinoma. A papillary transitional cell carcinoma (C) extends from the right lateral wall of the bladder. The tumor infiltrated the bladder wall but did not extend into the perivesical fat. Note the distinct fat plane separating the bladder from the pelvic sidewall. The bladder wall *(arrows)* is thickened owing to benign prostate hypertrophy.

2. Perivesical spread is seen as soft tissue density in the perivesical fat. Extension to the pelvic side wall precludes complete surgical resection.

3. Pelvic lymph nodes larger than 10 mm in short axis are considered positive for metastatic disease. Smaller nodes are unlikely to be involved.

Bladder Trauma

Rupture of the bladder occurs in 10% of patients with pelvic fractures. In most cases the bladder is lacerated by a spicule of fractured bone and urine (and contrast agent)

leaks into the extraperitoneal space. Intraperitoneal rupture of the bladder occurs as a result of a blow to the lower abdomen when the bladder is distended. Urine and contrast medium leak into the peritoneal cavity. Either type of rupture is effectively demonstrated by CT after contrast medium administration either intravenously or by bladder catheter. However, the bladder must be distended to at least 250 mL to demonstrate small ruptures With intraperitoneal rupture, contrast medium is seen within the peritoneal cavity surrounding bowel loops and extending into the pericolic gutters. Most extraperitoneal ruptures (Fig.

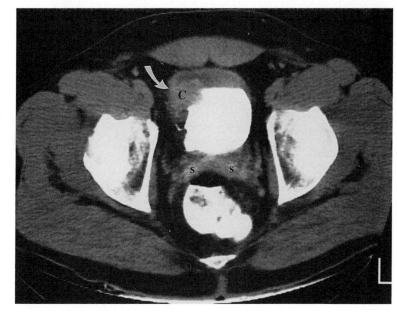

Figure 17–5. Bladder transitional cell carcinoma. CT scan of a 45-year-old man with gross hematuria demonstrates a transitional cell carcinoma (C) that extends *(arrow)* through the bladder wall into the perivesical fat. s = seminal vesicles.

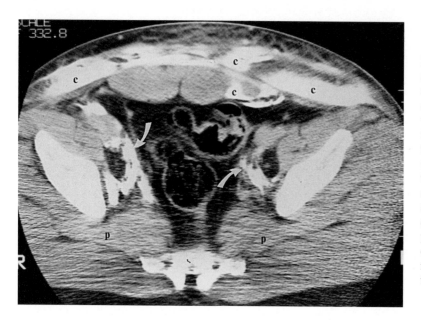

Figure 17–6. Extraperitoneal bladder rupture. CT slice at the level of the sciatic foramina in a patient with multiple pelvic fractures demonstrates the extraperitoneal dissection of contrast medium from a ruptured bladder. Contrast medium collections are seen along the iliac vessels *(arrows)* and in the fascial planes of the anterior abdominal wall (c). p = piriformis muscle coursing through the sciatic foramen.

17–6) leak into the retropubic space and may extend along fascial planes to the abdominal wall, to the retroperitoneal compartments of the abdomen, and into the scrotum and thigh.

UTERUS

Leiomyoma

Leiomyomas (fibroids) are found in up to 40% of women older than age 30. As fre-

quent incidental findings, their CT features should be recognized. Leiomyomas appear as homogeneous or heterogeneous masses that may be hypodense, isodense, or hyperdense relative to enhanced myometrium (Fig. 17–7). Coarse calcifications within the mass are common and characteristic. Cystic degeneration produces interior low density. Diffuse enlargement of the uterus and lobulation of its contour are common. Pedunculated leiomyomas may appear as adnexal rather than uterine masses. Leiomyomas

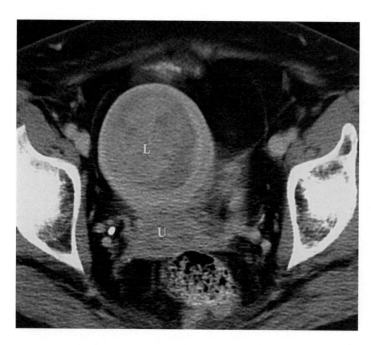

Figure 17–7. Leiomyoma. A large leiomyoma (L) extends anteriorly from the uterus (U).

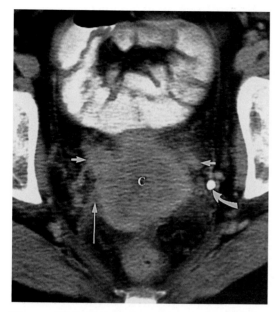

Figure 17–8. Cervical carcinoma. A cervical carcinoma, stage IIIb, replaces the cervix (C) and extends as nodular and stranding soft tissue densities *(short arrows)* into the paracervical fat, enveloping and obstructing the right ureter *(long arrow)*. The left ureter *(curved arrow)* remains uninvolved.

TABLE 17–2. **Staging of Cervical Carcinoma (FIGO)**

Stage	Description
0	Carcinoma in situ
I	Tumor confined to cervix
II	Tumor extends beyond cervix but not to pelvic sidewall or lower third of vagina
IIa	Invades vagina excluding lower third
IIb	Invades parametrium
III	Tumor extends to pelvic side wall or lower third of vagina and/or causes hydronephrosis
IIIa	Invades lower third of vagina
IIIb	Invades parametrium to pelvic side wall, and/or causes hydronephrosis
IVa	Tumor involves bladder or rectal mucosa
IVb	Tumor spreads to distant organs

apy, and to detect recurrence, MRI is preferable in most instances. Most cervical malignancies are squamous cell carcinomas that spread primarily by direct extension to adjacent organs and tissues. Lymphatic spread to regional nodes is common. Hematogenous spread to lung, bone, and brain is uncommon and occurs late in the course of disease. The accuracy of CT staging is in the range of 58% to 88% compared with 70% to 100% reported for MRI (Table 17–2). CT findings (Figs. 17–8 and 17–9) are

1. The primary tumor may enlarge the cervix (> 3 cm diameter) or be seen as a

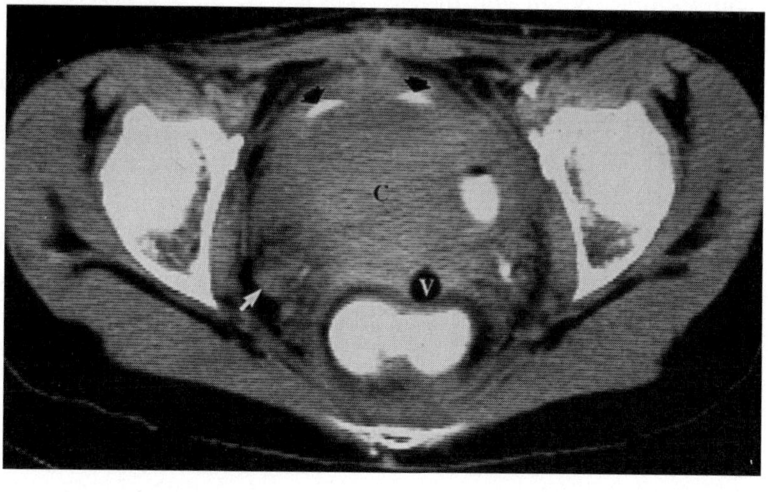

cannot be accurately differentiated from rare leiomyosarcomas by CT appearance alone. Rapid growth of a uterine mass in a postmenopausal woman suggests malignancy.

Carcinoma of the Cervix

Although CT has been used to stage cervical carcinoma, to document response to ther-

Figure 17–9. Cervical carcinoma. CT scan at the level of the cervix demonstrates a large cervical carcinoma (C) that has spread into the parametrium and upper vagina. The vagina is marked by a tampon (V). Enlarged internal iliac nodes containing metastatic tumor are also evident *(white arrow)*. The bladder *(black arrows)* is compressed and distorted by tumor.

hypodense mass within the normally homogeneous cervix. Fluid collections in the endometrial cavity are common due to tumor obstruction of the cervix.

2. Direct extension is seen as thick irregular tissue strands or masses fanning out from the cervix into the parametrium often encasing the ureters, into the vagina, or to the pelvic side walls (obturator internus). Normal broad, round, cardinal, and uterosacral ligaments should not be mistaken for tumor extension.

3. Enlarged lymph nodes (> 10 mm in short axis) are strong evidence of metastatic involvement, but cervical carcinoma will commonly involve nodes without enlarging them. These small but involved nodes cannot be differentiated from benign nodes by CT.

4. Recurrences appear as soft tissue masses anywhere in the pelvis but most commonly at the top of the vaginal vault in patients who have undergone hysterectomy. Enlarged nodes are also suggestive of recurrence. Percutaneous biopsy is usually needed to confirm the diagnosis.

Endometrial Carcinoma

Adenocarcinoma of the endometrium is the most common invasive gynecologic malignancy. CT evaluation is useful as an adjunct to clinical staging, especially in patients with advanced disease or who are difficult to examine. The tumor spreads first by invasion of the myometrium, then by lymphatic channels to regional nodes, or by direct extension through the uterine wall to parametrial tissues. When the uterine serosa is penetrated, diffuse peritoneal spread may occur. Hematogenous spread to lung, bone, liver, and brain is much more common with endometrial than cervical cancer. Because the tumor is isodense with uterine tissue on unenhanced CT, all studies should be performed with intravenous contrast medium enhancement. CT staging is reported to be 84% to 88% accurate compared with 83% to 92% accuracy for MRI (Table 17–3). CT features (Fig. 17–10) include

1. The primary tumor appears as a hypodense mass within the endometrial cavity or invading the myometrium. The uterine

TABLE 17–3. Staging of Endometrial Carcinoma (FIGO)

Stage	Description
0	Carcinoma in situ
I	Tumor confined to uterine corpus
II	Tumor invades cervix but does not extend beyond uterus
III	Tumor extends beyond uterus but not outside true pelvis
IVa	Tumor involves bladder or rectal mucosa and/or extends beyond true pelvis
IVb	Distant metastases

cavity is frequently fluid filled owing to tumor obstruction. The uterus may be greatly enlarged.

2. Parametrial invasion and sidewall extension has the same appearance as cervical carcinoma.

3. Enlarged pelvic lymph nodes indicate tumor involvement. However, as with other

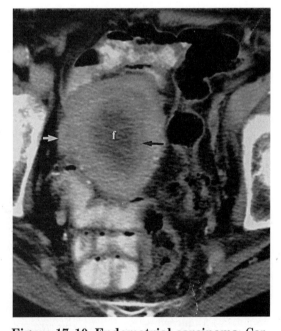

Figure 17–10. Endometrial carcinoma. Carcinoma arising from the endometrium causes a low-density rim of tumor *(black arrow)* surrounding low-density bloody fluid (f) within the endometrial cavity. Asymmetric thickening of the uterine wall *(white arrow)* is due to a small leiomyoma.

pelvic tumors, CT will miss microscopic nodal metastases that do not enlarge the nodes.

4. Tumor recurrences appear as pelvic soft tissue masses or nodal enlargement. Most recurrences happen within 2 years.

OVARY

Ovarian Cancer

Ovarian malignancy encompasses a wide range of histologic tumor types, but most share a common pattern of spread and similar range of CT appearances. Two thirds of ovarian cancers are cystic, 25% are bilateral, and 85% are endocrinologically nonfunctional. The primary route of tumor spread is diffusion throughout the peritoneal cavity. Direct extension to pelvic organs, lymphatic spread to nodes, and hematogenous spread to lung, liver, and bone also occur. Most patients will go directly to surgery for initial staging, hysterectomy, salpingo-oophorectomy, omentectomy, and tumor debulking without preoperative imaging. CT is, however, the imaging method of choice for documenting residual tumor response to therapy, and for detection of postoperative recurrence. MRI remains inferior to CT, primarily because of difficulty in differentiating intraperitoneal tumor from bowel. Staging accuracy of CT is 70% to 90% (Table 17–4). Important CT findings (Fig. 17–11) include

1. The primary tumor is usually cystic with thick irregular walls, internal septations, and prominent soft tissue components. Uniformly solid tumors and mixed cystic/solid tumors also occur. Calcifications may be evident in both the primary tumor and metastases.
2. Direct tumor extension commonly involves the uterus, colon, small bowel, and bladder.
3. Peritoneal implants are seen as soft tissue nodules on peritoneal surfaces or as "omental cake" separating bowel from the anterior abdominal wall (see Fig. 9–3). CT will commonly miss even extensive peritoneal seeding when the tumor nodules are small (<15 mm).

4. The presence of ascites usually indicates peritoneal spread even if peritoneal tumor nodules are not visualized.

5. Lymphatic metastases usually follow

TABLE 17–4. Staging of Ovarian Carcinoma (FIGO)

Stage	Description
I	Tumor limited to ovaries
Ia	Limited to one ovary
Ib	Limited to both ovaries
Ic	With malignant ascites
II	Tumor involves one or both ovaries with pelvic extension
IIa	Involves uterus/fallopian tubes
IIb	Extends to other pelvic tissues
IIc	With malignant ascites
III	Tumor involves one or both ovaries with peritoneal extension outside of the pelvis, and/or regional lymph node metastases
IV	Distant metastases

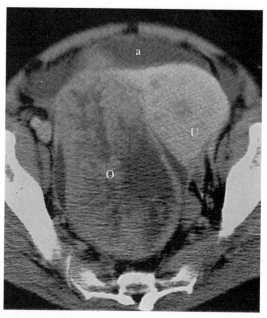

Figure 17–11. Ovarian carcinoma. A large mass (O) with prominent solid components arises from the right ovary and displaces the uterus (U) anteriorly and leftward. Ascites (a) is present, suggesting intraperitoneal spread of tumor.

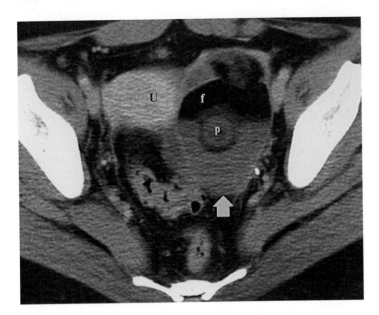

Figure 17–12. Benign cystic teratoma. A large cystic mass *(arrow)* arises from the left ovary and displaces the uterus (U) rightward. Layering fluid (f) is identical in CT density to intraabdominal and subcutaneous fat, confirming the diagnosis of benign cystic teratoma. A dermoid plug (p) is seen within the mass.

gonadal lymphatics, skipping pelvic nodes, to involve nodes at the renal hilum.

Benign Adnexal Masses

Although ultrasonography is the primary imaging modality for female pelvic masses, adnexal masses may be discovered incidentally on CT. CT may also be used to further characterize difficult examinations. A few conditions to consider are

1. *Functional ovarian cyst.* Benign ovarian cysts, including follicular and corpus luteum cysts, are common incidental findings. On CT they are well defined, are thin walled, and have homogeneous internal density near water. Atypical cysts can be followed with ultrasound to determine if they resolve after one or two menstrual cycles.

2. *Benign cystic teratoma.* The presence of fat-density fluid, teeth, bone formation, hair, or fat-fluid levels allows definitive CT diagnosis in most cases (Fig. 17–12). Dermoid plugs are conglomerations of tissue and hair seen as soft tissue nodules inside the cysts.

3. *Ovarian cystadenoma.* Benign ovarian tumors tend to have regular thin walls, fine septations, no solid components, and no associated ascites. Definitive differentiation of benign from malignant cystic ovarian tumors is not possible with CT.

4. *Endometriosis/tubo-ovarian abscess.* These two conditions have an identical CT appearance. Both cause complex cystic pelvic masses, frequently with high-density fluid components. Inflammation and fibrosis are prominent. Multiple pelvic organs may be incorporated into the mass. Differentiation from malignancy is usually not possible by imaging methods alone.

PROSTATE

Prostate Cancer

Prostate cancer is the second most common malignancy in males. Prostate carcinoma spreads by direct extension to periprostatic tissues and the seminal vesicles. Lymphatic spread is similar to bladder cancer with early involvement of internal iliac and obturator nodes and later involvement of paraaortic nodes. Hematogenous spread to the axial skeleton via vertebral veins is particularly characteristic. CT does not demonstrate intraprostatic architecture and is poor at demonstrating intraprostatic tumor. Benign prostatic hypertrophy cannot be differentiated from intraprostatic malignancy. CT is 65% to 75% accurate in demonstrating extraprostatic spread of tumor (Table 17–5). CT findings (Fig. 17–13) are

TABLE 17–5. **Staging of Prostate Carcinoma**

Stage	Description
A	Nonpalpable tumor
B	Palpable tumor confined to prostate
C	Tumor with capsular involvement
C1	Capsular invasion
C2	Capsular penetration
C3	Seminal vesicle involvement
D	Distant metastases
D1	Involvement of pelvic lymph nodes
D2	Metastases to bone/distant lymph nodes

1. Enlargement of the prostate is common and may be due to benign prostatic hypertrophy and/or tumor growth. Nodules or stranding densities in the periprostatic fat are signs of tumor extension outside the prostate gland.

2. Asymmetric size of the seminal vesicles and infiltration of fat between the bladder base, prostate, and seminal vesicles are signs of tumor involvement. Bladder involvement is very difficult to detect accurately. Rectal invasion is rare.

3. Nodes larger than 10 mm are usually involved with metastatic tumor.

Benign Prostatic Hypertrophy

Benign prostatic hypertrophy occurs in the periurethral transitional zone and results in nodular enlargement of the prostate with constriction of the urethra and obstruction to bladder emptying. CT findings include

1. The prostate is enlarged and commonly has a lobulated contour. Nodules may cause high- and low-density regions within the prostate with variable enhancement.

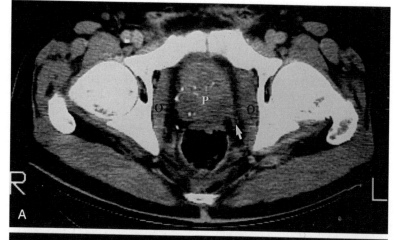

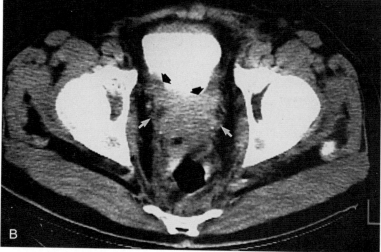

Figure 17–13. Prostate carcinoma. CT scans through the prostate gland *(A)* and through the bladder base *(B)* demonstrate signs of direct extension of prostate carcinoma into adjacent tissues. The prostate gland (P) is enlarged, is nodular, and has ill-defined margins. The tumor has invaded both seminal vesicles and the bladder base *(black arrows)*. Periprostatic stranding densities *(white arrows)* indicate invasion of adjacent fat. However the tumor does not extend into the obturator internus muscle (O). Calcifications in the prostate are associated with coexisting benign prostatic hypertrophy.

2. Cystic degeneration and course calcifications are common.

3. The bladder base is elevated and the prostate projects upward into the bladder lumen.

4. Bladder wall thickening and trabeculation result from bladder outlet obstruction. Diverticula may project through the bladder wall.

TESTES

Testicular Cancer

The long list of pathologic types of testicular germ cell tumors can be separated into seminomas and nonseminomas. Seminomas (40% to 50%) are treated with orchiectomy and radiation and generally do not require retroperitoneal node dissection. Nonseminomas are radioresistant, are treated with orchiectomy and chemotherapy, and generally do require retroperitoneal node dissection for staging. Lymphatic spread of tumor is most common, with nodal involvement following an orderly ascending pattern. Initial spread is along gonadal lymphatics following testicular veins to renal hilar nodes (Fig. 17–14). Alternatively, lymphatic metastases may follow the external iliac chain to the paraaortic nodes. Internal iliac and inguinal

TABLE 17–6. Staging of Testicular Carcinoma

Stage	Description
I	Limited to testis and spermatic cord
II	Metastases to lymph nodes below diaphragm
III	Metastases to lymph nodes above diaphragm
IIIa	Confined to lymphatic system
IIIb	Extranodal metastases

nodes are generally not involved. Lymphatic spread to the mediastinum and hematogenous spread to the lungs rarely occurs without paraaortic disease, except for choriocarcinoma, which spreads hematogenously early. CT is 73% to 97% accurate for initial tumor staging (Table 17–6) and for detection of recurrences:

1. Pelvic and retroperitoneal adenopathy is most pronounced on the side of involvement. Nodal enlargement near the ipsilateral renal hilum is particularly characteristic. Inguinal nodes are involved only when the scrotum is invaded by tumor. Bulky nodal mets may have low attenuation internally as a result of tumor necrosis.

2. Absence of the spermatic cord identifies the side of orchiectomy.

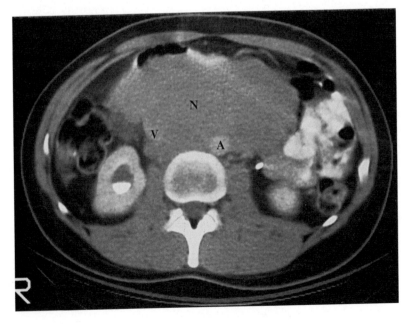

Figure 17–14. Metastatic testicular carcinoma. Teratocarcinoma of the testis metastatic to paraaortic nodes causes massive confluent adenopathy (N). The inferior vena cava (V) is anteriorly and laterally displaced by the adenopathy. The aorta (A) is surrounded by tumor. The right kidney is partially obstructed and demonstrates mild dilatation of the collecting system with a contrast medium–urine level.

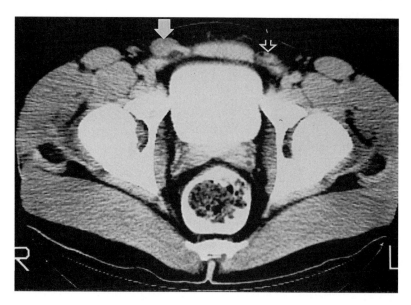

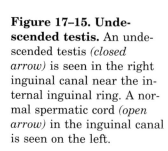

Figure 17–15. Undescended testis. An undescended testis *(closed arrow)* is seen in the right inguinal canal near the internal inguinal ring. A normal spermatic cord *(open arrow)* in the inguinal canal is seen on the left.

Undescended Testes

Undescended testes may be located anywhere along the course of testicular descent from the lower pole of the kidney to the superficial inguinal ring. Undescended testes are at high risk for development of malignancy (48× risk) and for torsion (10× risk). CT is reported 95% sensitive for detection of ectopic testes. The undescended testis appears as an oval soft tissue density up to 4 cm (Fig. 17–15). Undescended testes are usually atrophic. CT detection of intraabdominal testes requires optimal bowel opacification and intravenous contrast medium enhancement to opacify normal structures. Testes in the inguinal canal can be easily identified on CT as long as you know where to look. The inguinal canal runs an oblique, medially directed course through the flat muscles of the abdominal wall between the deep and superficial inguinal rings. The deep (internal) inguinal ring is located midway between the anterior-superior iliac spine and the symphysis pubis. The superficial (external) inguinal ring is located just above the pubic crest.

Suggested Reading

Casillas J, Joseph RC, Guerra JJ Jr. CT appearance of uterine leiomyomas. RadioGraphics 1990; 10:999–1007.

Dodd GD III, Budzik RF Jr. Lipomatous tumors of pelvis in women: spectrum of imaging findings. AJR 1990; 155:317–322.

Ellis JH, McCullough NB, Francis IR, et al. Transitional cell carcinoma of the bladder: patterns of recurrence after cystectomy as determined by CT. AJR 1991; 157:999–1002.

Forstner R, Hricak H, Occhipinti KA, et al. Ovarian cancer: staging with CT and MR imaging. Radiology 1995; 197:619–626.

Foshager MC, Walsh JW. CT anatomy of the female pelvis: a second look. RadioGraphics 1994; 14:51–66.

Kane NM, Francis IR, Ellis JH. The value of CT in the detection of bladder and posterior urethral injuries. AJR 1989; 153:1243–1246.

Karasick S, Lev-Toaff AS, Toaff ME. Imaging of uterine leiomyomas. AJR 1992; 158:799–805.

King BF, Williamson B Jr, Hattery RR, et al. Seminal vesicle imaging. RadioGraphics 1989; 9:653–676.

Lis LE, Cohen AJ. CT cystography in the evaluation of bladder trauma. J Comput Assist Tomogr 1990; 14:386–389.

Meyer JI, Kennedy AW, Friedman R, et al. Ovarian carcinoma: value of CT in predicting success of debulking surgery. AJR 1995; 165:875–878.

Nghiem HT, Kellman GM, Sandberg SA, Crain BM. Cystic lesions of the prostate. RadioGraphics 1990; 10:635–650.

Park JM, Charnsangavej C, Yoshimitsu K, et al. Pathways of nodal metastases from pelvic tumors: CT demonstration. RadioGraphics 1994; 14:1309–1321.

Richie JP. Detection and treatment of testicular cancer. CA Cancer J Clin 1993; 43:151–175.

Rozanski TA, Grossman HB. Recent developments in the pathophysiology of bladder cancer. AJR 1994; 163:789–792.

Sawyer RW, Walsh JW. CT in gynecologic pelvic diseases. Semin Ultrasound CT MR 1988; 9:122–142.

Steinfeld AD. Testicular germ cell tumors: review of contemporary evaluation and management. Radiology 1990; 175:603–606.

Sutton CL, McKinney CD, Jones JE, Gay SB. Ovarian masses revisited: radiologic and pathologic correlation. RadioGraphics 1992; 12:853–877.

Wilbur AC, Aizenstein RI, Napp TE. CT findings in tuboovarian abscess. AJR 1992; 158:575–579.

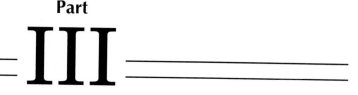

Part

III

The Musculoskeletal System

18

Musculoskeletal System

Clyde A. Helms, M.D.

The use of CT in the musculoskeletal system has been markedly affected by the introduction of MRI. Even though MRI has become the diagnostic modality of choice for many entities that were formerly imaged with CT, there continue to be areas where CT is superior and will remain appropriate. The advent of helical CT scanning has impacted the musculoskeletal applications, primarily in the setting of trauma and availability of rapid, thin sections for 3-D reconstructions. The future uses of CT in the musculoskeletal system will reflect not only the technologic advances of MRI but also the imagination of the radiologist. In this chapter the use of CT in the musculoskeletal system is examined, with the exception of diagnosis of lumbar spine disc disease and stenosis, which is presented in Chapter 19.

TRAUMA

CT has proven to be extremely important in trauma, both in the axial (central) and the appendicular (peripheral) skeleton. CT should be used in almost any instance of trauma in which plain films do not clearly depict the full extent of the bony pathologic process. Because of its ability to demonstrate cross-sectional anatomy and then display any additional plane with re-formations, CT has almost completely replaced conventional tomography in evaluating trauma to the skeleton.

Axial Skeleton (Spine)

All spinal trauma with neurologic deficits should be examined with CT to fully evaluate the amount of bony abnormality, regardless of what the plain films demonstrate. Obviously, the patient's condition will not always allow this; however, it should be considered in every case. If no neurologic deficits are present, plain films are usually sufficient. However, if the plain films are nondiagnostic or raise questions that cannot be answered by the clinical examination, CT should be performed.

It is not necessary to do a myelographic enhanced CT if MRI is available; however, it is usually recommended if no MRI can be obtained and the status of the cord is in question. In the lumbar spine CT myelography is rarely necessary.

Slice thickness varies depending on the anatomic location in the spine, the number of vertebral body levels to be examined, and the need for re-formations. In general, thin slices (1.5 mm) will allow for more acceptable re-formations but cannot be recommended over large areas of the spine owing to the enormous number of slices that would be taken unless spiral CT is available. Spiral CT enables rapid acquisition of multiple thin-section images over a large area.

Re-formations, including three-dimensional (3-D) re-formations, can be rapidly

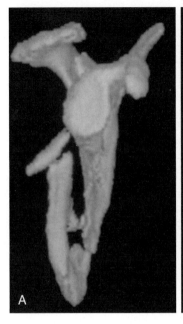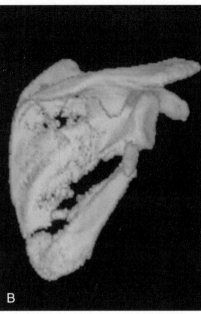

A

B

Figure 18–1. Three-dimensional (3-D) image of scapular fracture. *A* and *B,* Two views from a 3-D set in a patient with a scapular fracture show the fracture extending through the body of the scapula but not involving the articular portion of the labrum. Plain films and conventional CT showed the same diagnosis and extent of the fracture, but the clinician wanted the perspective of a 3-D image.

made with the currently available computer systems. In most instances of trauma, re-formations in at least one plane are recommended. Three-dimensional re-formations rarely aid in helping make the diagnosis, but many surgeons appreciate the overview and the different perspective that a 3-D image allows (Fig. 18–1). Two types of 3-D reformations exist: surface rendering and volume rendering. Surface rendering fails to show any detail deep to the surface of the bony structures and is believed by most to not produce as smooth or as true of a depiction as volume rendering. Different investigators seem to prefer one type of rendering over the other for a variety of reasons having much to do with personal preference as well as with which technique their computer software will allow. In general, volume rendering technique seems to be the more reliable method of 3-D re-formations.

When should 3-D re-formations be acquired? Because they do not increase diagnostic accuracy and they increase the cost, it is hard to justify them on a routine basis. If a clinician believes that 3-D re-formations help with his or her understanding of the diagnosis or treatment of an entity, then so be it.

A typical example of a cervical spine fracture that is more completely evaluated with CT is a Jefferson fracture, that is, a burst fracture of the C1 ring (Fig. 18–2). Any vertebral body fractures with bony fragments in the central canal should be examined with CT (Fig. 18–3).

It is not unusual to have an underlying

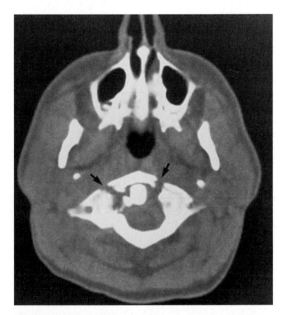

Figure 18–2. Jefferson fracture. An axial slice through the C1 vertebra in this patient with trauma shows several obvious fractures of the bony ring *(arrows)* that were not appreciated on the plain film. CT often reveals fractures not visible by conventional radiography and should be used in all spinal fracture cases.

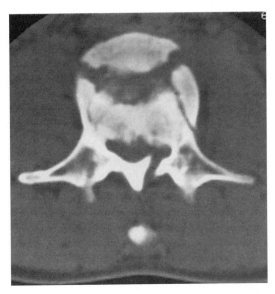

Figure 18–3. Vertebral body fracture. An axial cut through the L2 vertebral body in this victim of an automobile accident shows a stellate fracture of the body and, more importantly, shows a displaced fracture of the lamina with part of the lamina extending into the central canal.

bony abnormality that allows minor trauma to result in a fracture. An example of this is a pathologic fracture through a vertebral body with eosinophilic granuloma (Fig. 18–4). CT can demonstrate the extent of bony involvement as well as show the soft tissue mass. MRI would demonstrate these findings, but if life-support equipment or external stabilization is required, MRI might not be possible.

In the lumbar spine a common posttraumatic entity that is clearly shown with CT is spondylolysis. Although many claim it is necessary to use re-formations to identify the pars defects, they can be easily seen by examining the midvertebral body axial slice.

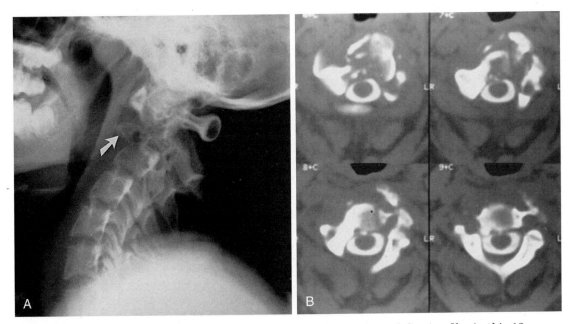

Figure 18–4. Eosinophilic granuloma with a fracture. *A,* A lateral C-spine film in this 12-year old with neck pain shows the C2 vertebral body to be disrupted with an apparent large fragment extending into the retropharyngeal space *(arrow). B,* An axial metrizamide CT slice through the C2 body shows a comminuted fracture of the body with some impression on the cord. This was secondary to eosinophilic granuloma.

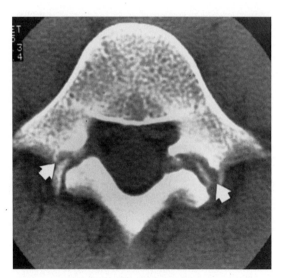

Figure 18–5. Spondylolysis. This axial CT slice through the center of the L5 vertebra reveals linear breaks in the lamina *(arrows)* bilaterally that can be mistaken for normal facets. On the mid-body cut, such as this, the lamina should be an unbroken bony ring. The facets are visible adjacent to the pars break on this image, a finding called the double facet sign.

This can be found by using the lateral "scout" view or by finding the basivertebral plexus, which is always in the posterior aspect of the midvertebral body. On this slice the lamina should be a continuous bony ring—any defect is a pars break (spondylolysis) (Fig. 18–5). Occasionally, the pars defect is very smooth and bilaterally symmetric so that it resembles normal facet joints and is overlooked. For this reason, any break in the bony ring that occurs on the slice that has the basivertebral plexus is a spondylolysis until proven otherwise.

A very uncommon but serious sequela of spondylolysis is a fibrocartilaginous buildup that can occur at the pars defect or fracture site to such a degree that it encroaches on the thecal sac or nerve roots (Fig. 18–6). If not recognized, a surgical fusion across that level would result in missing what could be the main cause of the patient's complaints. This fibrocartilaginous mass has been likened to excess callus across a fracture in a long bone that occurs if it is not immobilized. Whatever the cause, it is rare but should be searched for in every instance of spondylolysis that is studied with CT.

A fracture that can be mistaken for metastatic disease is a stress or insufficiency fracture of the sacrum. This is found primarily in two types of patients—patients with osteoporosis and patients with prior radiation. They present with low back or sacral pain and have patchy sclerosis of one or both sacral alae on plain films (Fig. 18–7A). A radionuclide bone scan is characteris-

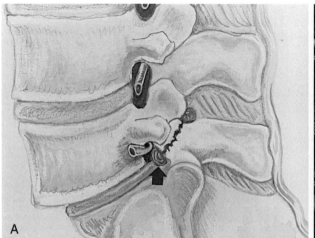
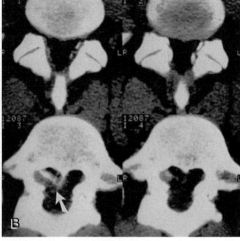

Figure 18–6. Fibrocartilaginous mass at pars break. *A,* This artist's drawing shows how a fibrocartilaginous mass *(arrow)* at a pars break can impinge on a nerve root in the neuroforamen. *B,* A CT slice through the L5 level in a patient with spondylolysis and spondylolisthesis shows a soft tissue mass in the central canal *(arrow)* that has encroached on the right lateral recess and the thecal sac. At surgery this was a large fibrocartilaginous mass that had emanated from the pars break.

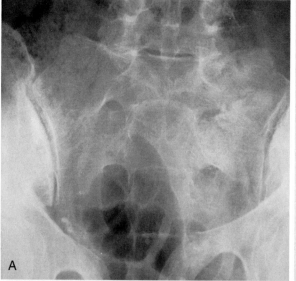

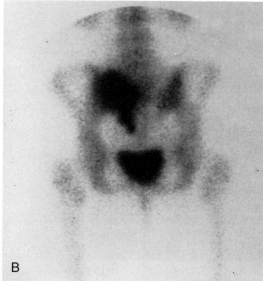

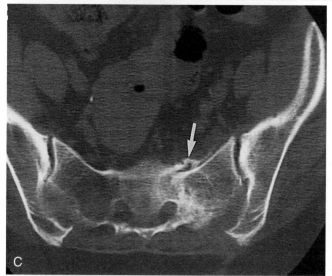

Figure 18–7. Sacral stress fracture. *A,* An anteroposterior plain film of the sacrum in this elderly woman with pain shows faint patchy sclerosis throughout the left sacral ala. This could easily represent metastatic disease. *B,* A posterior view of a radionuclide bone scan shows a geographic pattern of increased uptake corresponding to the left sacral ala and body. This is a characteristic appearance for a sacral stress fracture. *C,* A CT scan through the sacrum reveals a left-sided sacral fracture *(arrow)* with reactive sclerosis in the ala.

tic and should be pathognomonic because of its geographic appearance throughout half or all of the sacrum (see Fig. 18–7*B*). A CT scan is often done to confirm the diagnosis of a stress fracture or to convince a disbelieving clinician. CT will demonstrate a fracture in most cases (see Fig. 18–7*C*).

Appendicular Skeleton

Any complex joint, such as the hip or shoulder, can hide multiple fractures or loose bodies on routine plain film examination and should be considered for CT. The wrist and ankle are also imaged more completely with CT, as are the sacroiliac joints.

CT of the hip is routinely done in most centers when loose bodies are considered or when the position of fracture fragments needs to be precisely determined (Fig. 18–8). In instances where metal might be present in the joint (bullets, shrapnel, or fixation pins or screws from surgery), CT can still be employed, with useful information almost always obtained in spite of metallic streak artifacts (Fig. 18–9). Re-formations often diminish the metallic streak artifact, making interpretation less difficult.

Fractures of the shoulder, with or without dislocation, are studied with CT only if the plain films do not clearly show all the abnormalities or if it is thought that some aspect

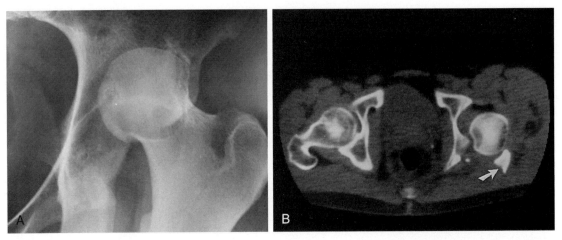

Figure 18–8. Hip dislocation with fracture fragments. *A,* A plain film of the hip in this patient with a history of trauma shows a dislocation of the hip with bony fragments just superior to the femoral head. *B,* A CT slice through the hip shows the posterior column is completely displaced *(arrow).* This is valuable information to the surgeon, who uses the amount of posterior column involvement to determine whether surgical fixation is necessary.

of the anatomy is not depicted (Figs. 18–10 and 18–11).

In the wrist, CT has been shown to be very adept at demonstrating fractures that are not seen on plain films (Fig. 18–12). It is helpful to image both wrists together so that a side-to side comparison can be made. A radionuclide bone scan can sometimes be helpful in pinpointing the area of concern, which can then be imaged in fine detail with thin-section CT slices as opposed to performing thicker slices through the entire wrist (Fig. 18–13).

A frequent use of CT in the ankle is in tarsal coalition. The most common site for coalition is at the calcaneonavicular joint.

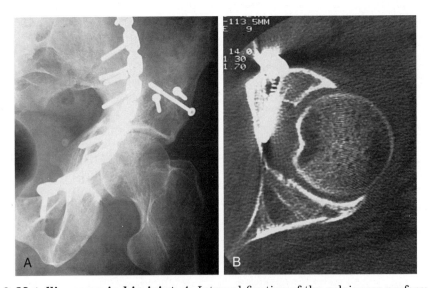

Figure 18–9. Metallic screw in hip joint. *A,* Internal fixation of the pelvis was performed on this patient after multiple fractures suffered in an automobile accident. He now presents with hip pain that was thought possibly to be secondary to one or more of the screws having been inadvertently placed into the joint. Plain films did not resolve the issue. *B,* A CT slice through the hip revealed one of the screws had indeed been placed in the joint. In spite of the metallic nature of the screws and plate and the streak artifacts, a diagnostic study was obtained.

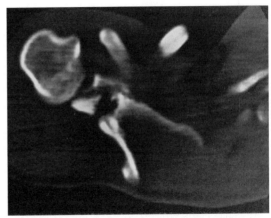

Figure 18–10. Glenohumeral joint fracture. An axial CT slice through a fractured scapula reveals that the fracture extends into the articular portion of the glenoid and to the anterior portion of the scapula. The plain films failed to show the full extent of the fracture.

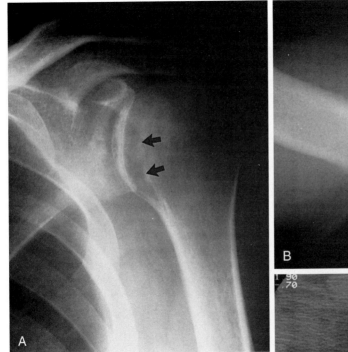

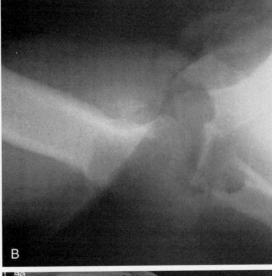

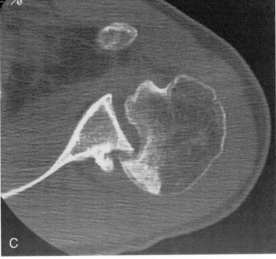

Figure 18–11. Posterior dislocation of the shoulder. *A,* An anteroposterior plain film of the shoulder in this patient with chronic shoulder pain reveals a vertical lucency *(arrows)* that has been termed a "trough" sign and indicates an impaction from a posterior dislocation. *B,* An axillary view shows that the humeral head is posteriorly dislocated and impacted on the glenoid. *C,* A CT scan through the shoulder gives a better look at the impacted humeral head and shows an avulsion off of the scapula.

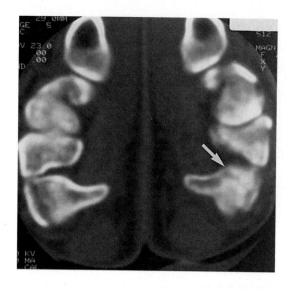

Figure 18–12. Fractured hamate bone. A CT of the wrist in this patient with wrist pain after a fall and a normal plain film shows a fracture of the body of the hamate bone *(arrow)* that extended through the entire hamate on several cuts. The normal opposite wrist is shown for comparison.

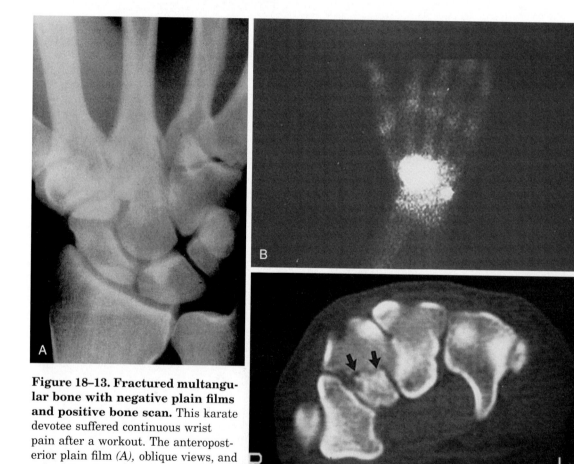

Figure 18–13. Fractured multangular bone with negative plain films and positive bone scan. This karate devotee suffered continuous wrist pain after a workout. The anteroposterior plain film *(A)*, oblique views, and conventional tomograms were negative. A radionuclide bone scan *(B)* showed increased radionuclide uptake over the pisiform and at the base of the second and third metacarpals. *C,* A CT scan of the wrist revealed a fracture of the lesser multangular bone *(arrows)*. The pisiform was normal.

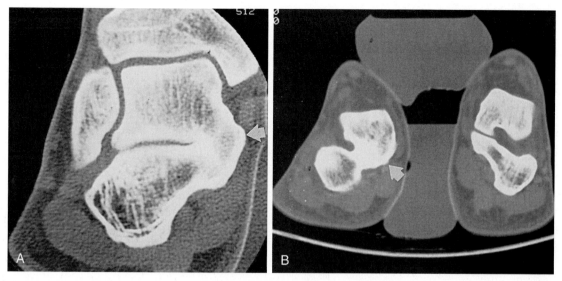

Figure 18–14. Tarsal coalition at the talocalcaneal joint. *A,* An axial CT scan through the ankle in this patient with painful flat feet shows a bony bridge between the talus and the calcaneus *(arrow)*. *B,* The coalition *(arrow)* is more easily appreciated when the opposite normal ankle is shown for comparison.

The next most common locations are at the talonavicular joint and the middle facet of the talocalcaneal joint (Fig. 18–14). It is often difficult to diagnose a coalition if there is a fibrous rather than a bony fusion, but usually there will be enough associated bony abnormalities to allow a diagnosis to be made (Fig. 18–15).

CT can be very helpful in ankle fractures and in evaluating displacement of the peroneal tendons from their normal position behind the fibula (Fig. 18–16). It has also been

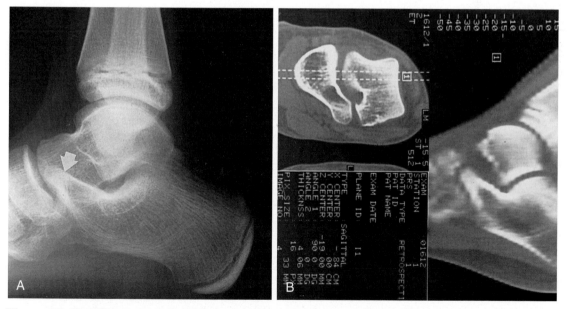

Figure 18–15. Fibrous tarsal coalition at the calcaneonavicular joint. *A,* A lateral plain film of the ankle in this patient with painful flat feet shows a prominent anterior process of the calcaneus *(arrow)*. *B,* CT through the ankle with a sagittal re-formation shows the prominent anterior process to better advantage. There is no bony ankylosis. This is consistent with a fibrous coalition.

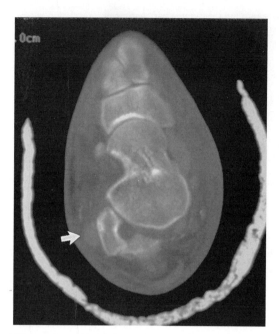

Figure 18–16. Dislocated peroneal tendons.
CT of the ankle in a patient with a fractured calcaneus shows the peroneal tendons *(arrow)* to be dislocated laterally from their normal position posterior to the fibula.

out fractures, LeFort fractures, and countless other types of facial fractures are often seen with CT and not appreciated on plain films. Mandibular and temporomandibular joint fractures should also be studied with CT when plain films are inconclusive.

TUMORS AND INFECTION

MRI is without question superior to CT in evaluating tumors of the musculoskeletal system. Although it is true that CT is better than MRI at evaluating subtle cortical abnormalities, in reality it is seldom necessary to improve on the resolution that MRI affords, with the exception, perhaps, of infection, when subtle cortical disruption is key in diagnosing osteomyelitis. In addition to passable bony evaluation, MRI is unsurpassed at showing the extent of tumors in the medullary bone and in the soft tissues. What then is the role of CT in tumors? Not much!

CT can be helpful in diagnosing bony involvement of multiple myeloma before plain film findings. CT of the spine will show a "Swiss cheese" pattern of lytic myeloma (Fig. 18–18). In long-standing myeloma the pattern is considerably different. The few remaining normal trabeculae undergo compensatory hypertrophy, and the resulting appearance is of thick, sclerotic bony struts with lytic areas in between (Fig. 18–19). This pattern resembles spinal hemangioma (Fig. 18–20) except that the hypertrophied trabecular struts in hemangioma are much more ordered and symmetric.

CT plays a very valuable role in cases of suspected osteoid osteoma. (Is it a tumor? Is it an infection? Is it a virus? Nobody really knows, but because it is most often confused with tumors and osteomyelitis it will be discussed with them.) CT can show the location of the nidus that will facilitate its removal by the surgeon. This is especially useful in complex joints such as the hip (Fig. 18–21) or in the spine (Fig. 18–22). Seeing a small lucency surrounded by sclerosis is not an absolute for the nidus of an osteoid osteoma. Osteomyelitis with a small abscess can have an identical appearance.

used to diagnose tendonitis or rupture of the posterior tibial tendon, usually seen in patients with rheumatoid arthritis. Most centers prefer MRI over CT for tendon evaluation.

An ankle fracture that can be confusing on plain films is avulsion of the anteroinferior tibiofibular ligament, called a fracture of Tillaux. A bony fragment off of the tibia is avulsed, but its location, as to whether it is anterior or posterior, can be difficult to ascertain on plain films (Fig. 18–17A through C). CT will demonstrate the fragment's position and can be performed quickly and inexpensively (see Fig. 18–17D). In children, the distal tibial physis fuses incrementally from medial to lateral with the lateral portion, which is attached to the anteroinferior tibiofibular ligament, susceptible to an avulsion injury called a juvenile Tillaux fracture. This is basically a Salter type 3 injury.

Facial trauma can be difficult to assess with plain films, and CT should be considered in almost all instances of facial trauma when fractures are suspected. Orbital blow-

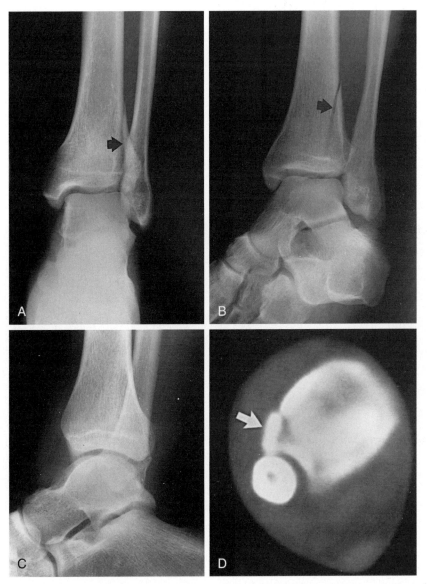

Figure 18–17. Fracture of Tillaux. Anteroposterior *(A)* and oblique *(B)* plain films of the ankle show a fracture of the lateral aspect of the distal tibia *(arrows),* but the lateral view *(C)* fails to show if it is anteriorly or posteriorly located. Because internal fixation was planned, it was believed to be essential to know the exact location of the fracture. *(D)* CT through the distal tibia shows the fracture to be anteriorly located *(arrow).* This is consistent with an avulsion of the anterior inferior tibiofibular ligament and has been termed a *fracture of Tillaux.*

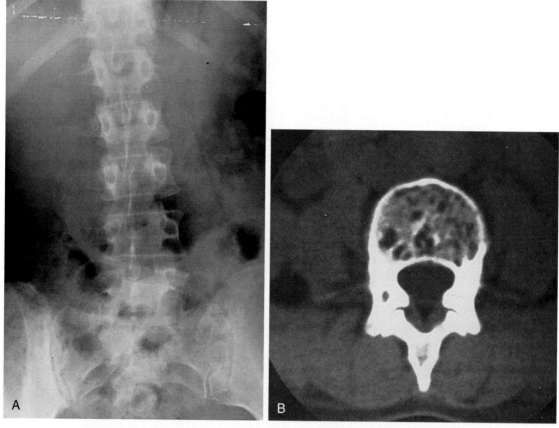

Figure 18–18. Multiple myeloma. *A,* An anteroposterior view of the lumbar spine was taken in this patient with known myeloma to see if bony involvement was present. The plain films were all considered normal except for mild osteopenia. *B,* CT through a lumbar vertebral body shows diffuse lytic lesions consistent with multiple myeloma. This is a typical appearance for multiple myeloma in the spine and almost always precedes plain film findings.

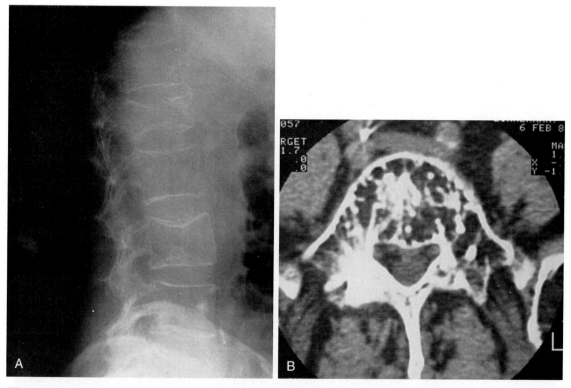

Figure 18–19. Chronic multiple myeloma. *A,* Lateral plain film of the spine in this patient with myeloma shows marked osteopenia and a partial collapse of the L2 vertebral body. *B,* CT scan through one of the noncollapsed lumbar bodies shows dense trabecular struts that are hypertrophied. They are separated by multiple cystic areas. This is a characteristic appearance for chronic myeloma with compensatory hypertrophy of the remaining trabeculae. It has a similar appearance to Paget's disease and to hemangioma.

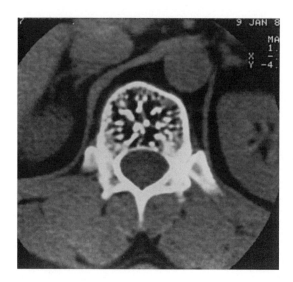

Figure 18–20. Hemangioma. CT through a vertebral body hemangioma reveals strikingly dense, hypertrophied trabeculae that are arranged in a columnar fashion. Note the symmetry to this pattern as compared with that of chronic myeloma.

The nidus of an osteoid osteoma often partially calcifies and can then resemble a sequestrum in osteomyelitis (Figs. 18–23 and 18–24). CT, plain films, and even MRI can appear identical in both osteoid osteoma and osteomyelitis, with or without a sequestrum; therefore, a differential diagnosis of both entities should be given when a lesion with this appearance is found. Radionuclide bone scan can usually differentiate between osteoid osteoma and osteomyelitis by noting a "double density" sign at the nidus of the osteoid osteoma. This is caused by the increased affinity for the radionuclide by the

hypervascular nidus. The surrounding reactive new bone takes up the radionuclide to a lesser degree than the nidus. In osteomyelitis a small abscess will be photopenic on radionuclide examination.

CT plays an important role in osteomyelitis by finding sequestrations (Fig. 18–25). The finding of a sequestration has both a diagnostic and a therapeutic significance. The diagnostic significance is that only a few entities have been described that commonly have a sequestration. These are osteomyelitis, eosinophilic granuloma (Fig. 18–26), and fibrosarcoma (Fig. 18–27). As

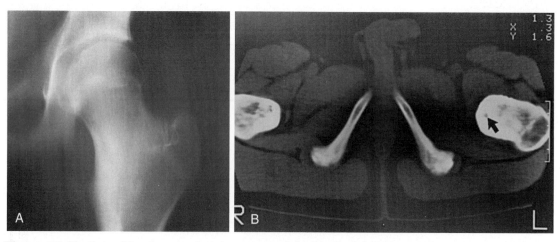

Figure 18–21. Osteoid osteoma. *A,* A tomogram of the hip in this 20-year-old man with hip pain shows cortical thickening and sclerosis about the medial aspect of the femoral neck. An osteoid osteoma was suspected, but the exact location of the nidus could not be determined. *B,* CT through the femoral neck revealed a focal lucency *(arrow)* surrounded by sclerosis. This was removed and found to be the nidus of an osteoid osteoma.

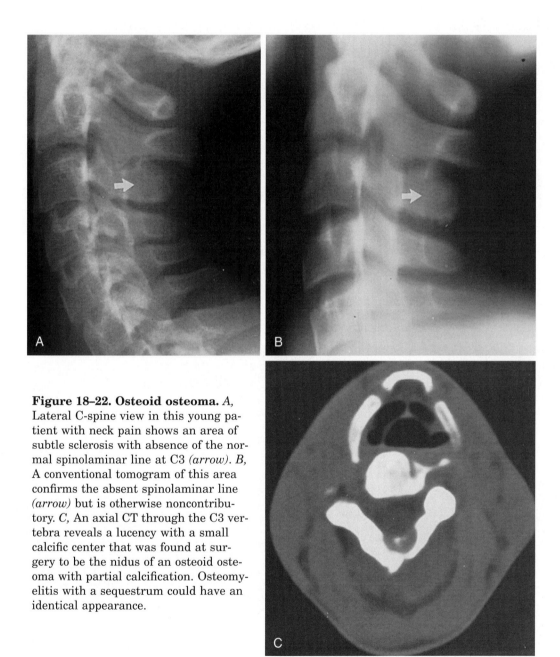

Figure 18–22. Osteoid osteoma. *A,* Lateral C-spine view in this young patient with neck pain shows an area of subtle sclerosis with absence of the normal spinolaminar line at C3 *(arrow). B,* A conventional tomogram of this area confirms the absent spinolaminar line *(arrow)* but is otherwise noncontributory. *C,* An axial CT through the C3 vertebra reveals a lucency with a small calcific center that was found at surgery to be the nidus of an osteoid osteoma with partial calcification. Osteomyelitis with a sequestrum could have an identical appearance.

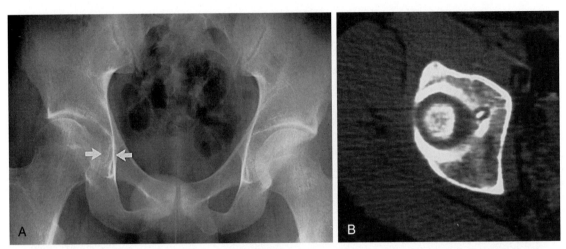

Figure 18–23. Osteoid osteoma with calcified nidus. *A,* This young patient presented with hip pain and a widened teardrop measurement *(arrows)* on the right as compared with the left. A hip aspiration ruled out an infectious process. *B,* Axial CT of the hip showed an acetabular lucency with a central calcific density consistent with either osteomyelitis with a sequestrum or an osteoid osteoma with a partially calcified nidus. At surgery this was found to be an osteoid osteoma.

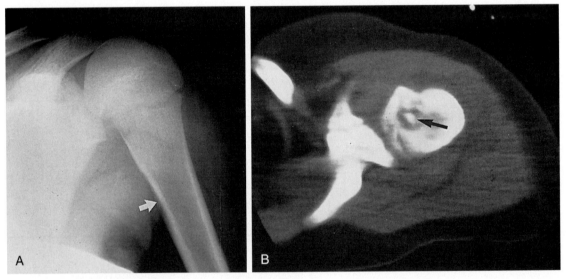

Figure 18–24. Osteomyelitis. *A,* Anteroposterior plain film of the upper humerus in this child with pain and swelling shows a faint permeative pattern in the bone with periostitis *(arrow)*. The differential diagnosis includes osteomyelitis, Ewing's sarcoma, and eosinophilic granuloma. *B,* CT of the humerus shows a lytic lesion with a bony sequestrum *(arrow)*. This narrows the diagnosis to osteomyelitis and eosinophilic granuloma, because Ewing's sarcoma will not have a sequestrum. Biopsy showed this to be osteomyelitis. Because a sequestrum was known to be present the surgeons opted to remove the sequestrum rather than just treat the condition with antibiotics.

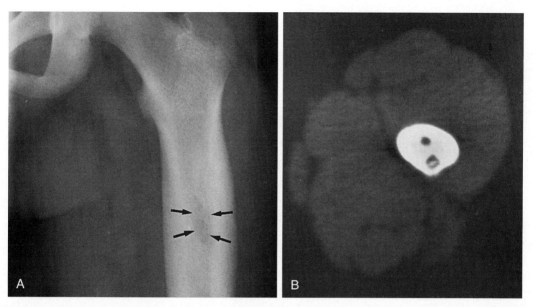

Figure 18–25. Sequestration in osteomyelitis. *A,* Anteroposterior plain film of the proximal femur in this child with pain shows an area of diffuse sclerosis and cortical thickening with a faint lucency in the intramedullary portion *(arrows). B,* CT of the femur reveals a lucency with a calcific central portion. Some believed this was a partially calcified nidus in an osteoid osteoma, whereas others thought it was a sequestration in osteomyelitis. Either process could have this appearance. At biopsy this was found to be a sequestration in osteomyelitis.

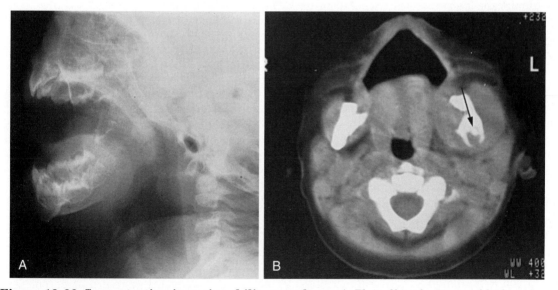

Figure 18–26. Sequestration in eosinophilic granuloma. *A,* Plain film of a 2-year old who presented with a painful, swollen jaw shows some destruction of the mandible near the angle of the jaw. Infection, Ewing's sarcoma, osteogenic sarcoma, neuroblastoma, and eosinophilic granuloma were diagnostic considerations. *B,* CT through the jaw revealed a destructive lesion that involved much of the mandible. A sequestration *(arrow)* was found that limited the differential diagnosis to osteomyelitis and eosinophilic granuloma. At biopsy this was found to be eosinophilic granuloma.

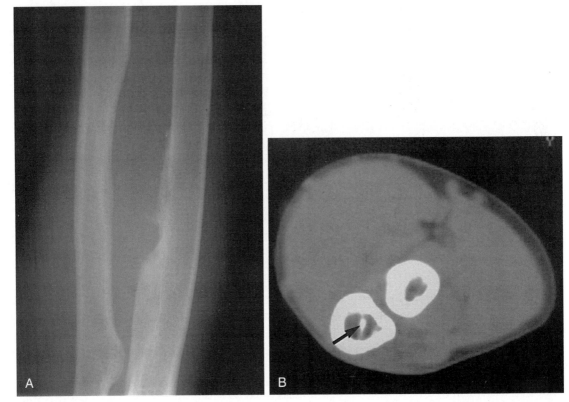

Figure 18–27. Sequestration in a desmoid tumor. *A,* A plain film of the forearm shows a destructive lesion of the ulna with some aggressive periostitis. Note the thick benign periostitis as well. *B,* CT through the lesion revealed a sequestrum *(arrow)* that limited the differential diagnosis to eosinophilic granuloma, fibrosarcoma, and osteomyelitis. At surgery this was sampled and initially reported to be a fibrosarcoma; however, it was subsequently found to be a desmoid tumor, which is a "half-grade" fibrosarcoma.

mentioned earlier, a partially calcified nidus of an osteoid osteoma can have an identical appearance as osteomyelitis with a sequestrum. All four entities should be considered when a sequestrum is encountered. The therapeutic significance is that the presence of a sequestrum usually requires surgical removal. Antibiotic therapy alone generally does not suffice because the sequestration does not have a blood supply and will not have the antibiotics delivered to it.

A "tumorous" condition that can be mistaken for a malignancy both radiographically and histologically is myositis ossificans. It is imperative that a biopsy not be performed if myositis ossificans is a consideration because it can resemble a sarcoma to the pathologist and result in unnecessary radical surgery. The plain film finding that is virtually pathognomonic for myositis ossificans is peripheral calcification (Fig. 18–

28). Often it is difficult to characterize the calcification as either central or peripheral on plain films; CT can help determine the location of the calcification and avert a biopsy in some instances (Fig. 18–29).

MISCELLANEOUS USES

There are several additional uses of CT in the musculoskeletal system that do not fall into any neat category. These include examination of the sacroiliac joints, measurements, temporomandibular joint examination, CT arthrography of the shoulder. and bone densitometry. Bone densitometry is not covered here because there are several different techniques employed and it is beyond the scope of this text.

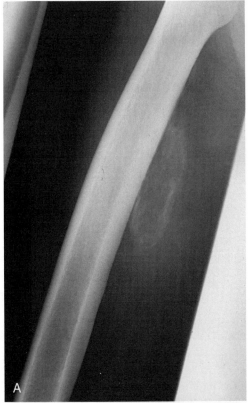

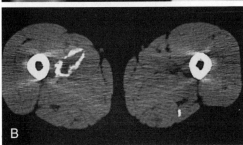

Figure 18–28. Myositis ossificans. *A,* A plain film of the thigh in this young surgeon with pain and swelling shows a calcific mass that could be myositis ossificans or a parosteal osteosarcoma. The patient could not recall any recent trauma to this area. *B,* CT through the mass shows definite peripheral, circumferential calcification that is characteristic of myositis ossificans. A planned biopsy was canceled, because myositis can mimic a sarcoma histologically.

Sacroiliac Joints

Plain film examination of the sacroiliac joints can be extremely difficult owing to the anatomic obliquity of the joints themselves and the thick overlying soft tissues.

If the diagnosis or treatment of the disorder rests on the appearance of the sacroiliac joints (and it is not always so), then CT is a more reliable imaging technique than plain radiography. It certainly is more reproducible, more sensitive, and more accurate than plain films and gives the patient less radiation. If the protocol is streamlined, it can be performed rapidly and at a relatively low cost, making it cost effective.

To streamline the protocol and diminish the number of cuts necessary to cover the sacroiliac joints, the gantry is reversed so that it is at a steep angle parallel to the sacroiliac joints (Fig. 18–30). This is just opposite to the direction the gantry is angled when trying to scan parallel to the L5-S1 disc. Eight to ten 3- or 5-mm thick slices are obtained that cover the sacroiliac joints as seen on the lateral scout film.

Sacroiliac joint sclerosis and erosions can be identified with much more clarity than on plain films (Fig. 18–31). The iliac side of the joint invariably has more sclerosis than the sacral side; however, this should not be confused with osteitis condensans ilii. Degenerative joint disease can also cause erosions in the sacroiliac joints and mimic a spondyloarthropathy or an infection (Fig. 18–32). It has been shown that erosions and sclerosis in the sacroiliac joints, as shown with CT, increase with aging to the point that patients older than 40 often have sacroiliac joint abnormalities.

Measurements

Almost any measurement that is done with plain films, such as pelvimetry and scanogram for leg-length discrepancy, can be done more accurately and with considerably less radiation by using CT. There are fewer more thankless tasks in skeletal radiology than trying to read a poorly exposed scanogram of the legs with a barely discernible ruler between the patient's legs and trying to give accurate measurements of leg length. The measurements can be easily and accurately obtained with CT by taking an anteroposterior scout film of the extremities and placing cursor points on the bony landmarks for measurement (Fig. 18–33). The computer gives the distance measurements between

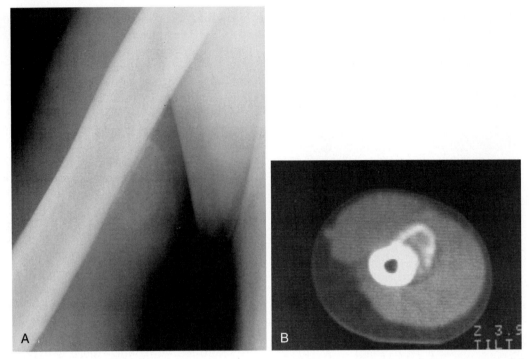

Figure 18–29. Myositis ossificans. *A*, A plain film of the humerus in this patient with a painful mass shows a faintly calcified mass adjacent to the humerus with some periostitis present. Myositis ossificans and parosteal osteosarcoma were believed to be the main considerations. *B*, CT through the mass shows definite circumferential calcification, which indicates myositis ossificans. No biopsy sample was taken because myositis can simulate a sarcoma histologically.

the chosen points. This technique has been shown to have reproducibility and accuracy, but it suffers from not being able to have the patient bear weight. Most of the time a weight-bearing examination is not necessary; however, if a weight-bearing examination is required, then a CT scanogram cannot replace the conventional scanogram. The radiation dose from the CT scanogram has been estimated at 50 to 100 times less than a conventional scanogram. The cost of a CT scanogram is less than a conventional

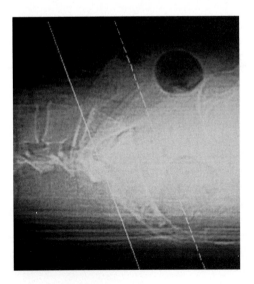

Figure 18–30. Scout film for sacroiliac joints. This lateral scout view of the sacrum shows how the cursors are angled parallel to the sacroiliac joints. Eight to ten 3- to 5-mm thick slices are then taken to cover the extent of the joints.

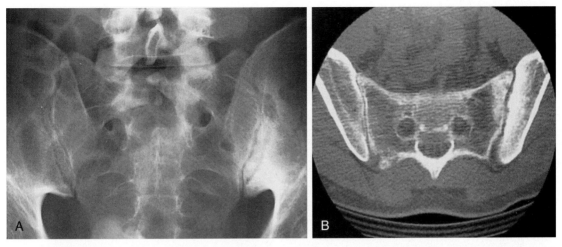

Figure 18–31. CT of the sacroiliac joints in psoriasis. *A,* An anteroposterior plain film of the pelvis demonstrates left-sided sacroiliac joint sclerosis and erosions. It was not clear if the right side was minimally involved or not. *B,* CT shows the left-sided changes nicely and shows that the right joint is definitely not involved.

scanogram because of the low cost of the scout views, which comprise the imaging portion of the examination.

Pelvimetry is a frequent source of consternation for many radiologists because of the difficulty seeing the bony landmarks and ruler markings, as well as the reluctance to order repeat films to improve the quality because of the radiation dose to this sensitive population. CT eliminates all these concerns. An anteroposterior and a lateral scout view are obtained. From these, the pelvic inlet can be measured (Fig. 18–34). A single axial CT slice is taken at the level of the fovea of the femoral heads that will

allow measurement across the ischial spines. This technique is accurate, is reproducible, and has a radiation dose 30 times less than conventional pelvimetry. The entire examination takes 10 minutes or less to complete; therefore, it should be cost effective.

Temporomandibular Joint

For several years CT was used to replace temporomandibular joint arthrography in multiple institutions. CT compares favorably with arthrography in diagnosing an anteriorly displaced disc. However, MRI is far

Figure 18–32. CT of the sacroiliac joints in degenerative joint disease. CT of the sacroiliac joints in this patient shows some minimal sclerosis and definite erosions in the right joint. A small erosion is also present in the left joint. These changes could be due to any inflammatory arthritis or a spondyloarthropathy, but these were due to degenerative joint disease. This patient has extensive osteoarthritis in his spine and large joints. This is a typical appearance of degenerative joint disease in the sacroiliac joints.

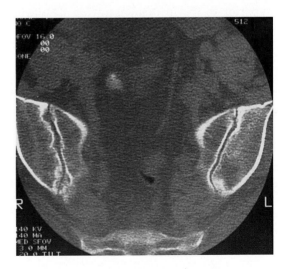

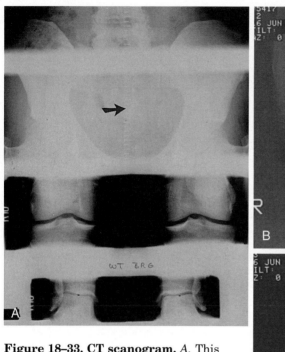

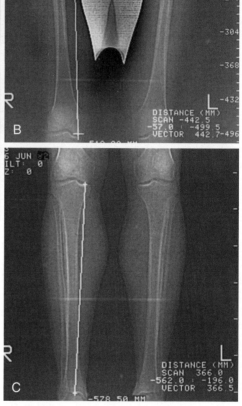

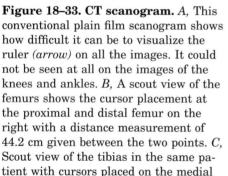

Figure 18–33. CT scanogram. *A,* This conventional plain film scanogram shows how difficult it can be to visualize the ruler *(arrow)* on all the images. It could not be seen at all on the images of the knees and ankles. *B,* A scout view of the femurs shows the cursor placement at the proximal and distal femur on the right with a distance measurement of 44.2 cm given between the two points. *C,* Scout view of the tibias in the same patient with cursors placed on the medial tibial plateau and on the plafond. The measurement of the distance between the cursors is 36.6 cm. These measurements are repeated on the opposite leg and compared.

superior to CT in demonstrating displaced discs as well as other joint pathology and is considered by most to be the procedure of choice for imaging the disc. CT is still very useful for imaging bony abnormalities of the temporomandibular joint.

The temporomandibular joint is very difficult to image with conventional techniques because of its position in the dense, bony glenoid fossa. With CT, the joint is clearly depicted and many joint abnormalities that are not appreciated on plain films are easily diagnosed.

Commonplace abnormalities such as degenerative joint disease and fractures are often not well visualized on plain films yet are shown clearly with CT. A less common abnormality that often goes undiagnosed because plain films fail to demonstrate it is coronoid process hyperplasia (Fig. 18–35). This is a congenital hypertrophy of one or both coronoid processes that can limit mouth opening by impinging against the zygomatic arch. Once recognized it can be surgically corrected.

Another abnormality that is occasionally seen in the temporomandibular joint and can go unrecognized on plain films is synovial osteochondromatosis (Fig. 18–36). This presents as a fullness or swelling in the joint and often goes to biopsy, where it can be confused with a chondrosarcoma. This

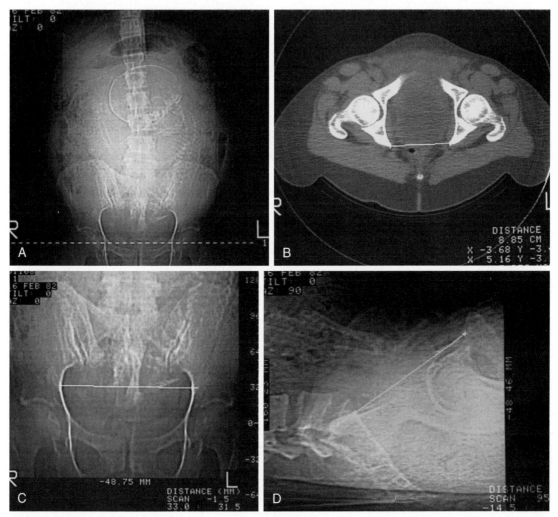

Figure 18–34. CT pelvimetry. For pelvimetry measurements it is necessary to take an anteroposterior and a lateral scout view of the pelvis and a single axial CT slice. The anteroposterior scout view is used to find the femoral head fovea, through which a cursor is placed *(A)* for a single axial slice. On the single axial slice through the fovea of the femoral heads the measurement of the ischial spines is made *(B)*. In this patient that measurement is 8.85 cm. The anteroposterior scout view is also used to measure the pelvic inlet *(C)*. In this patient the inlet measured 48.75 mm. The lateral scout view is then used to measure the pelvic inlet from the sacrum to the symphysis pubis *(D)*. This measured 48.46 mm in this patient.

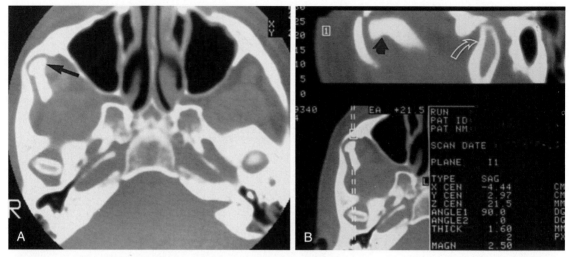

Figure 18–35. Coronoid process hyperplasia. *A,* An axial CT of the temporomandibular joints in this patient with joint pain and inability to fully open her mouth shows a large bony protuberance eroding the right zygomatic arch *(arrow).* This bony protuberance is a hypertrophied coronoid process and is mechanically impinging on the zygoma, thereby limiting mouth opening. *B,* A sagittal re-formation through the right temporomandibular joint shows the hypertrophied coronoid process *(black arrow)* to be larger than the condyle *(open white arrow).*

should be a radiologic diagnosis rather than a histologic one because it can resemble a sarcoma histologically. CT of synovial chondromatosis in the temporomandibular joint is characteristic and should be diagnostic.

CT Arthrography of the Shoulder

CT arthrograms of the shoulder are useful in examining the glenoid labrum in patients with shoulder instability. MRI has replaced the CT arthrogram in many institutions; however, the resolution and clarity of the labrum are not nearly so good with MRI as with CT. MRI can also diagnose abnormalities of the rotator cuff such as tendonitis and partial tears, whereas the CT arthrogram will only tell if there is a full-thickness cuff tear. For many surgeons, that is enough

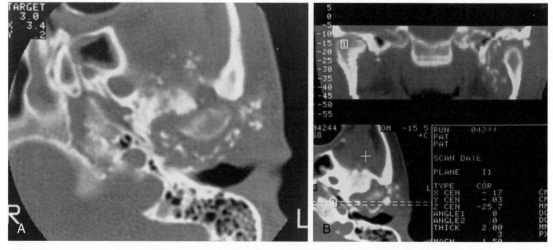

Figure 18–36. Synovial osteochondromatosis of the temporomandibular joint. *A,* Axial CT through the left temporomandibular joint reveals multiple calcific densities in the joint with some bony erosion of the temporal bone and condylar head. *B,* A coronal re-formation shows the multiple joint bodies in the left joint and the erosion in the joint as compared with the normal right joint. This is diagnostic of synovial osteochondromatosis.

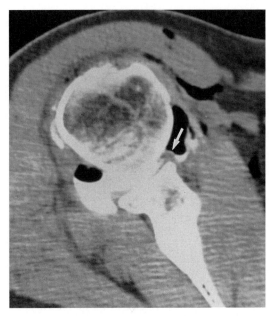

Figure 18–37. Normal shoulder CT arthrogram. This CT arthrogram of the shoulder demonstrates a smooth, rounded anterior labrum *(arrow)*. This is a normal appearance. The posterior labrum has a similar appearance in this patient.

information about the cuff, and the superior imaging of the labrum will make them prefer the CT arthrogram over the MRI examination.

The technique begins like a routine shoulder arthrogram with a needle placed into the glenohumeral joint near the axillary recess. Instead of the standard 10 mL of contrast medium placed into the joint, however, only 1.5 to 2 mL is instilled along with 0.25 mL of 1:10,000 epinephrine and 10 mL of air. The epinephrine will delay absorption of the contrast agent to allow for possible delays in completing the CT scan. The needle is removed and the patient is instructed to move the shoulder through a full range of motion to adequately coat the joint. Plain films are obtained and reviewed to look for leakage of air or contrast medium into the subacromial bursa, which would be diagnostic for a rotator cuff tear. The patient is then positioned at the CT scanner, and 3-mm

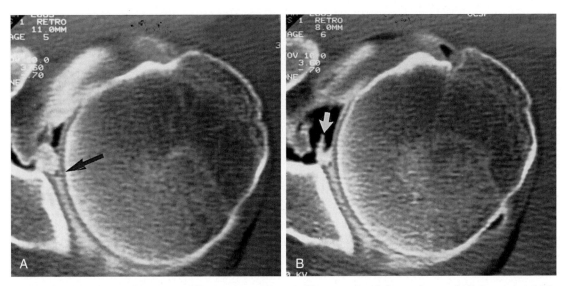

Figure 18–38. Torn labrum on CT arthrogram. *A,* The anterior labrum has a cleft *(arrow)*, which indicates a tear. *B,* CT slice shows the anterior labrum to be completely torn with a frayed piece remaining *(arrow)*.

thick contiguous slices are obtained through the glenoid. The normal glenoid has a smooth covering of cartilage that is slightly thicker and more triangular anteriorly (Fig. 18–37). A torn labrum will have an obvious irregularity (Fig. 18–38) or be absent or small.

Suggested Reading

Assoun J, Richardi G, Railhac JJ, et al: Osteoid osteoma: MR imaging versus CT. Radiology 1994; 191:217–223

Helms CA, Jeffrey RB, Wing VW: Computed tomography and plain film appearance of a bony sequestration: Significance and differential diagnosis. Skeletal Radiol 1987; 16(2):117–120

Link TM, Meier N, Rummeny EJ, et al: Artificial spine fractures: Detection with helical and conventional CT. Radiology 1996; 198:515–519

Ney DR, Fishman EK, Kawashima A, et al: Comparison of helical and serial CT with regard to three-dimensional imaging of musculoskeletal anatomy. Radiology 1992; 185:865–869

Chapter

19

Lumbar Spine

Clyde A. Helms, M.D.

DISC DISEASE

CT has proved to be of immense value in examining the lumbar spine. It gives us the capability of examining in detail not only the discs but also all of the bony and soft tissue structures in and about the spine, including the facets, the neuroforamen, the thecal sac and nerve roots as they exit the thecal sac, the ligamentum flavum, and the vascular structures. The discussion in this chapter shows how CT can be used to diagnose disc disease and spinal stenosis in the lumbar spine and explains why CT has made myelography obsolete.

Multiple comparison studies of CT versus myelography have been published that show that myelography and CT are both roughly 90% accurate in diagnosing disc disease. In fact, most of us who have been interpreting CT scans of the spine for a number of years know that CT is considerably better than myelography. Why doesn't the literature reflect this then? Several reasons account for this discrepancy that I will mention later in this chapter. Most of those comparison studies were performed in the early days of CT spine work—things have improved considerably since then. Also, more recent studies confirm that CT is around 95% accurate whereas myelography continues to be around 90% accurate. Even the older studies recommended that CT be the primary study of choice and that myelography be reserved for the nondiagnostic

CT examination. The current recommendation is to not perform the myelogram under any circumstances for routine disc disease or spinal stenosis. That's correct. Never! I can think of no clinical situation when a myelogram is warranted. If the CT examination does not answer the question, then an MRI is indicated.

How about CT myelography? This is unnecessary. Only a few studies have been performed comparing the accuracy of diagnosis of plain CT versus myelographic enhanced CT. These show no statistical differences between the two techniques. If there is no difference, then why put the patient through the extra expense and morbidity and, in some centers, hospitalization, when a plain CT will be as effective?

How does CT compare with MRI in the lumbar spine? Multiple papers have been published comparing CT of the spine with MRI. These are all showing that MRI is just as good as CT. I would certainly agree with that *if* the MRI examination is of high quality. The main point to make is that MRI is *no better* than CT unless it is done of a postoperative spine. Therefore, there is no good reason to switch from CT to MRI unless the cost of the MRI examination is less. It is interesting to hear many of the proponents of MRI claim that myelography is no longer necessary now that MRI is available. In fact, CT made myelography obsolete, but people have not caught on yet. Several articles on spine imaging concur with these statements, but it will take another 5 years or more before myelography is eliminated.

Technical Considerations

The proper imaging protocol for a diagnostic lumbar spine study is critical to lessen the chances of missing a lesion. The patient should be studied in the supine position with the knees flexed over a pillow or other similar object. Anteroposterior and lateral scout films are obtained. The anteroposterior scout film allows the radiologist to determine if transitional vertebrae are present. A significant number of operations are performed at the wrong level because of a mixup with labeling transitional vertebrae. The lateral scout view is used to place the cursors over the intended area of scanning. This should include contiguous slices, no thicker than 5 mm (I prefer 3- or 4-mm thick slices) from the midbody of L3 to the top of S1. Ten percent of disc protrusions occur at the L3-4 level, and they can clinically mimic protrusions from lower levels; therefore, the L3-4 level must be examined.

The early spine protocols recommended several angled-gantry slices parallel to each vertebral body end plate (Fig. 19–1). This is not advised for two reasons. First, this leaves spaces or gaps in the central canal that are not imaged that can result in missed free fragments. Second, it is not necessary to angle the gantry parallel to the end plate. I have seen thousands of levels imaged with both angled cuts and straight axial cuts and have yet to see a difference between the two. You simply cannot make a disc impress the thecal sac, or even appear to, with any degree of angling of the gantry. Therefore, why spend the extra time and radiation? My recommendation for a complete lumbar spine CT examination is 3-mm thick slices from the midbody of L3 to the top of S1 in a straight axial fashion (Fig. 19–2).

The completed study should be photographed with the images magnified in a manner so they are easily seen at arm's length. Each image should be photographed in a bone and a soft tissue window. I often see radiologists trying to diagnose facet disease or other bony abnormalities from a soft

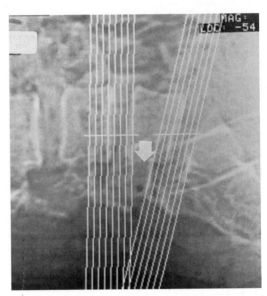

Figure 19–1. Inappropriate scanning protocol. This lateral scout view has the gantry angled parallel to the L5-S1 end plate with several slices above and below. This is repeated at the L4-5 level. A small but definite space or gap is present between the levels *(arrow)* where a free fragment or spinal stenosis could be missed. In addition, it is mandatory to study the L3-4 level, because up to 10% of disc protrusions occur at this level.

tissue window image, and it cannot be done with any accuracy. The anteroposterior and lateral scout views should be included on the hard copy film to allow the radiologist and the clinician to anatomically orient each image.

Pathology

When a disc bulges or protrudes beyond the end plate it takes on several names, some of which have more sinister connotations than others. The terms *herniated nucleus pulposus* and *bulging annulus fibrosus* are often mentioned, along with "contained," "extruded," and "sequestered" discs. How do we differentiate these various types of disc protrusions and what are the implications of each? First, radiologists are not very good at differentiating them, and, second, except for distinguishing a sequestration (a free fragment) it probably does not matter. The surgeons want to know if disc material of any kind is pressing against neural tissue,

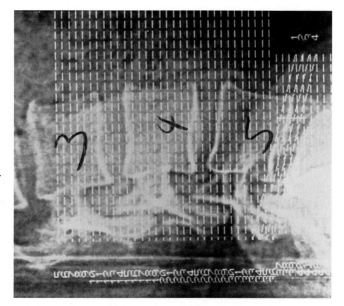

Figure 19–2. Proper scanning protocol. This lateral scout view has straight axial 3-mm thick slices from L3 to S1 without gaps. This is an adequate examination for disc disease or spinal stenosis.

and even then they know it might not be causing the patient's symptoms.

The early CT literature says that if a disc protrusion or bulge is broad based it usually represents a bulging annulus fibrosus, whereas if it is focal it usually represents a herniated nucleus pulposus (Fig. 19–3). If the early articles that compared CT to myelography are used, this morphologic classification was only correct about 85% of the time. It is not unusual to see a focal bulging annulus or a large, broad-based herniated

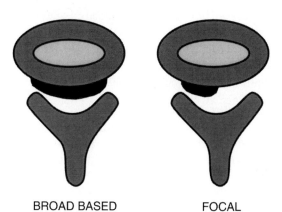

BROAD BASED   FOCAL

Figure 19–3. Schematic of focal versus broad-based disc protrusions. A broad-based disc protrusion has a uniform bulge that extends across the entire central canal. A focal protrusion extends only into a portion of the central canal.

nucleus pulposus. Also, most of the investigators did not require the myelogram to differentiate between the two entities—the myelogram only had to note an extradural bulge. Hence, the CT examinations were downgraded for accuracy unnecessarily. If this source of error is removed, CT is actually much more accurate at diagnosing disc protrusions than myelography.

If a disc protrusion does not impress the thecal sac or a nerve root, it will not be seen on a myelogram, yet the protrusion can be seen with CT. It would undoubtedly be asymptomatic and not deserving of surgical treatment. These were called "false positives" in the early comparison studies of CT and myelography, but they are no more false positives than a cervical rib on a chest film is a false positive. They are real findings, but they are not causing any symptoms. These are generally small disc protrusions (Fig. 19–4), and surgeons know that they are real but innocuous. If the disc does impress the thecal sac or a nerve root (Fig. 19–5), it may or may not be symptomatic, but surgeons know it has to be matched with the clinical findings. A very large disc protrusion with marked thecal sac impression (Fig. 19–6) is much more likely to be symptomatic.

A large disc protrusion should make one very suspicious for a sequestration or free fragment. The largest cause for failure of a

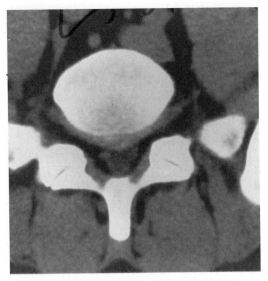

Figure 19–4. Small disc protrusion. This predominantly broad-based disc protrusion is not impressing the thecal sac or nerve roots. It is therefore a disc protrusion that would not be expected to be symptomatic.

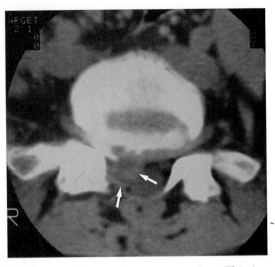

Figure 19–6. Large disc protrusion. This is an extremely large focal right-sided disc protrusion *(arrows)* that is impressing the right-sided nerve root and thecal sac. This disc also has a broad-based component that is not touching the thecal sac or nerve roots.

percutaneous discectomy procedure and a not infrequent cause for failed surgical microdiscectomy procedures is a missed free fragment. A free fragment should be suggested any time disc material is identified

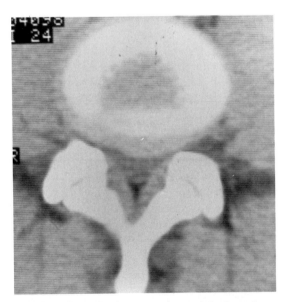

Figure 19–5. Disc protrusion with thecal sac impression. This broad-based disc protrusion is impressing the thecal sac moderately. This is therefore a disc protrusion that may or may not be symptomatic.

in the cut above or below the disc level (Fig. 19–7). If a soft tissue density is identified above or below the disc space, it should be determined if it is of a similar density as the thecal sac or if it is of a higher density. If it is clearly a higher density, it is disc material and should be considered a free fragment.

There are three methods to examine the density of the suspect tissue: (1) a region-of-interest box or cursor can be placed over the suspect area and the actual CT attenuation number can be compared with that of the thecal sac (Fig. 19–8); (2) the identity mode or "blink mode" can be set at disc density and compared with the questionable tissue (Fig. 19–9); the "blink mode" is a button on the scanner console that, when pressed, highlights in white all the tissue densities of a chosen CT number, allowing easy distinction of subtle density differences; and (3) the window width can be reduced to a very narrow setting and the density differences of various tissues will stand out. If a soft tissue density cannot be clearly distinguished visually as to its density compared with the thecal sac, one of these three methods should be tried.

If the soft tissue density above or below

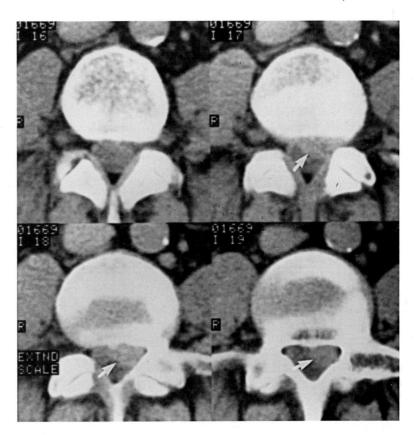

Figure 19–7. Free fragment. These four contiguous slices show a large focal left-sided disc protrusion on at least three adjacent cuts *(arrows)*. The lowest cut (#19) is below the disc space level and into the lateral recesses. This is consistent with a free fragment.

the disc space is isodense to the thecal sac it is not a free fragment and is most likely either a Tarlov cyst or a conjoined nerve root. A Tarlov cyst is merely an enlarged nerve root sheath. It is a normal variant and not a cause of any symptoms. It can get quite large and because of persistent pulsations from the cerebrospinal fluid can cause bony erosion (Fig. 19–10). It has also been termed a *perineural cyst.*

A conjoined root is a congenital anomaly of two nerve roots exiting the thecal sac together instead of separately (Fig. 19–11). The two roots run in the lateral recess together and appear as a soft tissue mass on CT (Fig. 19–12A). A free fragment can have the same appearance but will have an increased density as compared with the thecal sac (Fig. 19–12B), whereas a conjoined root will be isodense to the thecal sac (Fig. 19–13). The roots will invariably exit through their appropriate foramen; hence it is very unusual to have an "empty" foramen. Also, the conjoined roots are always associated with a slightly wider lateral recess than the opposite side. Conjoined roots occur in 1%

to 3% of all patients and are incidental findings with no reported symptomatology.

Many patients have had neural damage at surgery owing to failure to recognize two roots in an area where there is normally only one. Also, many patients have had explorations for "free fragments" when there was a conjoined root mimicking a free fragment. Because percutaneous discectomy is contraindicated in the presence of a free fragment and an open procedure requires a diligent search if a free fragment is suspected, it is critical for the radiologist to differentiate between a free fragment and a conjoined root or a Tarlov cyst. This is easily done by noting the density differences between the mass and the thecal sac. Therefore, it is inappropriate to list a differential diagnosis of free fragment, conjoined root, or Tarlov cyst when a soft tissue mass is found in a lateral recess.

A lateral disc is a disc protrusion that occurs lateral to the neuroforamen (Fig. 19–14). It is one of the more commonly missed disc protrusions simply because it is overlooked. The usual search pattern examines

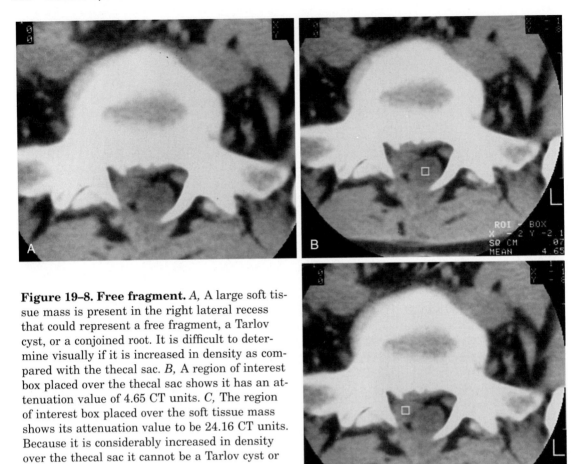

Figure 19–8. Free fragment. *A,* A large soft tissue mass is present in the right lateral recess that could represent a free fragment, a Tarlov cyst, or a conjoined root. It is difficult to determine visually if it is increased in density as compared with the thecal sac. *B,* A region of interest box placed over the thecal sac shows it has an attenuation value of 4.65 CT units. *C,* The region of interest box placed over the soft tissue mass shows its attenuation value to be 24.16 CT units. Because it is considerably increased in density over the thecal sac it cannot be a Tarlov cyst or a conjoined root—it is a free disc fragment.

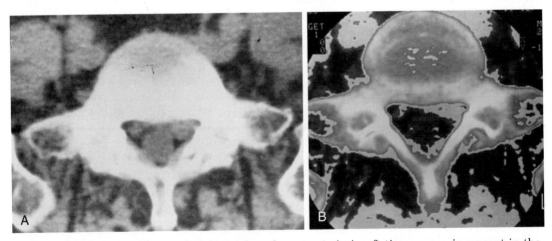

Figure 19–9. "Blink mode" identifying a free fragment. *A,* A soft tissue mass is present in the left lateral recess that could represent a free fragment, a Tarlov cyst, or a conjoined nerve root. It is difficult to tell visually if the mass is increased in density over the thecal sac. *B,* With the "blink mode" set at a level that allows the ligamentum flavum to light up, there is highlighting of the mass in the left lateral recess. This is diagnostic of a free fragment as a conjoined root and a Tarlov cyst would be lower in density than a free fragment. The ligamentum flavum is the same density as disc material and can be used to set the blink mode when the disc is not visible.

Figure 19–10. Tarlov cyst. Large dilatations of the nerve root sheaths are present that are causing some erosion into the vertebral body. The cysts are filled with cerebrospinal fluid and are the same density as the thecal sac. (From Helms CA, et al: Characteristic CT manifestations of uncommon spinal disorders. Orthop Clin North Am 1985;16:445.)

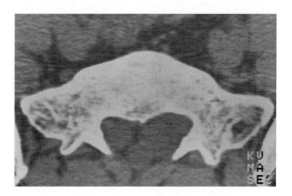

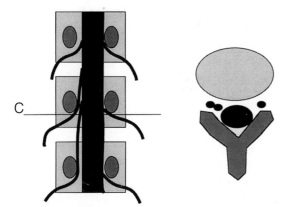

Figure 19–11. Drawing of a conjoined root. Two nerve roots have arisen from the thecal sac on the right side in an asymmetric manner as compared with the left. When a CT cut is made at the level of the cursor (C) two roots are visualized on the axial cut on the right side, one of which could be confused for a free fragment. They will be lower in density than disc material, however.

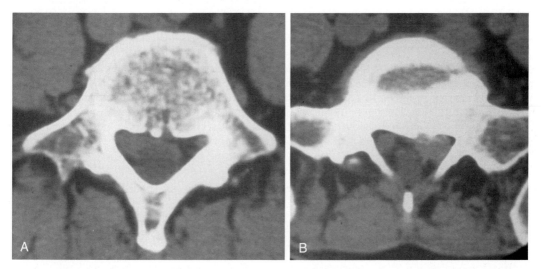

Figure 19–12. Conjoined root and free fragment at different levels in the same patient. *A,* A CT cut through the mid body of L4 shows a soft tissue density in the right lateral recess that is isodense to the thecal sac. This is a conjoined root. *B,* In the same patient, a CT cut through the L5-S1 disc level shows a soft tissue density in the left lateral recess that is denser than the thecal sac. This is a large free disc fragment.

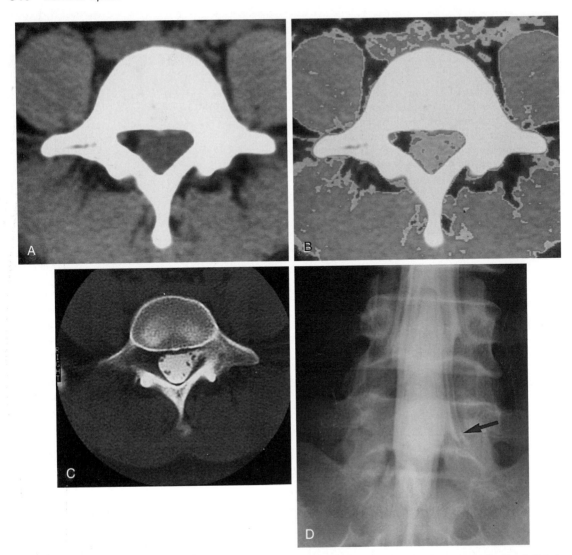

Figure 19–13. Conjoined root with blink mode. *A,* A soft tissue density is present in the left lateral recess that appears isodense to the thecal sac. *B,* The blink mode highlights the soft tissue mass at the same time the thecal sac is highlighted; therefore, this is isodense to the thecal sac and cannot be a free fragment. *C,* A CT myelogram shows the conjoined root sleeve filled with metrizamide in the left lateral recess. *D,* An anteroposterior view of the conventional myelogram shows two roots arising from the thecal sac on the left side at the L5 pedicle level *(arrow).*

the thecal sac/disc interface and not the area lateral to the foramen. A lateral disc has huge implications for the surgeon. First, a lateral disc will irritate a nerve root that has already exited the neuroforamen and will therefore mimic a disc protrusion at a more cephalad level (Fig. 19–14*C*). For instance, if a disc protrudes posteriorly at the L4-5 level it will usually press against the L5 root; therefore, if a patient presents with signs and symptoms of an L5 root irritation, the L4-5 level is usually the surgical

level. However, the L5 root can also be irritated from a lateral disc protrusion at L5-S1. Therefore, if overlooked, it can result in surgery at the wrong level, especially in a patient with disc abnormalities at multiple levels where the clinical presentation is relied on to determine which level should be operated on. Also, a lateral disc does not require a laminectomy because it can be approached from outside the bony central canal. A myelogram will not demonstrate a lateral disc, and an "exploration" is not

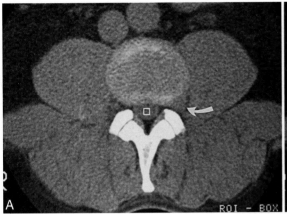
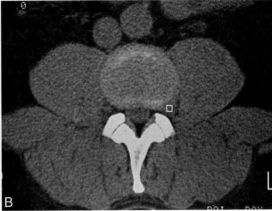

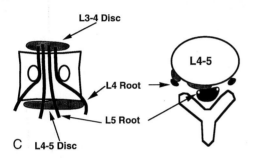

Figure 19–14. Lateral disc. *A,* A soft tissue mass that appears contiguous with the disc is present on the left side just lateral to the neuroforamen *(arrow).* A region of interest box placed on the thecal sac gives a density of 9 CT units. *B,* A region of interest box placed on the soft tissue mass shows its density to be 20.6 CT units. The increased density makes this mass diagnostic of a lateral disc. *C,* This drawing demonstrates how a posterior disc protrusion at L4-5 typically affects the L5 root, yet a lateral disc at the same level affects the L4 root. Because the L4 root is typically affected by a posterior L3-4 disc protrusion, a lateral disc at L4-5 could result in the L3-4 disc being inappropriately surgically removed.

likely to discover a lateral disc because it is not in an area the surgeon would normally explore. Lateral discs occur in less than 5% of cases but should be searched for in every case at each disc level.

SPINAL STENOSIS

Spinal stenosis has been classically divided into two types: congenital and acquired. Congenital stenosis includes achondroplasia, Morquio's disease, and idiopathic disease. Acquired stenosis includes degenerative joint disease with or without degenerative disc disease, posttraumatic stenosis, postsurgical stenosis, Paget's disease, and calcification of the posterior longitudinal ligament. In reality, almost no one ever presents clinically with spinal stenosis unless some component of acquired stenosis is present. Even the most severe form of congenital stenosis, achondroplasia, does not have clinical signs and symptoms until osteoarthritis or degener-

ative disc disease ensues in early adulthood secondary to an accentuated lordosis (Fig. 19–15).

A preferred classification for spinal steno-

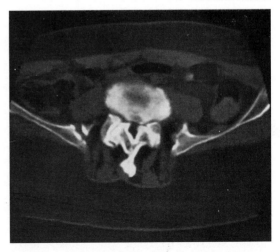

Figure 19–15. Achondroplasia with severe stenosis. Severe central canal stenosis occurs in patients with achondroplasia owing to their congenital stenosis combined with severe degenerative facet disease.

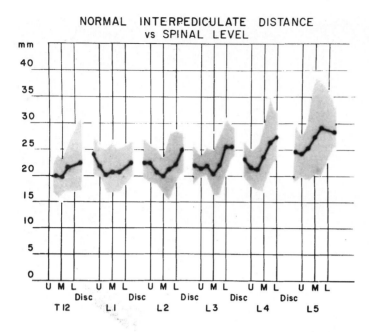

Figure 19–16. Spinal stenosis histogram. The normal interpediculate distance at each spinal level is marked with a heavy line, and a standard deviation above and below is shaded in gray. For example, the average L5 interpediculate measurement near the mid body would be 25 mm.

sis would be on an anatomic basis. This divides stenosis into central canal stenosis, neuroforaminal stenosis, and lateral recess stenosis. In each of these areas the most common cause is degenerative joint disease or degenerative disc disease.

Central Canal Stenosis

For decades radiologists have been asked to measure the central canal to diagnose spi-

nal stenosis. Many different histograms have been published to show which measurements are within normal limits for each anatomic level (Fig. 19–16). These do not take into account the fact that most people with small bony canals also have small neural structures and are, therefore, asymptomatic. We often encounter patients with bony measurements that are small but have small neural components as well (Fig. 19–17). For stenosis to be clinically manifest,

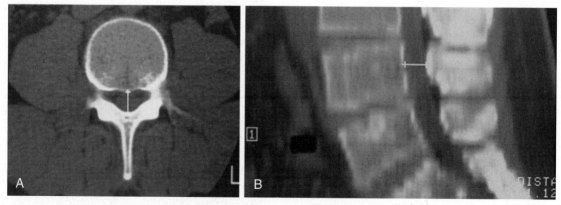

Figure 19–17. Small canal without stenosis. *A,* The anteroposterior diameter of the canal in this patient measures 11.5 mm, which is extremely small. Note that the thecal sac is not compressed and that the epidural fat is not obliterated. *B,* The anteroposterior measurement taken on a sagittal reformatted image is 11.2 mm. This patient had no clinical findings of spinal stenosis in spite of a very small central canal. The patient has a small thecal sac that is not compressed by the small bony canal; hence no symptoms are present. This patient has no spinal stenosis clinically, and measurements are not enough to make the diagnosis.

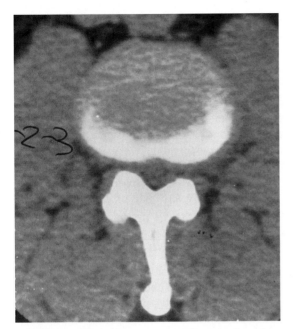

Figure 19–18. Obliteration of epidural fat.
This patient has central canal stenosis that is
compressing the thecal sac. The thecal sac is
not visualized because the epidural fat has been
obliterated. When the epidural fat is absent,
one should suspect spinal stenosis.

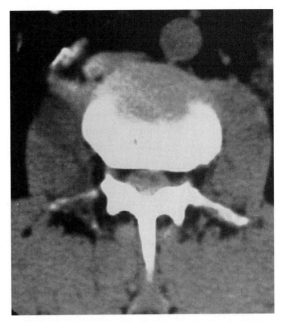

Figure 19–19. Flattening of the thecal sac.
The best CT sign for central canal stenosis is
flattening of the thecal sac. The patient may not
have clinical signs or symptoms of stenosis, but
the diagnosis is still suggested.

there must be a discordance in the size of
the bony canal and the thecal sac. Simply
measuring the central canal will not ad-
dress the "fit" of the thecal sac in that canal;
hence, measurements are virtually worth-
less. The only exception to this may be in
the cervical spine where a narrow central
canal has been correlated to an increased
risk of cord injury in football players.

The most useful CT criteria for diagnosing central canal stenosis are obliteration of
the epidural fat (Fig. 19–18) and flattening
of the thecal sac (Fig. 19–19). Both of these
findings can be present without symptoms
of spinal stenosis; therefore, stenosis can
only be proposed by the radiologist, with
clinical correlation required.

The most common cause of central canal
stenosis is secondary to facet degenerative
disease, which results in hypertrophy of the
facets and encroachment of the central canal and the lateral recesses (Fig. 19–20).
As mentioned previously, even patients with
the most severe example of congenital spinal stenosis, achondroplasia, rarely present

with clinical complaints until marked facet
degenerative disease occurs.

Another very common cause of central canal stenosis is hypertrophy of the liga-

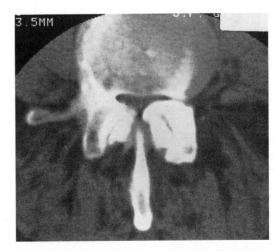

Figure 19–20. Facet hypertrophy. The most
common cause of spinal stenosis is due to facet
degenerative disease with hypertrophy. This is
best seen with bone windows because soft tissue
windows can be very misleading and make normal facets appear hypertrophied.

mentum flavum (Fig. 19–21). This is a misnomer because the ligamentum flavum does not actually hypertrophy but buckles inward owing to facet slippage and disc space narrowing. Since this is a soft tissue encroachment, measurements of the size of the bony canal would not reflect this process, which is another reason measurements are not reliable in detecting spinal stenosis.

Paget's disease with enlargement of the vertebral body can occasionally cause central canal stenosis (Fig. 19–22), as can ossification of the posterior longitudinal ligament (Fig. 19–23). Reportedly, up to 25% of the patients with diffuse idiopathic skeletal hyperostosis, a very common ailment of persons older than 50, will have ossification of the posterior longitudinal ligament. Other causes of central canal stenosis would include trauma and postoperative changes.

Neuroforaminal Stenosis

The causes of neuroforaminal stenosis, as in central canal stenosis, can be diverse but are usually due to degenerative joint disease. Osteophytes off of the vertebral body (Fig. 19–24) or off of the superior articular facet (Fig. 19–25) are most often the cause, but disc herniation and postoperative scar can also occur in the foramen.

The nerve root exits the central canal in the superior aspect of the neuroforamen; therefore, encroachment in the inferior aspect, near the disc space, is an infrequent cause of clinical problems. The nerve root is immobile in the neuroforamen, rather than free to move about; hence, even a small amount of stenosis in the superior aspect of the foramen can cause severe clinical symptomatology, whereas severe stenosis of the inferior aspect of the foramen may elicit no symptoms at all. For these reasons, the amount of narrowing of the neuroforamen often does not correlate clinically.

Although many believe that sagittal reformations through the neuroforamen are adequate to identify stenosis, axial images are by far more reliable in fully demonstrating the degree of neuroforaminal stenosis and its cause. The neuroforamen and the nerve root can be seen in its entirety with

the axial images whereas a single sagittal re-formation will show only a 3- to 5-mm slice (depending on the thickness of the re-formation).

A frequent cause of failed back surgery is failure to preoperatively note neuroforaminal stenosis in a patient undergoing disc surgery that results in an inadequate procedure being performed. It cannot be stressed enough that disc disease and stenosis, in any of its forms, often occur together and addressing only the disc often results in a case of failed back surgery.

Lateral Recess Stenosis

The lateral recess is the bony portion of the central canal that is just caudad and cephalad to the neuroforamen. When the neuroforamen ends as one proceeds caudad, the lateral recess begins. It is also called the nerve root canal because the nerve roots, after they leave the thecal sac and before they exit the central canal through the neuroforamen, run in this bony triangular space. In the bony lateral recess the nerve roots are vulnerable to being impinged by osteophytes (Fig. 19–26), disc fragments, and scar tissue from prior surgery.

Although measurements exist that define the normal lateral recess, they are very difficult to apply and have little practical meaning. As with the neuroforamen, the amount of stenosis often does not correlate with the clinical picture; therefore, it is best to just note that the lateral recess is or is not normal in appearance. Any narrowing must be correlated clinically.

SPONDYLOLYSIS AND SPONDYLOLISTHESIS

Spondylolysis can cause low back pain and sciatica but only occasionally causes spinal stenosis. As discussed in Chapter 18, Musculoskeletal System, on rare occasions a fibrocartilaginous mass builds up around a pars break that can extend into the central canal and impress on the thecal sac or nerve roots (Fig. 19–27). Although this is uncom-

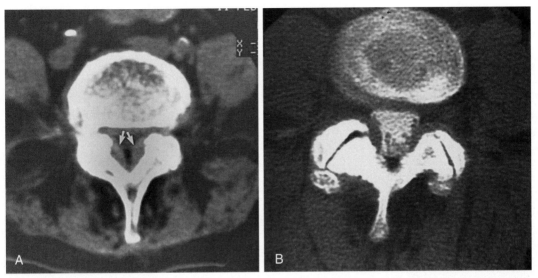

Figure 19–21. Ligamentum flavum hypertrophy. *A,* The ligamentum flavum *(arrows)* is bowing inward and encroaching on the central canal, causing spinal stenosis. The facets are hypertrophied, although this is a soft tissue window and does not show them well. *B,* This metrizamide CT scan shows a large impression on the right side of the thecal sac from ligamentum flavum hypertrophy. Note the facet degenerative joint disease.

Figure 19–22. Paget's disease. Bony overgrowth secondary to Paget's disease has caused central canal stenosis in this patient. This is a typical appearance of Paget's disease in a vertebral body, although it does not always cause stenosis. (From Helms CA, et al: Characteristic CT manifestations of uncommon spinal disorders. Orthop Clin North Am 1985;16:445.)

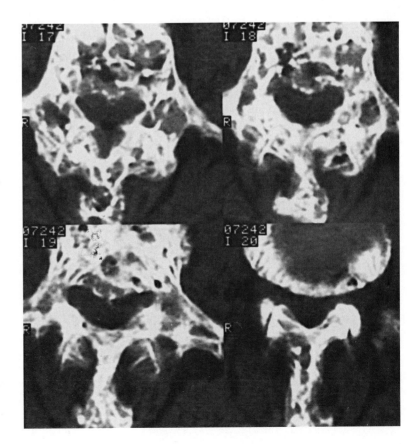

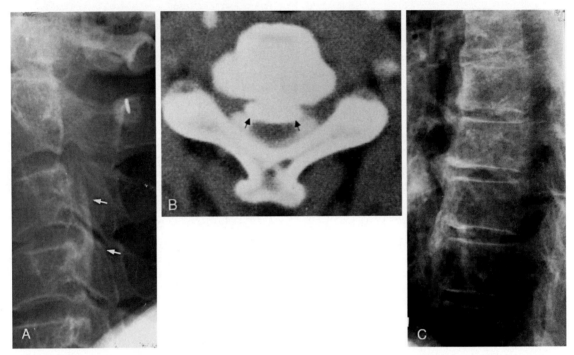

Figure 19–23. Ossification of the posterior longitudinal ligament. *A,* Calcification behind the C3 and C4 vertebral bodies *(arrows)* is seen on the plain film. *B,* A metrizamide CT at the C3 level shows a spherical calcific mass *(black arrows)* impressing the cord. This is a characteristic appearance of ossification of the posterior longitudinal ligament. *C,* A lateral T-spine plain film reveals hyperostosis consistent with diffuse idiopathic skeletal hyperostosis. Up to 25% of the patients with this disorder have ossification of the posterior longitudinal ligament. (From Helms CA, et al: Characteristic CT manifestations of uncommon spinal disorders. Orthop Clin North Am 1985;16:445.)

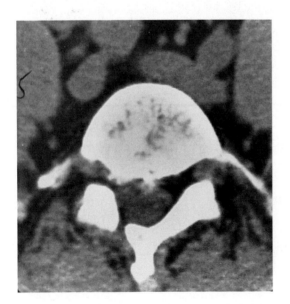

Figure 19–24. Neuroforaminal stenosis. An osteophyte off of the vertebral body is extending into the right neuroforamen causing neuroforaminal stenosis. The left neuroforamen is normal.

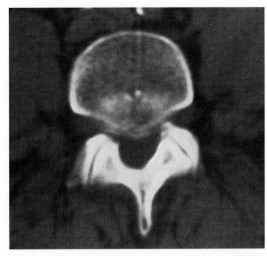

Figure 19–25. Neuroforaminal stenosis. An osteophyte off of the left superior articular facet is extending into the left neuroforamen causing neuroforaminal stenosis.

mon, it should be looked for in every case with a pars break so as not to have an unfortunate example of a fusion being performed without removal of the offending soft tissue mass in the central canal.

Spondylolisthesis can cause central canal stenosis or neuroforaminal stenosis. When one vertebral body slides forward on another, the thecal sac can be squeezed at the level of the slip. This rarely occurs with a grade 1 spondylolisthesis but is not uncommon with the more advanced grades. Occasionally, the broken pars will extend into the neuroforamen and impinge the nerve root (Fig. 19–28).

CONCLUSION

CT has replaced myelography for diagnosing lumbar spine disc disease. It can demonstrate disc protrusions that are central, lateral, and sequestered. The ability to fully evaluate both the bony and soft tissue structures is one of CT's greatest assets and has

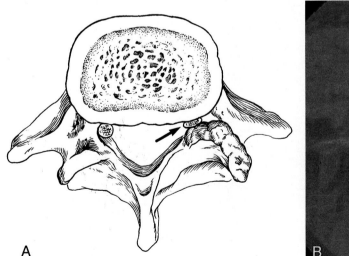
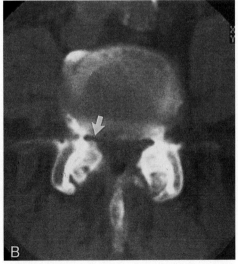

A   B

Figure 19–26. Lateral recess stenosis. *A,* This drawing illustrates how a nerve root *(arrow)* can get impinged in the lateral recess by bony overgrowth. *B,* The right lateral recess *(arrow)* is narrowed from bony overgrowth. The nerve root lies in the lateral recess and may or may not be impinged enough by this process to cause symptoms.

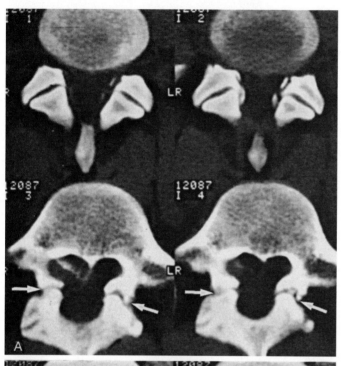

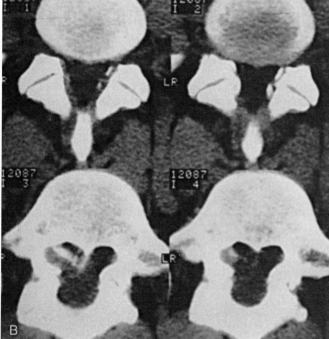

Figure 19–27. Spondylolysis with fibrocartilaginous mass. *A,* Bone windows through the L4-5 disc and the L5 vertebral body reveal a pars break *(arrows)* bilaterally. *B,* Soft tissue windows of the same slices show a large, partially calcified soft tissue mass in the right lateral recess that at surgery was found to arise from the pars break. This has been likened to callus around a fracture that increases when inadequate immobilization occurs.

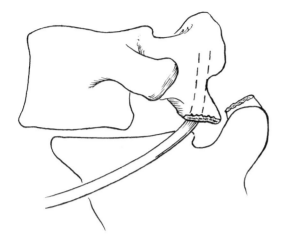

Figure 19–28. Spondylolisthesis. This drawing shows how the broken ends of the pars interarticularis can extend into the neuroforamen with spondylolisthesis and impinge a nerve root.

helped diminish the incidence of failed back surgery.

Spinal stenosis has many causes, congenitally and acquired, yet almost all clinically significant cases have degenerative joint disease and/or degenerative disc disease as the overriding cause. Measurements are not helpful in the lumbar spine and do not reflect the clinical picture in most instances. Spinal stenosis includes the neuroforamen and the lateral recesses as well as the central canal and is often present concomitantly with disc disease. Failure to note coexisting stenosis and disc disease is one of the leading causes of failed back surgery.

Suggested Reading

Goodman RE, Vander ZR, Kaiser GM, et al. Diagnosis of diseases of the lumbar spine: Correlation of computerized tomography with myelography and clinical findings. South Med J 1987; 80:855.

Hesselink JR. Spine imaging: History, achievements, remaining frontiers. AJR 1988; 150:1223.

Jackson R, Becker G, Jacobs R, et al. The neuroradiographic diagnosis of lumbar herniated nucleus pulposus: I. A comparison of computed tomography, myelography, CT-myelography, discography, and CT-discography. Spine 1989; 14:1356.

Modic MT, Masaryk TJ, Ross JS, Carter JR: Imaging of degenerative disk disease. Radiology 1988; 168:177.

Resnick D, Guerra J Jr, Robinson CA, Vint VC: Association of DISH and calcification and ossification of the posterior longitudinal ligament. AJR 1978; 131:1049.

Sartoris DJ, Resnick D: Computed tomography of the spine: An update and review. Crit Rev Diagn Imaging 1987; 27:271.

Schnebel B, Kingston S, Watkins R, Dillin W: Comparison of MRI to contrast CT in the diagnosis of spinal stenosis. Spine 1989; 14:332.

Index

Note: Page numbers in *italics* refer to illustrations;
page numbers followed by t refer to tables.

A

Abdomen, 171–177
CT scan of, angiographic, technique of, 175–176, *176*
approach in, 171–172
contrast in, gastrointestinal, 172
intravenous, 172–173
timing of administration of, 173, *173*
conventional, technique of, 174–175
helical, technique of, 173–174, *175*
image photography in, *176*, 176–177
patient preparation for, 173
technique of, 173–176
Abdominal abscess, 181, *182–183*, 183
Abdominal aorta, anatomy of, 183–184
aneurysms of, 184–187, *185–187*
classification of, 184, *185*
rupture of, 187, *188*
Abdominal cystic mass(es), 183
Abdominal wall, 191–193

Abdominal wall *(Continued)*
anatomy of, 191–192
hematoma of, 193
hernias of, 192, *192*
Abscess, colonic, *288*, 289
hepatic, amebic, 210, *210*
pyogenic, *209*, 209–210
intraperitoneal, 181, *182–183*, 183
pancreatic, 226, *227*, 231
pulmonary, 118, 120, *120*
empyema vs., *153*, 154–155
renal, 250, 253, *254*
splenic, 238–239, *239*, 239t
tubo-ovarian, 300
Accessory spleen, 236, *237*
Achondroplasia, with severe spinal stenosis, *341*
Acquired immunodeficiency syndrome (AIDS), intraabdominal opportunistic infections in, 189–190
splenic microabscesses in, 238–239, *239*, 239t
Addison's disease, 265–266
Adenocarcinoma, of Barrett's esophagus, 273
of pancreas, mucinous cystic, 231, *232*

Adenocarcinoma *(Continued)*
of small bowel, 280
of stomach, *277*, 277–278
Adenoid cystic carcinoma, vs. carcinoid tumors, 102
Adenoma, adrenal, 262–264, *263*
hepatic, 207
pancreatic, microcystic, 231, *232*
Adhesions, causing small bowel obstruction, 282
Adrenal glands, 259–269
adenoma of, 262–264, *263*
anatomy of, 259, *260–262*
calcifications of, causes of, 269t
carcinoma of, 264, *264*
CT scan of, technical considerations in, 259
cysts of, 267, *267*
endocrine syndromes associated with, 264–266, *265–266*
hemorrhage of, *268*, 269
hyperplasia of, 259, 262, *262*
metastases to, 266–267, *266–267*
myelolipoma of, *268*, 269
Agenesis, pulmonary, 108
Air, free, in peritoneal cavity, 180–181
in biliary tree, *214*

C